THE NEW
OXYGEN
PRESCRIPTION

THE NEW
OXYGEN
PRESCRIPTION

The Miracle of
Oxidative Therapies

Nathaniel Altman

Healing Arts Press
Rochester, Vermont • Toronto, Canada

Healing Arts Press
One Park Street
Rochester, Vermont 05767
www.HealingArtsPress.com

SUSTAINABLE FORESTRY INITIATIVE — Certified Sourcing
www.sfiprogram.org
SFI-00854

Text stock is SFI certified

Healing Arts Press is a division of Inner Traditions International

Originally published in 1995 by Healing Arts Press under the title *Oxygen Healing Therapies: For Optimum Health & Vitality*
Revised and expanded second edition published in 1998
Revised and expanded third edition published in 2007 under the title *The Oxygen Prescription: The Miracle of Oxidative Therapies*
Revised and expanded fourth edition published in 2017

Note to the reader: This book is intended as an informational guide. The remedies, approaches, and techniques described herein are meant to supplement, and not to be a substitute for, professional medical care or treatment. They should not be used to treat a serious ailment without prior consultation with a qualified health care professional.

Library of Congress Cataloging-in-Publication Data
Names: Altman, Nathaniel, 1948- author.
Title: The new oxygen prescription : the miracle of oxidative therapies / Nathaniel Altman.
Other titles: Oxygen prescription
Description: Revised and expanded fourth edition. | Rochester, Vermont : Healing Arts Press, 2017. | Preceded by The oxygen prescription / Nathaniel Altman. Rev. and expanded 3rd ed. 2007. | Includes bibliographical references and index.
Identifiers: LCCN 2016045986 (print) | LCCN 2016046924 (e-book) | ISBN 9781620556078 (pbk.) | ISBN 9781620556085 (e-book)
Subjects: | MESH: Hydrogen Peroxide—therapeutic use | Ozone—therapeutic use
Classification: LCC RM666.H83 (print) | LCC RM666.H83 (e-book) | NLM QV 229 | DDC 615.8/36—dc23
LC record available at https://lccn.loc.gov/2016045986

Printed and bound in the United States by Lake Book Manufacturing, Inc.
The text stock is SFI certified. The Sustainable Forestry Initiative® program promotes sustainable forest management.

10 9 8 7 6 5 4 3 2 1

Text design by Deborah Glogover and layout by Priscilla Baker
This book was typeset in Garamond Premier Pro with Goudy

To send correspondence to the author of this book, mail a first-class letter to the author c/o Inner Traditions • Bear & Company, One Park Street, Rochester, VT 05767, and we will forward the communication, or contact the author directly at **www.oxygenprescription.com**.

This book is dedicated to the memory of
Adelson de Barros.

Disclaimer

The author of this book is not a physician. The following material is presented in the spirit of historical, philosophical, and scientific inquiry and is *not* offered as medical advice, diagnosis, or treatment of any kind.

Although studies have attested to the safety of oxidative therapies at established therapeutic dose levels, it should be remembered that ozone and hydrogen peroxide are powerful oxidizers. They can be dangerous if not stored, handled, and utilized properly. Oxidizers like food-grade hydrogen peroxide should always be correctly labeled and kept out of reach of children. The author and publisher advise against self-treatment with oxidative therapies. Any medical treatment should be done under the supervision of a qualified health practitioner.

Contents

PART THREE

A Holistic Protocol

Foreword to the Third Edition

I am glad that Nathaniel asked me to write a few words for his new book: he has been a pioneer in writing about oxygen and ozone therapy. In this third edition of *Oxygen Healing Therapies,* he includes all the available information without overemphasizing either results or practical implications.

He has proved to be a very precise journalist, retrieving and reporting a great number of studies, some of them unknown to me. It was a pleasure to read this latest edition, particularly those chapters dealing with nutrition and the powerful influence of our mind on our body.

Nathaniel has reported all the results of the laboratory and clinical studies that have been done on oxygen therapies, even though some data seem too good to be true. I know too well that owners of private clinics often want to sell gold for copper because of their personal interest. Both Nathaniel and I are convinced that boosting untruthful results is wrong, and we hope that the reader will discern "the wheat from the chaff," because we do not want desperate patients to believe that ozone is a miraculous drug able to "cure" the very worst illnesses.

Biological and clinical experience acquired in the last fifteen years has taught me that, up to now, the pathology where ozonated auto-hemotherapy has a unique advantage is the dry form of age-related macular degeneration. Even though distinguished ophthalmologists do not admit this, I can assure them that about two-thirds of patients (except those advanced cases whose photoreceptors are already dead) will notice an improvement of their visual acuity, enough to become self-sufficient and improve their overall quality of life. Orthodox ophthalmologists have no therapy, except the administration of antioxidants like lutein, which neither harm nor help the macular ischemia.

Other diseases such as vascular ischemias (limb and heart) improve markedly with autohemotherapy, particularly when used in conjunction with, when necessary, topical therapy with ozonated water and ozonated oil. In my experience, these treatments yield better results than the orthodox prostanoid infusions usually prescribed, without adverse side effects. A preparation of ozonated oil, which is the only way to "stabilize" ozone as a triozonide, displays marvelous disinfectant and stimulatory activities in chronic purulent ulcers, bedsores, and other skin problems. When the benefits of ozonated oil become more widely known and accepted by the medical community, this treatment will become a valuable resource for millions of patients. However, in vascular pathologies (such as atherosclerosis, high blood pressure, and angina), I advise patients to also take advantage of the idoneous drugs (such as statins, antihypertensives, and anticoagulant drugs) provided by the medical establishment.

I would like to take the opportunity to remark upon the very intense and foolish antagonism between orthodox and complementary medicine over whether there is only one medicine or form of treatment that is able to restore a patient's health. To claim that treatments such as ozone therapy, homeopathy, or acupuncture are better than conventional medicine because they are less toxic (but not necessarily cheaper) is incorrect and naive; common sense and experience tell us that it is better to select and take advantage of the most available and effective treatments. Physicians must be acquainted with all useful options and cannot behave like religious sectarians.

There are certainly other relevant pathologies, such as chronic bacterial, fungal, and viral infections, that can be treated proficiently and cured when we use an appropriate combination of ozone therapy along with antibiotics and/or antivirals. We have learned the hard way that attacking serious diseases with a combination of approaches is the winning strategy, because these diseases are always sustained by a variety of causes.

Do ozone therapy and oxidative therapy have some limits? They certainly have, and the patient must be better informed about them because they are not trivial. Owing to the chemical instability of ozone, self-treatment is not recommended. Patients should always go to a hospital or medical clinic for treatment. There is often the need for venipuncture and, particularly in women, venous access tends to deteriorate over time. Moreover, after a first therapeutic cycle, ozone therapy must be continued practically for life, even though a less frequent schedule is required.

Unfortunately, recent clinical papers claiming the superiority of ozone therapy in patients with a diabetic foot condition neither mention the need for follow-up treatments nor discuss the absolute need for continuing treatments for years. The papers only mentioned that the treatments were performed over three weeks with about fifteen rectal insufflations of gas versus antibiotic therapy.

My experience has taught me that ozone therapy does not improve diabetes in three weeks. In addition, rectal insufflation of gas, although safe, simple, and economical, is an imprecise and only modestly effective method. If a patient were to acquire an ozone generator, he or she might be able to perform the therapy at home under a physician's supervision, but this rarely happens because of the expense and limited availability of the necessary equipment.I have mentioned these drawbacks because we are hoping to soon find new, valid options that will overcome these limitations.

The beauty of ozone is that when this molecule, almost as old as primordial life, is applied in small and precise doses, it is able to simultaneously trigger or reactivate many functional activities that have gone astray during a chronic disease. Among complementary medical approaches, ozone therapy is the only one where the chemistry, the mechanisms of action, and the biological effects (hence the therapeutic effects) have been delineated well enough to be considered a scientifically based discipline. From a neurophysiological point of view, acupuncture has also reached a similar stage of scientifically documented effectiveness. By contrast, homeopathy remains undefined, perhaps because we do not yet have the appropriate technology to demonstrate the pharmacological effect, if any, transmitted by water.

I am still fighting with some chemists who state that ozone is always toxic and should not be used in medicine. Their opinion is based on a lack of understanding about biology and medicine. In addition, they prefer to ignore that any drug, including crucial molecules (O_2, NO, CO, H_2S) or a compound like glucose, depending upon its concentration and the time period of action, can be either toxic or physiologically valid. There is no doubt that continuous exposure to tropospheric ozone is noxious. But those who make the generalization that ozone therapy is also toxic show that they do not understand anything about these two completely different situations. I hope that, by continuing to explain in detail this profound difference, we will eventually win the battle and stop others from comparing apples with oranges.

Nathaniel's book offers a very responsible, balanced, and broad view of how we should live and care about our health and the valuable uses of oxidative therapies in treating health concerns. I am sure that the material he has gathered here will be very useful for years to come.

Velio Bocci, M.D.

Velio Bocci, M.D., is a specialist in respiratory diseases and clinical hematology. He is emeritus professor of physiology at the University of Siena, Italy, and the author of *Oxygen-Ozone Therapy: A Critical Evaluation* and *Ozone: A New Medical Drug.*

Preface to the Fourth Edition

Since the first edition of this book was published in 1995 under the title *Oxygen Healing Therapies,* hundreds of clinical studies around the world have resulted in an impressive amount of new information about the continued safety and effectiveness of therapeutic ozone and hydrogen peroxide. New developments in administering oxidative therapies have also been introduced, from intraperitoneal applications to injecting ozone into muscles and joints. And several important websites dealing with oxygen therapies have been established on the Internet, making information instantly available to people all over the world.

Dr. Velio Bocci's breakthrough discoveries on how ozone works in the human body in the early part of this century have been built upon by other researchers and practitioners around the world. Research into the therapeutic uses of ozone has accelerated dramatically in medical and dental clinics as well as university research centers, resulting in a growing number of clinical findings published in peer-reviewed medical and scientific journals. Many of these clinical studies will be cited in this new edition. The use of oxygen therapies in dentistry and veterinary medicine continues to grow in popularity as well.

Probably the most exciting development in recent years was the establishment of the International Scientific Committee of Ozone

Therapy (ISCO3) in 2010. Made up of Dr. Bocci and other preeminent experts in the field of oxygen therapies, ISCO3 created the landmark *Madrid Declaration on Ozone Therapy,* first written in 2010 and updated in 2015. The result of months of collaboration (and twenty-two separate drafts), the Madrid Declaration is the first document of its kind to present unified recommendations by leading experts on the scientific basis, medical uses, and therapeutic applications of ozone therapy. It not only has set the standards for the safest and most effective methods of patient care but has elevated the level of clinical training for practitioners throughout the world.

Acknowledgments

I would like to thank the following people who assisted in the creation of this book. This assistance took the form of providing information, reviewing the chapters, helping me locate other sources of information, and offering advice and/or encouragement.

For the first edition: Michael Carpendale, M.D.; Silvia Gra Menendez, Ph.D.; Geoffrey Rogers; Toby Freedman, M.D.; Alison Johnson; Mildred Aissen; Gerard Sunnen, M.D.; Stuart Rynsburger, D.C.; Michael E. Shannon, M.D.; Jose Alberto Rosa, M.D.; Carlos Hernandez Castro, Ph.D.; Sigfried Rilling, M.D.; Horst Kief, M.D.; Jon Greenberg, M.D.; Dr. Juliane Sacher; Lilya Zevin; John C. Pittman, M.D.; and Frank Shallenberger, M.D.

Special thanks go to Siegfried Rilling, M.D., and Haug Publishers for permission to reproduce graphics from his book *The Use of Ozone in Medicine;* to Horst Kief, M.D., for permission to use his photographs of patients; to Charles H. Farr, M.D., Ph.D., for permission to use his chart on the effects of hydrogen peroxide on Shanghai influenza; to Mark Konlee for permission to use material from his book *Immune Restoration Handbook;* and to Dr. Juliane Sacher for permission to reproduce the information found in her article on vitamin and mineral supplementation.

For the second edition, thanks to Zdenek (Den) Rasplicka of Ozone Services for suggesting changes in the original text and for providing new information and graphics and to Dr. Guy Savoie for offering suggestions and information about his personal experiences with ozone. Thanks also go to Bryan McAllister, R.N., for his sound overall advice as well as his practical instruction in the art of ozone applications.

For the third edition, thanks to Den Rasplicka and Bryan McAllister, R.N., for their encouragement and constructive ideas, as well as Frank Shallenberger, M.D.; Dr. Silvia Gra Menendez; Prof. M. Nabil Mawsouf; Lyle Hassell; Bernard Kirshbaum, M.D.; Robert Smatt, D.V.M.; Dr. Siegfried Schulz; and Norman Goldstein for their guidance, information, and inspiration. I thank Dr. Julian Holmes for permission to use his photos of the HealOzone dental device. Finally, I would like to thank Dr. Velio Bocci for his foreword and for taking the time to carefully read over the manuscript and offer valuable suggestions and generous advice, despite a very busy schedule. Like many individuals within the "oxygen community," I consider Dr. Bocci the world's foremost ozone investigator, whose research and writings will continue to bring ozone therapy more into the medical mainstream. I believe that his assistance has helped make this book the best it can possibly be.

For this fourth edition, I would like to again thank Dr. Silvia Gra Menendez for her helpful guidance and advice. I am also grateful to the following practitioners and researchers for sending me their articles: Dr. Rola Alhabashneh, Dr. Mariana Aparecida Brozoski, Dr. Walter Dukić, Dr. Gregorio Martínez Sánchez, Dr. William C. Domb, Dr. Marko Samardzija, Dr. Pepa Osvaldo, Dr. Matteo Bonetti, Dr. Emma Borrelli, Dr. M. T. Crockett, Dr. Lamberto Re, Dr. F. J. Hidalgo Tallon, Dr. Massimo Dall'Olio, Dr. Leonid Khodasevich, and Dr. Heinz Konrad. I also thank Dr. Margo Roman for permission to use her images of ozone therapy in veterinary practice.

Introduction

My personal interest in oxidative therapies is the result of having been the primary caregiver for a friend with very advanced AIDS who was sent home from the hospital to die.

During the final weeks of my friend's life, I administered daily infusions of diluted 35 percent food-grade hydrogen peroxide under a physician's supervision. To my surprise, it was one of the only therapies that seemed to help. Although my friend did not survive, we were impressed at how the infusions gave him energy, inner peace, and optimism. He experienced far less discomfort than he had before the infusions began and was able to sleep better. He also applied undiluted hydrogen peroxide directly to a Kaposi's sarcoma lesion on his foot, and it shrank by half within three weeks.

Having been interested in complementary and natural therapies for over twenty years, I became intrigued with the healing potential of hydrogen peroxide. If it could make such a difference in the quality of life of a person dying from AIDS-related diseases, how could it help people who were not at death's door?

Ozone—another oxidative therapy—has been used extensively in Europe for over fifty years to treat a wide variety of medical conditions, including heart disease, cancer, and AIDS. However, medical doctors in the United States and Canada who use oxidative therapies have often been persecuted by state medical authorities and

1

medical societies. Some have even had their practices closed down.

Ozone and hydrogen peroxide are two chemical substances that could have a major impact on our health and are inexpensive, relatively safe, and easy to administer. Thousands of practitioners have used them in Europe on millions of patients, but they have been legal to use (as an experimental therapy) in only a handful of states and Canadian provinces. In fact, hundreds of people leave the United States and Canada every year to receive these therapies—especially ozone therapy—elsewhere. They pay for care out of their own pockets, since health insurance does not cover experimental treatments. At the same time, the mainstream press largely ignores oxidative therapies, with the exception of sensational stories of unqualified quack physicians offering oxygen therapies to desperate patients with promises of miracle cures for cancer or AIDS, often at a cost of tens of thousands of dollars.

I soon began reading what I could about hydrogen peroxide and ozone. I attended an International Bio-Oxidative Medicine Foundation conference and several conferences of the International Ozone Association, where I participated in workshops, attended presentations, and reviewed the medical literature offered by dozens of physicians, chemists, and other researchers.

Although I had been writing about holistic and alternative healing for more than twenty years, I had not come across any information about oxidative therapies until the late stages of my friend's illness. Several self-published books were available and a number of people like Ed McCabe, Gary Null, and Walter Grotz had been struggling to educate the public for years, but many others (including myself) had never heard about these therapies.

I was also surprised to find that a tremendous volume of scientific and medical literature on the medical use of ozone and hydrogen peroxide had been published since the 1920s. Although a few articles were published in well-known journals like *Science, Lancet, Cancer,* and the *Journal of the American Medical Association,* most were published in obscure scientific journals that are rarely read by the general public.

For a medical writer, this represented a treasure trove of information. I soon realized that there was much more to learn about ozone and hydrogen peroxide, especially in their possible application in preventive health care. I learned that some of the most exciting work in the field of medical ozone therapy is being done in Cuba and Russia, but that little information was known outside those countries.

In 1993, I decided that an objective, scientifically documented, yet readable book was needed for both practicing physicians and the general public. I have always believed that information is vital to enabling us to make intelligent decisions about our health, and I wanted to assemble the latest and most reliable information about oxidative therapies—what they are, how they work, and what they can do to promote the healing process. I also wanted to introduce these therapies as part of a holistic approach to health, in which body cleansing, diet, and exercise could enhance the therapeutic qualities of hydrogen peroxide and ozone.

The first edition of this book was published in 1995, and it was very well received. Medical doctors who were involved with oxidative therapies often recommended the book to their patients as an educational tool. The book went through several printings and was followed by a second edition, expanded and updated, a few years later. It's now time for a fourth edition that not only is updated and enlarged but highlights several major developments from the last few years that will change the face of oxidative therapies forever.

Writing this book over the years has been an incredible experience. My research has taken me to Germany, France, Cuba, and all over the United States. I've been privileged to meet and correspond with scientists and physicians from Italy, Russia, France, Cuba, Canada, and throughout the United States, including Charles H. Farr, Velio Bocci, Frank Shallenberger, Horst Kief, Den Rasplicka, and Lyle Hassel, many of whom have contributed material to this book. I have read hundreds of articles and have spoken to many patients who have received oxidative therapies.

As I complete this fourth edition, I continue to be astonished, although not surprised, at the continued opposition of the United States' medical establishment and government agencies toward researching these therapies, let alone allowing their use under medical supervision. While they are not always a "miracle cure," the proven safety, effectiveness, and varied medical applications of hydrogen peroxide and ozone warrant far more attention.

The fact that ozone and hydrogen peroxide cannot be patented, are inexpensive, and are useful in treating dozens of diseases plays a primary role in this situation. Unlike expensive pharmaceuticals, surgery, and other advanced medical modalities, these simple therapies are not going to line the pockets of physicians, drug companies, medical equipment manufacturers, insurance companies, and hospitals. Since those interests influence—primarily through professional, trade, and political action organizations—the direction of health care policy in this country (along with media outlets that receive their abundant advertising dollars), research in oxidative therapies will probably never be initiated by them.

The future of alternative and complementary therapies like ozone and hydrogen peroxide is in the hands of the health care consumer. About 50 percent of us consulted nontraditional practitioners in the past five years. We support the health care industry through taxes and by purchasing its products and services. We should demand to have the freedom to choose the healing modalities that we want for ourselves and our families without having such personal decisions made by others. At the same time, we should insist on receiving the highest-quality care from certified oxidative practitioners who are recognized experts in their field.

I didn't write this book in order to persuade anyone to use ozone or hydrogen peroxide. I am not affiliated with any clinic, physician, or company that manufactures equipment, supplies, or nutritional supplements related to hydrogen peroxide or ozone. Except for the modest royalties I earn from sales of this book, I do not make any commissions from physicians, clinics, or manufacturers. This financial independence allows me not only to be a more objective writer but also to offer constructive criticism without fear of financial hardship.

I believe that the field of oxidative therapies is worth learning about. My primary goal is to present the facts about these therapies, highlight new scientific findings, and show how they are being used in hospitals and clinics around the world. I hope that this book will stimulate discussion and even controversy. Eventually, perhaps, it can lead both the public and the medical and scientific communities to take a more serious look at the therapeutic potential of hydrogen peroxide and ozone. As a result, consumers can make more educated and intelligent decisions regarding our health care options.

PART ONE

Foundations

I n an age of increasing medical specialization, complex and sometimes questionable medical procedures, and expensive, often ineffective medications, many health care consumers are interested in getting back to basics. They are looking for safe and effective medical therapies that will naturally enhance their body's innate healing powers. They are looking for therapies that cause a minimum of negative side effects and will not bring about their financial ruin.

Most of us feel that such therapies don't exist. However, there are two simple, natural substances whose clinical use has been well documented in medical literature. Health care practitioners who have used these substances in this country have been threatened, harassed, and persecuted by state medical associations and the federal government, despite the fact that the substances have proved safe and effective in treating some of our most common serious health problems, including heart disease, cancer, diabetes, and HIV. Overlooked by the mainstream medical and dental professions, ignored by the government, and feared by the pharmaceutical industry, the substances are now being used by a rapidly growing underground of health care consumers. A small number of physicians who are tired of the expensive, dangerous, invasive, and often useless medical procedures used to treat these and other diseases are also turning to these substances, known as hydrogen peroxide and ozone, using them in a health-enhancing context known variously as bio-oxidative therapies, oxidative therapies, or simply oxygen therapies. Oxygen therapies have been used for over 120 years. They first appeared in mainstream medical journals in 1888. Since that time, they have been studied in many major medical research centers throughout the world.

Hydrogen peroxide is involved in all of life's vital processes and must be present for the immune system to function properly. The cells in the body that fight infection (known as *granulocytes*) produce hydrogen peroxide as a first line of defense against invading organisms like parasites, bacteria, viruses, and fungi. It is also required for the metabolism of protein, carbohydrates, fats, vitamins, and minerals. As a hormone regulator, hydrogen peroxide is necessary for the body's production of estrogen, progesterone, and thyroxine. It also helps the body regulate blood sugar and the production of energy in cells. Hydrogen peroxide has long been known medically as a disinfectant, antiseptic, and oxidizer. Clinically, it has been used to successfully treat a wide variety of human diseases—including circulatory disorders, pulmonary diseases, parasitic infections, and immune-related disorders—with few harmful side effects.

Ozone is one of three forms, called *allotropes,* of the element oxygen. Electrical sparks and ultraviolet light can cause ordinary oxygen to form ozone, which is probably why many people call ozone an energized form of oxygen. Ozone was first used therapeutically to disinfect wounds during World War I. It was later found that ozone can "blast" holes through the membranes of viruses, yeast, bacteria, and abnormal tissue cells before killing them. Ozone was the focus of considerable research during the 1930s in Germany, where it was successfully used to treat patients suffering from inflammatory bowel disorders, ulcerative colitis, Crohn's disease, and chronic bacterial diarrhea. As we will see later on in this book, there is evidence that ozone can destroy many viruses and abnormal tissue cells, including those related to hepatitis, Epstein-Barr, cancer, herpes, cytomegalovirus, and HIV.

Hydrogen peroxide and ozone hold great promise in helping to treat some of the most devastating diseases confronting humanity today. Together, they form the cutting edge of a new healing paradigm involving safe, effective, natural, and inexpensive forms of medical therapy. In the following section, I will introduce oxidative therapies and examine their theoretical basis.

1
Foundations of Oxidative Therapies

Oxygen is essential for life. Over 62 percent of Earth's crust (by mass) is made up of oxygen. Compounds containing oxygen form a major part of oceans, rocks, and all living things. Oxygen also is found in 65 percent of the elements of our body, including blood, organs, tissues, and skin.[1]

Like all matter, oxygen comprises atoms. A substance that is made up of only one type of atom is known as an *element* (of which there are 108); a substance that is made up of more than one element is called a *compound*. Scientists have discovered literally millions of compounds, and new ones are being discovered and produced in laboratories every year.

Oxygen is a clear, odorless gas that can easily be dissolved in water. Each *molecule* (the smallest amount of a chemical substance that can exist by itself without changing or breaking apart) of oxygen is composed of two atoms of oxygen and is known by the chemical formula O_2.

We require a continual supply of oxygen in order to survive. The average person needs some 200 milliliters (about 1 cup) of oxygen per minute while resting, and nearly 8 liters (approximately 2 gallons) per minute during periods of strenuous activity. The brain—which makes up about 2 percent of our total body mass—requires over 20 percent of the oxygen taken in by the body. While we can go without food for several months and survive without water for a couple of days, we cannot live without oxygen for more than a few minutes.

Oxygen makes up approximately 21 percent of the air we normally breathe.* Smokers or people who live in heavily polluted environments are likely to consume a smaller percentage of oxygen.

The oxygen in the air we breathe reacts with sugars in our systems (from the food we eat and from the breakdown of fats and starch in the body) to produce carbon dioxide, water, and energy. The energy from this process, a form of combustion, is stored in a compound called ATP (adenosine triphosphate). ATP is essentially the fuel we need to live, think, and move. According to Sheldon Saul Hendler, M.D., in his book *The Oxygen Breakthrough,* oxygen is the most vital component of ATP within our cells: "ATP is the basic currency of life. Without it, we are literally dead. Imbalance or interruption in the production and flow of this substance results in fatigue, disease and disorder, including immune imbalance, cancer, heart disease and all of the degenerative processes we associate with aging."[2]

The lungs, heart, and circulatory system deliver sufficient amounts of oxygen to the entire body. This oxygen creates the energy we need to survive and thrive. At the same time, the lungs take carbon dioxide (CO_2), a waste product, from the blood and discharge it back into the air. It is estimated that we breathe in 2,500 gallons of air each day. Trees take in carbon dioxide and convert it into oxygen through the process of photosynthesis, sending it back into the atmosphere for us to enjoy once more.

We all know how tired and sluggish we feel when we are in a closed room full of people. Although the room is filled with air, that air is high in carbon dioxide and deficient in oxygen. A number of studies have linked the high CO_2 level in the cabins of commercial jet aircraft (which is almost double the minimum comfort standard for indoor air) to a variety of temporary health problems, including headaches, exhaustion, and eye, nose, and throat discomfort.[3] When passengers arrive

---

*The other principal component of air is nitrogen; air consists of four volumes of nitrogen to one of oxygen.

at their destination and leave the aircraft, and oxygen consumption returns to normal, symptoms often disappear within a couple of hours.

Oxygen is absolutely essential for healthy cells, as it acts against foreign toxins in the body. Many such toxins, like viruses and bacteria, are mostly *anaerobic,* meaning that they thrive in a low-oxygen environment. Cancer viruses are among those that are anaerobic. In 1966 Nobel Prize winner Dr. Otto Warburg confirmed that the key precondition for the development of cancer is a near lack of oxygen on the cellular level.[4]

HOW DO HUMANS
BECOME OXYGEN DEFICIENT?

In a perfect world, we would easily get enough pure oxygen for our body's needs. However, in modern society, there are several major factors that make this difficult.

Polluted Air

Perhaps the most important contributor to oxygen deficiency is air pollution. Automobile exhaust, factory emissions, and burning garbage are the three greatest causes of lowered oxygen content in the air we breathe. The oxygen content of the air for those who smoke or are unfortunate enough to breathe in secondhand smoke is even lower.

Devitalized Foods

As we will see later, fresh fruits and vegetables contain an abundance of oxygen that is dissolved in water. When we eat generous amounts of fresh, raw vegetables and fruits, we benefit from increased oxygen intake as well as from the valuable vitamins and minerals these foods contain.

However, foods that have been heavily processed, cooked, and preserved through canning tend to be very low in oxygen. High-fat foods like meat, eggs, and dairy products tend to be lower in oxygen as well.

The standard American diet (known appropriately as SAD) tends to be very low in oxygen content. It should be no surprise that this type of diet has been linked to a wide variety of degenerative diseases like arteriosclerosis, cancer, and diabetes.

Poor Breathing

Healthy breathing involves deep, rhythmic breaths that fill the lungs with air and then exhale that air fully back into the atmosphere. Due to pollution, stress, or simply habit, most people do not breathe fully. For example, many of us were taught to breathe relying only on the muscles of the upper chest, which tends to ventilate just the upper part of the lungs. By using the diaphragm as well as the upper chest to breathe, we are able to take fuller breaths and incorporate more of the available oxygen in our lungs. We'll examine the subject of breathing later on.

OXIDATION

The primary effect that breathing has on the body is *oxidation*. Oxidation is simply a natural process that involves oxygen combining with another substance, resulting in changes in the chemical composition of both substances. Technically speaking, oxidation includes any reactions in which electrons (tiny particles smaller than an atom that have an electrical charge) are transferred. Most oxidation produces large amounts of energy in the form of light, heat, or electricity. The products of oxidation include corrosion, decay, burning, or respiration.[5] By exposing certain metals to oxygen, for example, the metal is oxidized, producing rust. When butter is left out in the open air for long periods of time, the process of oxidation turns the butter rancid.

Oxidation is also a primary component of combustion. When we light a fire in the fireplace, we are causing the wood to be oxidized. When we start our car engine in the morning, gasoline combines with oxygen and is oxidized to water and carbon dioxide.

Oxidation occurs as combustion within the body when oxygen turns sugar into energy. Our body uses oxidation as its first line of defense against harmful bacteria, viruses, yeast, and parasites. Oxidation breaks down the toxic cells into carbon dioxide and water, and they are removed from the body through its normal processes of elimination.

OXYGENATION

After oxidation, the most important effect of breathing is *oxygenation*. Oxygenation involves saturation with oxygen, as in the aeration of blood in the lungs. Breathing in oxygen is a major source of oxygenation. Although hydrogen peroxide and ozone are best known as oxidizers, they are also powerful oxygenators.

If the oxygenation process within the body is weak or deficient, the body cannot eliminate poisons adequately and a toxic reaction can occur. In minor cases, a toxic buildup can lead to fatigue, dullness, and sluggishness. However, when poor oxygenation is chronic, our overall immune response to germs and viruses is weakened, making us vulnerable to a wide range of diseases.

OXIDATION AND FREE RADICAL PRODUCTION

One of the medical establishment's chief reservations about the use of oxidants like ozone and hydrogen peroxide in medicine is the production of *free radicals*. A free radical has been defined as "any molecule that possesses an unpaired electron, an electrically-charged particle spinning in lonely orbit and searching for another electron to counterbalance it."[6]

Stable molecules have electrons in pairs. To become stable, a free radical will steal an electron from a stable molecule, which then becomes a free radical itself. Free radical formation follows a chain reaction, with one free radical causing important structural changes in many other molecules. Cell damage, including mutations, often results.

Yet free radicals are not necessarily "bad." In fact, many are essential to life. Physiological amounts of some free radicals (including superoxide and hydroxyl radicals) are produced by the body to deliver energy to the body's cells. In addition, free radicals have a crucial role in killing bacteria, fungi, and viruses—without them, we could not survive on Earth. For example, when exposed to a flu virus, the body creates free radicals to destroy it. Free radicals also play an important role in regulating the chemicals the body needs for its survival, such as hormones.

Free radicals are manufactured by the body (they are produced in extra-high amounts during vigorous exercise, but people who are in good physical shape are easily able to detoxify them) and are formed by certain medications. Free radicals are also produced in the environment. Air pollution (including ozone-laden smog, motor vehicle exhaust, and cigarette smoke), toxic waste, certain food additives, pesticide residues, and radiation (such as radiation from X-rays and airplane travel) all produce free radicals that can affect us in different ways.

When we have too many free radicals in our bodies, cell damage can occur. In his book *Free Radicals and Disease Prevention,* David Lin lists how excess free radicals can cause harmful effects to cells. They can

- Break off the membrane proteins, destroying a cell's identity
- Fuse together membrane lipids (fats) and membrane proteins, hardening the cell membrane and making it brittle
- Puncture the cell membrane, allowing bacteria and viruses easy entry
- Disrupt the nuclear membrane, opening up the nucleus and exposing genetic material
- Mutate and destroy genetic material, rewriting and destroying genetic information
- Burden the immune system with the above havoc and threaten the immune system itself by undermining immune cells with similar damage[7]

As a result, free radical damage has been linked to a number of degenerative diseases, including atherosclerosis, cancer, cataracts, diabetes, allergies, mental disorders, and arthritis. Excess free radicals also play a role in the aging process and decreased immune response, opening the door to a variety of immune disorders, including the onset of AIDS.[8]

SEEKING BALANCE:
THE BODY'S "ANTIOXIDANT" SYSTEM

The human body is more than a machine; it is a highly complex living organism that is constantly striving to achieve a dynamic state of self-healing. Healing involves the constant interaction among the myriad aspects of the immune system. One of the most complex and yet powerful components of body healing is the so-called "antioxidant" system. Antioxidants are enzymes (such as catalase, superoxide dismutase, and glutathione peroxidase) that protect cells from free radicals by chemically changing them into harmless compounds like oxygen and water.

In their book *Antioxidant Adaptation,* Stephen A. Levine, Ph.D., and Parris M. Kidd, Ph.D., write about the ability of the body's antioxidant defense system to fight off free radical attacks by providing greater tolerance to oxidative stress to selected tissues:

> The system is flexible: individual antioxidant factors can interact to donate electrons on to another, thereby facilitating the regeneration of optimally active (fully-reduced) forces. The system is also versatile and can respond adaptively to abnormal oxidative challenges subject to source and site availability of required factors. . . . The adaptability of the antioxidant defense system appears to be rather remarkable.[9]

Nutritional Antioxidants
Because excess free radical activity can seriously deplete our body's antioxidant reserves, nutritionists recommend that we augment those supplies with foods rich in antioxidants. Three common vitamins—

beta-carotene (vitamin A), vitamin C, and vitamin E—are important dietary antioxidants, as are minerals like zinc and selenium. According to Natalie Angier, writing in the *New York Times Magazine*:

> Vitamin E and beta-carotene both are used in the fatty membranes of the cell, sponging up free radicals before the vagrants can poke holes in the cellular sheath. Vitamin C, a water-soluble compound, works in the aqueous innards of the cell, coupling with radicals and allowing them to be flushed away in the urine.[10]

These natural antioxidants can help inhibit or control excessive oxidation. They help protect proteins, fats, and other substances in the body from oxidative damage. They can help stabilize cell membranes. Antioxidants have also been found to influence chemical "messengers" both within and between body cells.

Many of the foods we eat—green and yellow vegetables, fruits, nuts, and seeds—contain antioxidant vitamins and minerals in abundance and are recommended as a major part of all healthy diets. Many people take nutritional supplements rich in antioxidants for additional protection. We'll discuss the role of nutrition as an adjunct to oxidative therapies later on.

A Problem of Language

Though still widely used in scientific and medical literature like the sources quoted above, some practitioners feel that the word *antioxidant* is really a misnomer. Why? They claim that because oxidation is essential for both life and for healing, it should not be seen as a negative process. They correctly point out that our minds often think in terms of "good" and "bad," with oxidation viewed as bad and antioxidants as good. Yet neither is bad nor good; instead, together they are essential for healing. For this reason, some physicians feel that the term *reduction* is a more appropriate term. We'll see how this amazing process works in the following chapter.

2

What Are Oxidative Therapies?

A major aspect of free radical activity involves oxidizing the pathogenic by-products of modern living: environmental pollution, dietary toxins, stress, and radiation. This is part of the body's normal healing process and is essential for our survival and well-being. However, a growing number of physicians believe that if the body's antioxidant/ reduction requirements are met, adding certain oxidative substances to the body is safe as long as these substances are of the right kind and are introduced in the proper manner.

Utilizing the principles of oxidation to bring about improvements in the body is known as *bio-oxidative* therapy. This term was first introduced in 1986 by Charles H. Farr, M.D., Ph.D., in his monograph *The Therapeutic Use of Intravenous Hydrogen Peroxide*. Although some practitioners still use Dr. Farr's term, these therapies are also popularly known as *oxidative therapies* or simply *oxygen therapies*.

While aerobic-type exercises; deep, rhythmic breathing; and high-oxygen foods (like fresh fruits and vegetables) promote the normal oxidation process in the body, two natural elements—ozone and hydrogen peroxide—are among the most powerful oxidizers available to humanity and form the essence of oxidative therapy today.

OXIDATIVE STRESS FOR HEALTH?

We mentioned earlier that air pollution and other environmental contaminants, food toxins, smoking, lack of exercise, poor diet, and psychological stress can, over time, overwhelm the body's oxidation/reduction system. The result is commonly known as chronic *oxidative stress,* which has been linked to a wide range of degenerative diseases including diabetes, cancer, heart disease, yeast problems, and infections. Medical research has also connected chronic oxidative stress to premature aging.

Mainstream physicians tend to believe that oxidative stress is always harmful to health. They cannot understand how a powerful oxidizer like ozone or hydrogen peroxide could possibly be safe, let alone promote healing for a wide variety of health problems including cancer, eye problems, diabetes, wound healing, heart disease, and circulatory problems. Though an apparent contradiction, the medical potential for oxygen therapies like hydrogen peroxide and ozone is based on both transient and long-term biochemical reactions that take place when introduced to the body.

Velio Bocci, M.D., emeritus professor of physiology at the University of Siena in Italy and author of two groundbreaking medical texts on ozone therapy, believes that transient oxidative stress is the reason why oxygen therapies work. In *Ozone: A New Medical Drug,* he writes: "*Blood exposed to ozone undergoes a transitory oxidative stress* absolutely necessary to activate biological functions without detrimental effects. The stress must be adequate (not subliminal) to activate physiological mechanisms, *but not excessive* [enough] to overwhelm the intracellular antioxidant system and cause damage."[1]

So how does this work? Ozone is a form of superactive oxygen. When it comes in contact with blood inside an ozone-resistant glass bottle ex vivo (that is the preparative phase of autohemotherapy), it *immediately reacts* with blood plasma and other body fluids, such as those found in the skin and the mucous membranes, thus generating a number of chemical "messengers" like antioxidants and polyunsaturated fatty acids.

This reaction yields two results: the production of hydrogen peroxide (along with other chemicals collectively known in scientific literature as *reactive oxygen species* or ROS) and *lipid oxidation products* (LOPs). The ROS are believed to be responsible for immediate negative biological effects, such as free radical production. However, within a few seconds the oxidized antioxidants are recycled back in reduced form, leading to more positive biological effects. Over the longer term, the ROS target the erythrocytes (red blood cells containing hemoglobin with the main job of transporting oxygen), resulting in improved oxygen delivery to the body; the leukocytes (blood cells whose main job is to engulf and digest bacteria and fungi), thus stimulating immune system activation; and the blood platelets, which stimulate the release of growth factors, substances made by the body that regulate cell division and cell survival.

The biological effects of their "partner" LOPs are both positive and more long term. Through the continual circulation of blood, LOPs can reach virtually any organ of the body and stimulate important biological functions like the generation of cells with improved biochemical characteristics ("supergifted erythrocytes" with the ability to deliver more oxygen to ischemic tissues) and the upregulation of antioxidant enzymes in the blood. Antioxidant enzymes have been found to neutralize oxidative stress, perhaps explaining some of the extraordinary clinical results of ozone therapy. Dr. Bocci believes that LOPs can also mobilize endogenous stem cells (stem cells already inside the body), which can promote regeneration of ischemic heart tissue (tissues of the body damaged by heart disease) and other tissues.[2]

Through both transient oxidative stress and the biochemical reactions that take place within the body over time, therapeutic ozone and hydrogen peroxide stimulate the body's immune system. Because they are not designed to treat specific symptoms, these modalities enjoy numerous and varied clinical applications, often with unexpected beneficial side effects. For example, a person undergoing ozone therapy for Lyme disease may discover that his or her chronic asthma symptoms have improved as well.

As we'll see in laboratory and clinical studies later on, ozone and hydrogen peroxide therapy can help achieve a multitude of therapeutic outcomes that would be unthinkable with a single drug or mainstream medical procedure. Simply put, oxidative therapies can help accelerate oxygen metabolism and stimulate the release of oxygen atoms from the bloodstream to the cells. When levels of oxygen increase, the potential for disease decreases. Germs, parasites, fungi, bacteria, and viruses are killed along with diseased and deficient tissue cells. At the same time, healthy cells not only survive but are better able to multiply. The result is a stronger immune system and improved overall immune response.

Although ozone and hydrogen peroxide are highly toxic in their purified state, they are safe and effective when diluted to therapeutic levels for medical use. When administered in prescribed amounts by a qualified and experienced medical practitioner, the chances of experiencing adverse reactions to oxidative therapies are extremely small. For example, a German study evaluating the adverse side effects of over five million medically administered ozone treatments found that the rate of adverse side effects was only 0.0007 per application. This figure is far lower than that of any other type of medical therapy.[3]

However, this figure can be deceiving. Outside of Germany, many practitioners—particularly in the Americas, with Cuba being the exception—have received only minimal education and hands-on training in the correct use of oxidative therapies. In addition, there is presently no single medical, scientific, or government organization that provides standards of training, certification, or oversight. Finally, some patients opt to treat themselves, whether out of necessity, for convenience, or because they believe that ozone and hydrogen peroxide can be administered by anyone, regardless of training. As a result, both the safety factor and effectiveness of oxidative therapies can be severely compromised.

LONG HISTORY

Although few of us have ever heard of them, oxidative therapies have been around for a long time. They have been used clinically by European physicians for more than a century and were first reported by Dr. I. N. Love in the *Journal of the American Medical Association* in 1888.[4] Since that time, they have been studied in many major medical research centers throughout the world, including Baylor University, Yale University, the University of California at Los Angeles, and Harvard University in the United States, as well as in medical schools and laboratories in Great Britain, Italy, Germany, Russia, Canada, Japan, Cuba, Mexico, and Brazil. Today, between fifty and one hundred scientific articles about the chemical and biological effects of ozone and hydrogen peroxide are published each month.

HOW ARE OXIDATIVE THERAPIES USED?

Tiny amounts of ozone or hydrogen peroxide, added to a base of oxygen or water, are used to introduce active forms of oxygen into the body by intravenous, oral, intradermal, or rectal means. Once in the body, the ozone or hydrogen peroxide breaks down into various oxygen subspecies that contact anaerobic viruses, bacteria, fungi, microbes, and diseased and deficient tissue cells. Through oxidation and the other chemical reactions described earlier, these disease microorganisms and deficient cells are killed and eliminated from the body.

It has been estimated that over twelve million people (primarily in Germany, Russia, and Cuba) have been given oxidative therapies over the past ninety years to treat more than fifty different diseases, including heart and blood vessel diseases, diseases of the lungs, infectious diseases, and immune-related disorders. In some cases, oxidative therapies are administered alone; in others, they are used in addition to traditional medical procedures (such as surgery or chemotherapy) or as adjuncts to alternative health practices like megavitamin therapy, acupuncture, chelation, ultraviolet light therapy, or herbal medicine. According to the International Bio-Oxidative Medical Foundation, the following conditions or diseases have been treated with ozone and hydrogen peroxide with varying degrees of success:

Heart and Blood Vessel Diseases

    Cardiac arrhythmias (irregular heartbeat)
    Cardioconversion (heart stopped)
    Cardiovascular disease (heart disease)
    Cerebral vascular disease (stroke and memory loss)
    Coronary spasm (angina)
    Gangrene (of fingers and toes)
    Peripheral vascular disease (poor circulation)
    Raynaud's disease ("white finger")
    Temporal arteritis (inflammation of the temporal artery)
    Vascular and cluster headaches

Pulmonary Diseases

    Asthma
    Bronchiectasis (dilatation of bronchus or bronchi)
    Chronic bronchitis
    Chronic obstructive pulmonary disease
    Emphysema
    Pneumocystis jiroveci (PCP or AIDS-related pneumonia)

Infectious Diseases

    Acute and chronic viral infections
    Chronic unresponsive bacterial infections
    Epstein-Barr virus (chronic fatigue syndrome)
    Herpes simplex (fever blister)
    Herpes zoster (shingles)
    HIV-related infections
    Influenza

Parasitic infections
Systemic chronic candidiasis (candida)

Immune Disorders

Diabetes mellitus type 2
Hypersensitive reactions (environmental and universal reactors)
Multiple sclerosis
Rheumatoid arthritis

Other Diseases

Alzheimer's disease
Cancers of the blood and lymph nodes[5]
Chronic pain syndromes (due to multiple causes)
Migraine headaches
Pain of metastatic carcinoma
Parkinson's disease

In the *Madrid Declaration on Ozone Therapy* (June 2015), the authors divided the range of diseases that have been treated with ozone therapy into three "levels" according to their degrees of documented clinical success reported in peer-reviewed journals, with Level A as the highest.

Diseases in Level A include:

• Spinal diseases, including herniated disc and spondylolysis

Diseases in Level B include:

• Orthopedic diseases and localized osteoarthritis
• Painful disorders of musculoskeletal soft tissue
• Gonarthrosis
• Patellar chondromalacia
• Pathologies of the tendons (including tennis elbow and jumper's knee)
• Carpal tunnel syndrome

- Diabetes, diabetic foot
- Chronic fatigue syndrome and fibromyalgia
- Ménière's disease
- Advanced ischemic diseases; lower limb arterial ischemia
- Age-related macular degeneration
- Dental cavities, particularly in children
- Osteomyelitis
- Pleural emphysema
- Abscesses with fistula
- Infected wounds
- Bedsores
- Chronic ulcers
- Burns
- Acute and chronic infectious diseases, including hepatitis, HIV-AIDS, herpes, papilloma virus infections, nail fungus, candida, giardia, athlete's foot

Diseases in Level C include:

- Cancer-related fatigue (when ozone therapy is integrated with conventional cancer treatment)
- Asthma

In addition, the *Madrid Declaration on Ozone Therapy* includes a number of diseases where ozone therapy has been used successfully either alone or in combination with other therapies, both orthodox and unorthodox. Because many of the reports on the success of these treatments are anecdotal, they may not be considered scientifically reliable. These diseases include:

- Autoimmune diseases (multiple sclerosis, rheumatoid arthritis, Crohn's disease, chronic inflammatory bowel disease)
- Lung diseases (emphysema, chronic obstructive pulmonary disease, idiopathic pulmonary fibrosis, acute respiratory distress syndrome)

- Skin diseases (psoriasis, eczema, atopic dermatitis)
- Cancer metastasis (when ozone therapy is used as an adjuvant therapy or to reduce the effects of radiation or chemotherapy)
- Severe sepsis and multiple organ dysfunction
- Reynaud's syndrome
- Chronic kidney failure
- Liver diseases, including hepatitis A, B, and C
- Thyroid nodule
- Alzheimer's disease and senile dementia[6]

HOW DO THESE THERAPIES WORK?

According to Frank Shallenberger, M.D., H.M.D., one of America's most respected oxidative practitioners and president of the American Academy of Ozonotherapy, ozone and hydrogen peroxide therapies have been found to have the following effects on the human body:

1. They stimulate the production of white blood cells, which are necessary to fight infection.
2. Ozone and hydrogen peroxide are virucidal.
3. They increase oxygen and hemoglobin disassociation, thus increasing the delivery of oxygen from the blood to the cells.
4. Ozone and hydrogen peroxide are antineoplastic, which means that they inhibit the growth of new tissues like tumors.
5. They oxidize petrochemicals.
6. They increase red blood cell membranes' distensibility, thus enhancing their flexibility and effectiveness.
7. They increase the production of interferon and tumor necrosis factor, which the body uses to fight infections and cancers.
8. They increase the efficiency of the antioxidant enzyme system, which scavenges excess free radicals in the body.
9. They accelerate the citric acid cycle, which is the main cycle for the liberation of energy from sugars. It also breaks down proteins, carbohydrates, and fats to be used as energy.

10. Oxidative therapies increase tissue oxygenation, thus bringing about patient improvement.[7]

Later in this book, we'll focus in detail on the many health effects of ozone and hydrogen peroxide therapies under a wide variety of conditions and clinical applications.

UNKNOWN, IGNORED, AND FORGOTTEN

Although ozone and hydrogen peroxide therapy have been proven in both clinical trials and regular clinical practice to be safe and effective in countries such as Germany, Cuba, Mexico, Russia, Italy, Spain, France, China, and Australia, very few people have heard about oxidative therapies in the United States and Canada. Even though an estimated fifteen thousand European practitioners legally use oxidative therapies in their practices, the number of physicians using these therapies in North America is small, due in part to the fact that information about ozone and hydrogen peroxide is not provided in medical schools, which are largely funded by pharmaceutical companies. In addition, the medical establishment does not advocate the use of oxidative therapies and often discourages or prevents licensed physicians from using them in their medical practice. In the United States, medical doctors have been threatened with having their licenses revoked if they administer hydrogen peroxide or ozone. Clinics have been closed down and practitioners have been threatened with jail.

Perhaps the best-known victim of government persecution was the late Robert Atkins, M.D., the developer of the Atkins diet and author of *Dr. Atkins' Diet Revolution* and other books. As director of the Atkins Center for Complementary Medicine in New York City, Dr. Atkins had his medical license revoked because he was treating patients with ozone. After he regained his license in court, Dr. Atkins's 1993 lawsuit against the state of New York helped bring about the passage of a law permitting physicians to use ozone and other modalities not approved by the U.S. Food and Drug Administration (FDA).

Yet even before the government attempted to take away Dr. Atkins's license, the FDA harassed him through his supplier of ozone equipment. During an interview with Geoffrey Rogers in the award-winning film *Ozone and the Politics of Medicine,* Dr. Atkins said:

> Well, I had an ozone generator, and we used it on all our AIDS patients, [on] just about all our cancer patients, and we used it on the yeast patients, which was really the largest group. Generally, we gave it intravenously, [via] autohemotherapy, where we pull the blood out, mix the blood with ozone, and in a few minutes gave ozonated blood back to the patient.
>
> We found that our cancer protocol, which includes ozone, was effective and was keeping people alive, and without ever having to require pain medicine, without losing weight, without any sign of deterioration. And then when we lost our ozone machine, the patients began to go downhill. The FDA saw to it that our manufacturer had to take away the business end of the machine, so we no longer had an effective ozone-generating machine. That's where we are right now currently. I'm right now trying to figure out how to get around that, because I believe that my patients need ozone.[8]

A major reason for this bias against oxidative therapies is that ozone and hydrogen peroxide are *nonpatentable* substances that are very inexpensive to manufacture and use. There is simply no financial incentive to incorporate them into traditional medical practice.

In addition, these substances are being used to treat a broad spectrum of health problems at a low cost. And when compared to chemotherapy or surgery, medical ozone and hydrogen peroxide are extremely cheap. Typically, oxidative therapies properly administered in a medical setting cost up to 50 percent less than traditional therapies, especially for chronic and degenerative diseases. As we will see later on, there are successful case histories involving patient-administered treatments under proper medical supervision that can cost far less. For these reasons, ozone and hydrogen peroxide pose a threat to the continued dominance of the medical establishment, which includes the pharmaceutical industry, medical centers, and physicians who are accustomed to providing expensive drugs, complex medical procedures, and long hospital stays.

Because U.S. government agencies like the FDA and the National Institutes of Health (NIH) are influenced by the pharmaceutical industry and the medical lobby, objective investigation and development of effective protocols for oxidative therapies have been difficult to undertake. According to the late Michael T. F. Carpendale, M.D., a pioneer ozone researcher and professor of orthopedic surgery at the University of California School of Medicine:

> In the FDA, the drug companies have representatives on nearly all the committees. If there's something which may be very effective but may undersell the average drug company, of course they are not going to be very pleased if it gets developed. It might be very difficult for them to compete with that. And ozone is obviously inexpensive to produce; it is very potent [and] if it works half as well as the Germans claim it does, everyone should be using it.[9]

Dr. Horst Kief, one of the first physicians in the world to successfully treat HIV-infected patients with ozone, commented on why so little government-sponsored and drug company research is taking place regarding ozone therapy: "Nobody in the pharmaceutical industry can sell ozone. That's the main reason. When we can find a way to sell ozone, I am sure that ozone [will be] the most important drug in the world."[10]

WHERE PATIENTS COME FIRST?

Now that pharmaceutical companies can legally promote their products in newspapers, in magazines, on television, on highway billboards, on the radio, and over the Internet, we are saturated by drug advertising.

Industry propaganda is constantly provided to radio and television stations as either news reports or public service announcements to highlight what appear to be positive outcomes of drugs and surgical procedures (long-term follow-up results, often with negative outcomes, are rarely announced to the public). In addition, the pharmaceutical industry hires physicians as spokespeople to promote their products using the media and gives them free drug samples to distribute to patients in their medical offices.

Through such carefully crafted publicity campaigns, the pharmaceutical industry has tried to cultivate the image of a benign, humanitarian organization whose primary goal is to serve humanity, cure disease, and end human suffering. This image has been tarnished over the past few years with the multibillion-dollar lawsuits surrounding the deaths of patients taking COX-2 inhibitor drugs like Vioxx, Bextra, and Celebrex, which are commonly used to treat arthritis symptoms, as well as other scandals where concerns about drug company profits have far outweighed those about public safety.

On June 10, 2005, the *New York Times* published a front-page story about the drug Propulsid, manufactured by Johnson & Johnson to treat heartburn. In July 1998, after more than a hundred patient deaths and injuries, Johnson & Johnson issued a new warning label, but the label did not contain all the warnings and qualifications originally sought by the FDA (because pharmaceutical companies are not required by law to change their warning labels, they often can negotiate changes with the FDA). According to the article:

> Propulsid's history has striking parallels with the painkillers now at the center of controversy. Dozens of studies sponsored by Johnson & Johnson that might have warned doctors away were never published, just as the pharmaceutical manufacturer Pfizer failed to publish an early study of Celebrex that indicated a heart risk. And Johnson & Johnson was able to delay and soften some proposed label changes, just as Merck later did with Vioxx.[11]

Looking After the Bottom Line

Although many scientists employed by the pharmaceutical industry are true humanitarians who are seriously committed to fighting disease and relieving human suffering, we should never forget that the main goal—the bottom line—of the drug companies is to *make as much money as possible.*

In 2014 the global drug industry was estimated to be a $1 trillion business. With an average net profit margin of 18.1 percent, the American pharmaceutical industry is one of the most profitable sectors of all industry groups.[12]

As an extremely powerful economic and political force in the United States and around the world, these giant multinationals play a major role in determining government policy and influencing medical schools through educational grants, which often disguise efforts to further marketing aims. In 2015 alone, the pharmaceutical industry coordinated a massive $178,863,490 effort by 1,320 lobbyists to protect its interests in Washington. This was led by a $14,565,000 campaign by the Pharmaceutical Research and Manufacturers of America (PhRMA), an industry organization composed of no fewer than fifty-five manufacturers of drugs and medical devices. Many of its members—like Amgen, Novartis, Bayer, and Johnson & Johnson—also spent millions of dollars on lobbying efforts on their own. For details and updates, visit the website of the Center for Responsive Politics (www.opensecrets.org).[13]

Physicians are also influenced by all-expenses-paid junkets to posh resorts in cities like Las Vegas and Honolulu, generous free samples of selected drugs, kickbacks, and advertising in medical journals. The October 20, 2015, issue of the *Journal of the American Medical Association* contained no fewer than seventeen pages of drug advertising.[14] Drug companies also advertise heavily in mainstream consumer magazines (the November 2015 issue of *Family Circle* contained just over forty-three pages of drug advertising),[15] leading editors to avoid running objective articles that may educate readers about alternative modalities like oxygen therapies.

Given the tremendous influence and power of the drug companies, it is amazing that oxidative therapies are practiced to even the modest extent that they are today. As these inexpensive, nonpatentable and multidisease therapies become better known, we can be certain that the pharmaceutical industry will strengthen its resolve to make medical ozone and hydrogen peroxide unavailable to the general public and continue to lobby to prevent research and clinical application.

The sixteen biggest drug companies trading on the New York Stock Exchange reported 2016 sales and profits and 2018–2020 estimates as seen in table 2.1.

Table 2.1. Annual Estimated Sales and Profits of the Largest Publicly Traded Pharmaceutical Companies

Name	Sales ($billion)		Net Profit ($billion)		Net Profit Margin (percent)
	2016	2018–2020	2016	2018–2020	2018–2020
Abbvie	27.0	33.0	8.36	11.5	34.8
Allergan	25.0	31.0	8.82	12.6	40.6
AstraZeneca	24.0	25.0	3.75	5.5	22.0
Biogen	11.37	15.91	4.17	4.91	30.1
Bristol-Myers Sqibb	16.8	20.3	3.795	4.87	24.0
Eli Lilly	21.0	25.0	3.89	5.78	23.1
Gilead Sciences	31.2	35.1	16.8	16.9	48.3
GlaxoSmith-Kline	38.0	41.0	4.8	8.4	20.5
Johnson & Johnson*	74.5	89.55	7.8	22.1	24.7
Merck	41.0	44.0	10.64	12.88	29.3
Novartis AG	53.0	56.0	10.6	14.0	25.0
Novo Nordisk	17.69	24.95	5.95	8.22	32.9
Pfizer	47.5	50.0	10.37	3.34	26.7
Sanofi	43.0	46.0	6.2	7.9	17.2
Teva	19.0	19.6	4.46	4.65	23.7
Valeant	13.0	16.5	5.1	7.5	45.5

The Value Line Investment Survey (August 21, 2015). Figures include sales of medical devices.
Source: *The Value Line Investment Survey* (October 9, 2015): 1605–1634.

LEGAL STATUS (2016)

In many European countries and in Cuba, bio-oxidative therapies can be legally administered by a licensed health care professional, although each country has regulations governing the licensure of practitioners and limitations, if any, of specific therapeutic procedures. As we will see later on, these therapies are being used by licensed practitioners in many other countries around the world, including China, India, Japan, and Turkey.

At the time of this writing, ten U.S. states (known as "health freedom states") have laws that protect patient access to alternative therapies (such as oxidative therapies) if they are administered by a licensed physician: Arizona, California, Colorado, Idaho, Louisiana, Minnesota, Nevada, New Mexico, Oklahoma, and Rhode Island. For updates, visit the website of the National Health Freedom Coalition: www .nationalhealthfreedom.org.

USELESS AND UNSAFE?

Nevertheless, there is still considerable prejudice against the use of oxidative therapies from within the medical mainstream, especially in the United States.

Barrie R. Cassileth, Ph.D. (sociology), is the founder and director of the Integrative Medicine Service at the Memorial Sloan-Kettering Cancer Center in New York City. She is also a staunch opponent of oxygen therapies. Writing in *Oncology,* she declared:

> Oxygen therapies are unproven alternatives promoted as a cure for cancer, acquired immune deficiency syndrome (AIDS), and other degenerative diseases. These "therapies" are offered at clinics in Mexico, the United States, and Europe. Proponents claim that many diseases, including cancer, are caused by oxygen deficiency and that oxygenation can restore health by destroying cancer cells,

eliminating pathogens, stimulating metabolism, and by producing "oxidative detoxification." There is no scientific evidence to support any of these claims. . . . The use of oxygen therapies has resulted in serious adverse events and several deaths.[16]

Despite Dr. Cassileth's pronouncements on the reputed dangers of ozone therapy, the fact is that traditional medical therapy is far from safe. Although rarely discussed by the mainstream media—which receives billions of dollars in yearly advertising by pharmaceutical manufacturers, clinics, and hospitals in the United States alone—traditional medical therapy causes injury, illness, and death to millions of people each year.

Medications: Prescribed or Otherwise

On the one hand, all medications—whether over the counter or prescription—can produce adverse side effects. Even though they are among the most popular, drugs designed to relieve pain are among the most dangerous. They are also subject to abuse, because many people who take them become addicted and tend to overdose, which often leads to death. A big part of the overdose problem results from prescription painkillers called opioids; the other drug family of concern is the benzodiazepines. The U.S. Centers for Disease Control and Prevention (CDC) warns that people who take prescription painkillers can become addicted with just one prescription.

One of the most serious dangers of painkilling drugs is that they often lead to heroin addiction. According to the National Institute on Drug Abuse, a part of the National Institutes of Health, "Nearly half of young people who inject heroin surveyed in three recent studies reported abusing prescription opioids before starting to use heroin. Some individuals reported taking up heroin because it is cheaper and easier to obtain than prescription opioids."[17]

The amount of painkilling drugs consumed in the United States is staggering. Despite the fact that that there has not been an overall change in the amount of pain that Americans report, the CDC noted in a 2015 paper that the amount of prescription painkillers dispensed in the United States quadrupled between 1999 and 2013, when 207 million prescriptions were written for prescription opioid pain medications. During this fourteen-year period deaths from prescription painkillers also quadrupled, killing more than sixteen thousand people in the United States. It also reported that nearly two million Americans aged twelve or older either abused or were dependent on opioids alone in 2013. The CDC report added that drug misuse and abuse caused about 2.5 million emergency department (ED) visits in 2011. Of these, more than 1.4 million ED visits were related to prescription drugs.[18]

This is merely a part of a worldwide epidemic of opioid addiction and abuse, a health problem that affected an estimated 26.4 million and 36 million people by 2014.[19]

Hospital-Acquired Conditions
According to the Agency for Healthcare Research and Quality, a part of the U.S. Department of Health & Human Services, health care–associated infections (HAIs) result in 1.7 million infections and 99,000 deaths each year. HAIs are the result of medical care administered in either a doctor's office or a hospital.[20]

Another specific area of concern involves hospital-acquired conditions (HACs). A 2015 report by the Agency for Healthcare Research and Quality reported almost *four million* cases of HACs in American hospitals in 2014 alone. Often expressed in euphemistic technical terminology, the report listed:

- Adverse drug events (ADEs): 1,360,000
- Catheter-associated urinary tract infections: 250,000
- Bloodstream infections associated with central venous catheters: 5,000
- In-hospital patient falls: 260,000
- Obstetric adverse reactions (trauma in vaginal delivery): 77,000
- Pressure ulcers: 1,010,000

- Surgical-site infections: 79,000
- Ventilator-associated pneumonia: 38,000
- Postoperative venous thromboembolic events (embolism): 16,000
- "All other HACs": 872,000

The "good" news is that American hospitals reported that HACs had declined 17 percent from 2010 levels, largely due to more careful safety and patient monitoring practices.[21]

No medical therapy is 100 percent safe. However, as we will see later on, oxygen therapies—when properly administered according to established protocols—are far safer than medicine, surgery, and most other traditional medical modalities.

A VIABLE ALTERNATIVE?

In an age of increasing medical specialization, complex and sometimes questionable medical procedures, and expensive, often ineffectual and dangerous medications, people want to get back to basics. Interest is high in medical therapies for both major and minor health problems that are safe and effective and that can naturally enhance our innate healing powers. We are looking for therapies that will cause a minimum of side effects and that will not bring about financial ruin.

The use of oxygen therapies—particularly ozone and hydrogen peroxide—holds great promise in treating both minor health problems and some of the most devastating diseases confronting humanity today, including cardiovascular disease, arthritis, and diabetes. Together, they form the cutting edge of a new healing paradigm involving safe, effective, natural, and less costly forms of medical therapy. In the following chapters we will examine ozone and hydrogen peroxide in greater detail.

3
Ozone:
Properties and Uses

Ozone is an elemental form of oxygen occurring naturally in Earth's atmosphere. It is created in nature when ultraviolet energy causes oxygen atoms (which are normally found in pairs, forming oxygen molecules) to temporarily recombine in groups of three. Ozone is also formed by the action of electrical discharges on oxygen, so it is often created by thunder and lightning. After a thunderstorm, the air seems to smell like freshly mown hay because of the small quantities of ozone generated by the storm. Ozone is also produced commercially in ozone generators, which involves sending an electrical discharge through a specially built condenser containing oxygen. Figure 3.1 on page 38 shows the principle behind ozone generation. Because it is made up of three atoms of oxygen, ozone is known chemically as O_3. The newly formed molecule is quick to react with other substances.

Ozone surrounds the earth at an altitude of between 50,000 and 100,000 feet in the form of a pale blue gas that condenses to a deep blue liquid at very low temperatures.[1] When it occurs in the upper atmosphere, ozone forms a protective layer that absorbs much of the sun's ultraviolet radiation. If it were not for the ozone layer, animal and plant life on this planet would not survive. The depletion of the ozone layer caused by the use of chlorofluorocarbons (CFCs)—released into the atmosphere by refrigerators, air conditioners, and aerosol containers— has become a grave concern to scientists and physicians the world

Figure 3.1. Principle of ozone generation. (From Siegfried Rilling and Renate Viebahn, *The Use of Ozone in Medicine* [Heidelberg: Haug Publishers, 1987]. Reprinted courtesy of Dr. Siegfried Rilling and Haug Publishers.)

over. The dangerous ultraviolet light that is ordinarily blocked by the ozone layer has been linked to a wide variety of human health problems, including skin cancer and immunosuppression. Ultraviolet radiation has also been a factor in poor crop growth for certain species of grains. After many years of study and much procrastination on the part of industry and government, efforts are finally being made to phase out the use of CFCs completely.

In the lower atmosphere, ozone combines with hydrocarbons (like carbon dioxide) and nitrogen oxide from vehicle exhaust and other sources to create photochemical smog. As a result, new and often highly corrosive pollutants are formed. The number of possible chemical reactions that can occur when ozone is combined with these oxides can reach into the hundreds. Ozone-laden smog has been linked to acid rain; a variety of lung-, eye-, and nose-related diseases; and the oxidation of buildings and monuments, especially in smoggy cities like Mexico City, Los Angeles, and São Paulo.

Many people feel that ozone is toxic because it is associated with these reactions. Yet the ozone index published in the newspapers and announced during the evening weather report is only an assay to estimate the amount of toxic nitrous oxide and hydrocarbons present in the atmosphere. As a powerful oxidizer, ozone actually helps clean the atmosphere of hydrogen monoxide, nitrous oxide, sulfur dioxide, and dozens of other dangerous compounds. Rather than warn only of the dangers of breathing ozone (and even breathing pure ozone can be harmful), weather reporters should focus more on the effects of breathing these other (far more dangerous) elements of smog, formed primarily by vehicle exhaust and factory emissions.

Scientific and medical studies have emphasized the negative consequences ozone has on breathing, while ignoring the benefits of a transitory, precisely calculated medical application of a tiny amount of ozone that is never inhaled by the patient. This may be the main reason why physicians and others feel that ozone is not only medically useless but also a dangerous substance to take into the body under any circumstances, despite recent scientific findings at the Scripps Research Institute in La Jolla, California, that the human body can produce its own ozone for healing.[2]

HISTORY

Ozone's distinctive odor was first reported by Van Mauren in 1785, but the gas was not actually "discovered" by German chemist Christian Frederick Schonbein at the University of Basel in Switzerland until 1840. Schonbein decided to name the gas *ozone* (from the Greek word for "smell") because of its pungent odor. In 1860, the Swiss chemist Jacques-Louis Soret concluded that the ozone molecule was made up of three atoms of oxygen. However, it was the Irish chemist Thomas Andrews, a member of the Royal Society of London, who demonstrated many of ozone's oxidating and disinfecting properties for the first time in a laboratory.

In 1856, ozone gas was used for the first time to disinfect operating rooms, and in 1860, the first water treatment plant to use ozone to purify municipal water supplies was built in Monaco. After a severe cholera epidemic in Hamburg killed thirty thousand people, the first waterworks to use ozone in Germany was constructed by chemist and inventor Werner von Siemens (the company he founded has evolved into the huge German conglomerate that bears his name) in Wiesbaden in 1901, followed by one in the Westphalian city of Paderborn a year later.[3]

Since the early part of the twenty-first century, many advances have been made in ozone technology. Sophisticated ozone generators and related technologies that incorporate ozone in a wide range of industrial and scientific applications have been developed. Over the last few years, a number of ozone-resistant materials have been developed for use with ozone generators. In addition to custom-blown glass components, modern substances like Teflon, a form of plastic known as PVDF or Kynar, a rubberlike substance called Viton, and silicone for flexible tubing are becoming increasingly available.

MUNICIPAL WATER TREATMENT

Ozone is a powerful oxidizer that can kill a wide variety of viruses, bacteria, and other toxins. It also oxidizes phenolics (poisonous compounds of methanol and benzene), pesticides, detergents, chemical manufacturing wastes, and aromatic (smelly) compounds more rapidly and effectively than chlorine without chlorine's harmful residues.[4] For this reason, ozone has become the element of choice for disinfecting and purifying drinking water and wastewater through a wide variety of applications.

More than a hundred different viruses that are excreted in human feces can be found in contaminated drinking water. Viruses such as those associated with hepatitis infect thousands of people a year and can survive for a long period of time in potable water. As a potent virucide, ozone is seen as an effective alternative to chlorine, which (in addition to its undesirable taste and odor) may yield chloroform and other compounds that are potentially carcinogenic.[5] According to *The Encyclopedia of Chemical Technology:* "Chlorination as it is practiced in potable-water treatment plants cannot adequately remove viruses to an acceptable level. The complete control of viruses by ozone at low dosage levels is well documented."[6]

As a potent oxidizer, ozone kills bacteria by rupturing the cell wall. Among the harmful microorganisms that ozone can oxidize are *Escherichia coli* (*E. coli*), *Enterococcus faecalis, Mycobacterium tuberculosum, Bacillus megaterium* (spores), *Cryptosporidium parvum,* and *Entamoeba histolytica. The Encyclopedia of Chemical Technology* reports, "Ozone displays an all-or-nothing effect in terms of destroying bacteria. This effect can be attributed to the high oxidation potential of ozone. Ozone is such a strong germicide that only a few micrograms per liter are required to measure germicidal action."[7]

The process of purifying water with ozone is a simple one: a small amount of ozone is added to oxygen and mixed with the drinking water. Not only does it kill viruses and bacteria, but it also removes the microorganisms that cause bad taste and odor in the water. Today, over 2,500 municipalities around the world use ozone to purify their drinking supplies, including Amsterdam, Brussels, Florence, Helsinki, Kiev, Los Angeles, Manchester, Marseilles, Montreal, Moscow, Singapore, and Turin.[8] The technique seems to be most popular in western Europe, including France, with over 700 units, and Switzerland, with over 100.[9]

An advice column in a weekend supplement to the *Los Angeles Times* spoke highly of using ozone in swimming pools, adding that ozone purifiers are easy to install and use in residential pools. Speaking of the advantages of ozone over chlorine, the author wrote:

Activated oxygen, ozone, is one of the best and safest swimming pool and spa purifiers. An ozone purifier can cut chemical usage by 80% and eliminate burning eyes, faded and bleached bathing suits, dry skin, etc. Many major cities use ozone to purify their drinking water. . . . A very low concentration of ozone gas in water is not harmful to people or pets, but it destroys bacteria, viruses and tiny particles. Within several minutes, ozone converts back to pure oxygen. Ozone gas breaks down bacteria and virus cell-walls in seconds and kills them. Chlorine takes hours to slowly penetrate these cells. Chlorine can react with common compounds in the pool to create cancer-causing chemicals.[10]

Ozone has also been used to purify the water in public swimming pools since 1950. During the Olympic Games held in Los Angeles during the summer of 1984, the European teams insisted that the water in the swimming pools be treated with ozone, not chlorine, or they would not participate in the events.

OZONE IN INDUSTRY

Ozone is used by the bottling industry to disinfect the inside of soda and beer bottles. The ozone later disappears as it decomposes to oxygen. Brewers use ozone to remove any residual bad taste and odor from the water used in beer production. Ozone is also employed by the pharmaceutical industry as a disinfectant and in the manufacture of electrical components to oxidize surface impurities. Ozone concentrations of one to three parts per million are used to inhibit the growth of molds and bacteria in stored foods like eggs, meat, vegetables, and fruits.[11]

WASTEWATER POLLUTION CONTROL

Ozone can break down industrial wastes like phenol and cyanide so that they become biodegradable. It is often utilized to oxidize mining wastes, wastes from the photographic industry, and harmful compounds like heavy metals, ethanol, and acetic acid.[12]

Ozone is also used to disinfect municipal wastewater and to clean up lakes and streams that have become polluted by sewage and other pollutants. Unlike chlorine, ozone can clean up a lake or stream without killing the resident animal life or leaving potentially harmful chemical residues in the ecosystem.

AIR AND ODOR TREATMENT

In the United States, over one hundred ozone generators are used by both municipalities and private companies to remove noxious odors from treated sewage. Sewage contains high amounts of foul-smelling chemicals like sulfides, amines, and olefins. Ozone gas does not mask their odors; instead, it oxidizes these compounds and leaves them odor-free.

Ozone is also used to reduce odors in rendering plants, paper mills, compost operations, underground railways, tunnels, and mines. The food industry uses minute amounts of ozone to treat odors in dairies, fish processing plants, and slaughterhouses.[13]

FOOD SANITATION

In addition to controlling odors, the potential use of ozone in ensuring food sanitation, eliminating pesticide residues, and killing harmful fungi is now being recognized by food technologists, with industry leaders like Ozone Safe Food Inc. (see the resources—appendix 2, page 438) developing sophisticated ozonation equipment for use in farms, slaughterhouses, dairies, fish processing plants, and fruit and vegetable processing facilities.

During the past few years, increasing attention has been focused on the importance of food safety, not only related to food growing in the field but also in food processing and storage. Cases of food-borne diseases have increased over recent years, and spoilage in the fruit and vegetable industry has been estimated to be as high as 30 percent.[14]

The most popular sanitizing agent has been water, used either alone or with added chemicals like chlorine. However, not only has chlorine been found to have limitations as an effective sanitizer, but it also forms by-products like trihalomethanes (THMs), dioxins, and other harmful chemical residues formed in wastewater. When returned to the environment, these by-products lead to water pollution and other ecological damage.

However, ozone is being increasingly regarded as a safe and effective alternative to chlorine, especially in the washing, sanitizing, and storing of produce. It can also destroy pesticides and chemical residues, as well as kill bacteria like *E. coli,* listeria, cryptosporidium, giardia, and other pathogens far more efficiently than chlorine. Ozone leaves no chemical residues: it completely decomposes within minutes into simple oxygen. And best of all, ozonated wastewater can be easily recycled without causing environmental damage of any kind.[15]

Studies have found that ozone, whether applied as gas or as ozonated water, reduces spoilage of fresh fruits and vegetables, including foods like blackberries, which are very prone to fungal decay.[16] Ozone has also been found to be a cheap and effective method of decontaminating food-processing equipment, storage rooms, food containers, food contact surfaces, and rooms where food is processed.[17]

Ozone has been found especially effective in controlling aflatoxin, a naturally occurring cancer-causing chemical that is produced by the fungus *Aspergillus flavus.* Found primarily in corn, cottonseed, and peanuts, aflatoxin can find its way into the products of animals that feed on corn (such as meat and dairy products) and foods made from corn and cornmeal (such as corn chips, muffins, and breakfast cereal). A study published in the *Journal of Food Science* found that ozone reduced aflatoxin levels by 92 percent, with no reversion to the parent compound observed.[18]

Reducing Pesticide Residues

Although numerous research studies dedicated to the sanitization of food products with ozone have been conducted over the years, it appears that few have focused specifically on how ozone can reduce the presence of pesticide residues in food of plant origin.

A study was undertaken by researchers at the University of Rzeszów in Poland to see if ozone could reduce pesticide residues in foods. The results, published in *Roczniki Państwowego Zakładu Higieny* [*Annals of the National Institute of Hygiene*], reported that washing with ozonated water was very effective in degrading pesticide residues present on fruit surfaces: "Even as low concentration as 0.25 ppm ozone in water enabled reduction of over 50% of residue levels of substances like azinphos-methyl (OFI), captan (phthalimide fungicide) and formetanate hydrochloride in fresh apples and their products. . . . [An] aqueous solution containing 2 ppm of ozone enabled 60% reduction of initial residue level of diazinon (OFI), parathion (OFI), methyl-parathion (OFI) and cypermethrin (PI) in vegetables." They also reported that ozone is effective in much lower concentrations than other agents used for washing food products.

The researchers concluded:

1. Ozone used in storage facilities was proven to inhibit the development of microbial infection in food products. This fact alone is sufficient to reduce levels of fungicides in food products.
2. Ozone can also play an active role in cleaning food products contaminated with pesticide residues.
3. No evidence of research on the degradation of pesticide residues with gaseous ozone in food products being conducted in the past was found.[19]

OZONE, ANTHRAX, AND HOMELAND SECURITY

In addition to aflatoxin, ozone can also kill *Erwinia,* a pathogen found in potatoes and other vegetables that causes rot after harvesting. After the bioterrorist attacks with anthrax on U.S. Postal Service facilities in 2001, scientists at the U.S. Department of Energy's Idaho National Engineering and Environmental Laboratory (INEEL)—who had tested ozone on potato crops—discovered that ozone can also kill anthrax spores. Ken Watts, a manager of the National Security Division of INEEL, reported that ozone "basically oxidizes the anthrax into a carbon dioxide compound. But the actual kill mechanism of the spore itself, no one knows for sure."[20]

In addition to being safer than chlorine dioxide and electron beam irradiation—which can destroy computer memory, photographic film, some medicines, and seeds—ozone is also much less expensive than electron beam irradiation. The price of a radiation machine is in the neighborhood of $5 million, while a comparable ozone generator costs about $120,000. Scientists like Watts believe that ozone can play an important role in national security, but more research needs to be carried out to see how best to proceed.[21]

"GENERALLY REGARDED AS SAFE"

On June 23, 2001, the FDA officially granted GRAS (generally regarded as safe) status to ozone for use in food contact applications. Whether working to limit food-borne illness or to address concerns over food contamination (either by accident or as a result of terrorist activity), ozone offers exciting possibilities for enhancing the safety of our food supply.

STERILIZATION OF MEDICAL DEVICES

A major challenge in medical practice has been to keep medical devices and products sterile and free from harmful contaminants such as fungi, viruses, spores, and bacteria, including "superbugs." Over the years, a number of methods have been developed to sterilize medical instruments, including autoclave stream sterilization, gamma ray sterilization, and the use of chemical disinfectants like ethylene oxide (EtO) and chlorine dioxide.

Ozone has been utilized to sterilize medical devices in hospitals, clinics, and research laboratories for decades. Specialized ozone sterilizers have been in use since the 1990s and were licensed for use in Canada in 2002 and in the United States by the FDA in 2003. Sterilization with ozone is as effective as chemical methods, yet it is more than seventy times more cost-efficient that using chemicals like EtO. Since the ozone sterilizer produces its own sterilizing agent, ozone does not require physical contact with or transportation by technicians; EtO is potentially explosive and difficult to handle. Ozone releases only oxygen and water vapor into the environment, while EtO residues in the environment must be carefully monitored.[22]

4
Ozone in Medicine

Toward the beginning of the twentieth century, interest began to focus on the uses of ozone in medical therapy. In September 1896, Nikola Tesla, the electronics genius and inventor of the radio, patented his first ozone generator, and in 1910 he formed the Tesla Ozone Company with a capital of $400,000. He hoped to apply his invention to a number of commercial uses, including refrigeration. It is said that Tesla sold his machines to doctors for medical use, and he is believed to have been the first person to manufacture ozonated olive oil to be sold to naturopathic physicians.

A recent discovery at the historical collection of the College of Physicians and Surgeons in Philadelphia shows that ozone was first used therapeutically by surgeon Samuel R. Beckwith, M.D., a member of the American Institute of Homeopathy and the Medical Society of Ohio. His book, *A New Therapeutics for the Cure of Disease by Sending Ozone, Oxygen and Medicine into Diseased Tissues,* was published in New York City in 1899.[1]

In Germany, physician Albert Wolff first utilized ozone to treat skin diseases in 1915, and the German army used ozone extensively during World War I to treat a wide variety of battle wounds and other anaerobic infections.

However, it was not until 1932 that ozone was seriously studied by the scientific community, when ozonated water was used as a disinfectant by Dr. E. A. Fisch, a German dentist. One of his patients was surgeon Erwin Payr, who immediately saw the therapeutic possibilities of ozone in medical therapy. Dr. Payr, along with French physician P. Aubourg, was the first medical doctor to apply ozone gas through rectal insufflation to treat mucous colitis and fistulas. In 1945, Payr pioneered the method of injecting ozone intravenously for the treatment of circulatory disturbances.

Other German pioneers in medical ozone include physician Hans Wolff (1924–1980), who wrote *Medical Ozone (Das medizinische Ozon)* and collaborated with physicist Joaquim Hansler (1908–1981) to establish the Medical Ozone Society (now the Medical Society for Ozone Application in Prevention and Therapy) in 1972.[2] Hansler designed and built the first medical ozone generator (the "OZONOSAN") that could make accurate dosages of oxygen and ozone. The company he founded still bears his name and is one of the largest and most trusted manufacturers of medical ozone generators in the world. A picture of a modern medical ozone generator is reproduced in figure 5.1 on page 58.

World War II brought about major setbacks for German research into medical ozone, because many clinics and laboratories were destroyed in Allied air raids. It was not until the 1950s that clinics reopened and research was begun once more.

The first physician to treat cancer with ozone was Dr. W. Zable in the late 1950s, followed by Drs. P. G. Seeger, A. Varro, and H. Werkmeister. During the next twenty years, hundreds of German physicians began using ozone in their practice to treat a wide variety of diseases (both alone and as a complement to traditional medical therapy) through a number of applications. Horst Kief is believed to have been the first physician to use ozone therapy to successfully treat patients infected with HIV. He also pioneered the development of autohomologous immunotherapy (AHIT) using ozone and other elements, which can be used to treat a wide variety of diseases that are resistant to traditional medical therapy.

Today some eight thousand licensed health practitioners

(including medical doctors, homeopathic physicians, and naturopaths) in Germany use ozone in their practices, while some fifteen thousand practitioners use ozone on the European continent, either alone or as a complement to other therapies. It is estimated that over twelve million ozone treatments have been given to over one million patients in Germany alone over the last fifty years. Although medical uses of ozone are still considered experimental by North American scientists, they are well known and well established outside the United States.

PSEUDOSCIENCE?

Some critics of ozone therapy have condemned it as a "pseudoscience" that has no solid medical foundation. Although prejudice can be a factor, this view may in part be a reaction to proclamations from overenthusiastic supporters of oxidative therapies who have claimed that ozone and hydrogen peroxide are "miracle drugs" that can cure any disease known to humankind. In addition, many reports on cures have never been documented by objective medical and scientific sources. While personal case histories have value, a major challenge among oxidative practitioners is the careful documentation of their clinical findings and collaboration with others to expand their research.

It's important to remember that while the clinical findings related to ozone and hydrogen peroxide are often impressive, oxidative therapies only *assist the body to heal itself.* Not every disease will respond to oxidative therapy, and many patients will find that these therapies will not relieve their health complaints. This is why we must focus not only on claims of miracle cures but also on documented clinical and laboratory findings that show why and how these therapies can work.

RESEARCH IN MEDICAL OZONE

Since the end of World War II, literally hundreds of laboratory and clinical studies in the medical uses of ozone have been done, primarily in Europe, and their findings have been published in a variety of scientific and medical journals. Many have been published in German, with the exception of those findings first reported at international medical conferences sponsored by the International Ozone Association, which were presented in English. At the present time, the bulk of scientific research in the medical uses of ozone is being undertaken in Cuba, Russia, Germany, and Italy, where researchers receive cooperation and support (in varying degrees) from the government and major universities. Research is going on to a far lesser extent in the United States, France, Mexico, and Canada.

However, one recent American study by scientists at the Scripps Research Institute in La Jolla, California, received worldwide attention. Published in the respected journal *Science* and other publications, it showed that in addition to hydrogen peroxide, ozone may be naturally produced in the human body to help kill bacteria, viruses, and other pathogens. These antibodies may not only kill pathogens directly but might also promote inflammatory and other immune responses.[3] Unfortunately, the article's authors emphasize the point that, particularly when ozone seems to be located in atherosclerotic plaques, ozone is always an unwelcome compound. Their report certainly does not explain how ozone works in the human body to both prevent and cure disease. Yet commenting on these surprising findings in another issue of *Science,* Dr. Carl Nathan, an immunologist at the Weill Cornell Medical Center in New York City, commented, "It will be hard to think of antibodies in the same way [as before]."[4]

More clear evidence that ozone works in this way is necessary. However, if true, this could be a significant discovery for several reasons. First, the fact that ozone is naturally produced by the human body removes from it the stigma of being classified as a "foreign element" that is harmful under all circumstances. It can also answer the critics of ozone therapy by helping explain how ozone works naturally in the human body to both prevent and cure disease.

Another important North American study receiving wide

publicity was published in the *Canadian Medical Association Journal* when fears of AIDS-related blood transfusions were at their height. It showed that ozone can kill HIV, the hepatitis and herpes viruses, and other agents in blood used for transfusion in vitro. The article's author added: "The systemic use of ozone in the treatment of AIDS could not only reduce the virus load but also possibly revitalize the immune system."[5]

Other research in ozone therapy is taking place in two unlikely countries: Russia and Cuba. In Russia, physicians, chemists, biologists, and other scientists have been working with the support of the Ministry of Public Health at major institutions like the Interregional Cardiosurgical Center and the Central Scientific Laboratory at the Medical Academy in Nizhny Novgorod (Gorky), the Sechenov Medical Academy and the Central Scientific and Research Institute of Dermatology and Venereology in Moscow, and the Institute of Photobiology in Minsk, Belarus. Ozone therapy is becoming part of the medical mainstream in Russia, and physicians from around the country come to Nizhny Novgorod for training.

Medical ozone research has been carried out since 1985 in Cuba under the auspices of the National Center for Scientific Research (in the former Ozone Research Center, which closed in 2011). In addition to investigations in medical ozone under the leadership of Dr. Silvia Menendez, director of research, the center was involved in the use of ozone for sanitation, wastewater treatment, and the design, construction, and installation of ozone generators. The National Center for Scientific Research also worked closely with physicians throughout the country as part of the National Program for Ozone Therapy and offered training for physicians from Cuba as well as from other countries. The National Center for Scientific Research sponsored the International Symposium on Ozone Applications every few years, which was attended by physicians, researchers, and others from all over the world. Since 1985, over one million patients have been treated with ozone at clinics and hospitals throughout the country, and many foreigners travel to

Cuba for ozone therapy at the International Ozone Therapy Clinic and other institutions, mostly in Havana.

By 2007, the National Center for Scientific Research and a staff of more than fifty-five chemists and laboratory technicians were located at a modern campus on the outskirts of Havana. The facility includes two laboratories, two ozone clinics (one for Cubans and one for foreigners), and an administration building. A 180-bed four-star hotel for foreign patients and their families, complete with an ozonated swimming pool, is located across the street.

It is important to view ozone therapy in the context of the Cuban health care system. One of the primary goals of the Cuban revolution of the 1950s was to provide free and universal health care to all Cuban citizens. Although subjected to a crippling economic blockade by the U.S. government since 1961, Cuba has nonetheless been able to position itself in the vanguard of medical research characteristic of many developed nations, including genetic engineering (the Center for Genetic Engineering and Biotechnology is the first of its kind in Latin America), organ transplant technology, the development of an artificial heart, vaccines for hepatitis B and meningococcal meningitis B, neural brain implants to treat Parkinson's disease, and the use of epidermal growth factor to aid burn victims.[6]

In contrast to his devastating eyewitness account of the disintegration of Castro's Cuba in his book *Castro's Final Hour*, Andres Oppenheimer had the following to say about the Cuban health care system:

> In fact, the revolution's greatest success had been in providing a first-class health care system for free. Whatever health needs Cubans had, whether a pregnancy test or a heart-bypass operation, they could have it for the asking. And because health care was the revolution's greatest pride, the state's magnanimity was unlimited: even cosmetic surgery and orthodontic treatments were performed without charge.[7]

Despite severe ongoing problems with transportation, agriculture, and economic development, Cuba has consistently maintained one of the highest levels of health care in all of Latin America. The results of much of the Cuban research will be presented here in this book.

Why are the Cubans and Russians so interested in ozone? Citizens of both countries have enjoyed socialized medicine for decades, so private drug manufacturers and private hospitals and clinics have traditionally played a small or nonexistent role in determining the direction of the health care system. As mentioned before, ozone cannot be patented, it is extremely cheap to produce, and it can be used effectively in a wide range of therapeutic applications. In countries like the United States, where large drug companies provide funding for medical schools, are directly or indirectly involved in all medical research, and lobby to influence governmental policy, there is simply no interest in researching the possibilities of ozone therapy. And even when private funding is offered for scientific or clinical research, hospitals have been known to refuse it. Yet in countries where the profit motive has traditionally been absent from health care, physicians, chemists, and other researchers enjoy government support and funding for their work.

The Bocci Breakthrough

One of the most tireless researchers in the therapeutic applications of ozone has been Velio Bocci, M.D., specialist in respiratory diseases and hematology and emeritus professor of physiology at the University of Siena in Italy. Since 1988, when Dr. Bocci first began to study ozone, he has collaborated with numerous researchers in Europe and has authored or coauthored more than fifty published articles on the subject. He is also the author of two respected scientific texts on ozone therapy: *Oxygen-Ozone Therapy: A Critical Evaluation,* followed by *Ozone: A New Medical Drug.* Both books were primarily written for the scientific and medical communities, but the newer book is more easily understood by the lay reader.

Although German researcher J. Washuttl and colleagues wrote about immunoactivation through ozone in the 1980s, Dr. Bocci was the first to scientifically explain how ozone actually works when added to blood removed from the body and then reinfused into the patient. As described in chapter 2, rather than merely kill bacteria and viruses directly through oxidation, ozone induces a cascade of complex immunological reactions within the body that promote health and healing. According to Renate Viebahn-Haensler in the fourth English edition of *The Use of Ozone in Medicine,* these findings, first published in a 1990 edition of the medical journal *Haemalotogica,*[8] represent "a major milestone in ozone therapy."[9]

ONE GAS,
MANY APPLICATIONS

Because ozone works primarily to stimulate the body's immune reactions through transient oxidative stress, and because blood is composed of a number of cells with different functions, the range of human health problems that can respond favorably to ozone therapy is quite broad. According to *The Use of Ozone in Medicine* (considered to be the basic reference book for physicians who work with ozone therapy), ozone has been used therapeutically in the areas of allergology, angiology (blood vessels), dermatology, gastroenterology, gerontology, gynecology, intensive care, neurology, odontology (dental medicine), oncology, orthopedics, proctology, radiology, rheumatology, surgery (including vascular surgery), and urology.[10] As the Canadian report cited earlier indicated, ozone has also been proven to effectively purify human blood supplies.

The European Cooperation of Medical Ozone Societies (made up of national affiliates in Germany, Austria, Italy, and Switzerland) and the National Center for Scientific Research in Cuba report that physicians are currently treating the following diseases listed on page 56 with different forms of ozone therapy.

abscesses

acne

AIDS

allergies (hypersensitivity)

anal fissures

arthritis

arthrosis

asthma

cancerous tumors

cerebral sclerosis

circulatory disturbances

cirrhosis of the liver

climacterium (menopause)

constipation

corneal ulcers

cystitis

decubitus (bedsores)

diarrhea

fistulas

fungal diseases

furunculosis

gangrene

gastroduodenal ulcers

gastrointestinal disorders

giardiasis

glaucoma

hepatitis

herpes (simplex and zoster)

hypercholesterolemia

mucous colitis

mycosis

nerve-related disorders

osteomyelitis

Parkinson's disease

polyarthritis

Raynaud's disease

retinitis pigmentosa

rheumatoid arthritis

scars (after radiation)

senile dementia

sepsis control

sinusitis

spondylitis

stomatitis

Sudeck's disease

thrombophlebitis

ulcus cruris (open leg sores)

vulvovaginitis

wound healing disturbances[11]

5
How Is Ozone
Therapy Applied?

Over the past sixty years, more than a dozen methods have been developed in the medically therapeutic application of ozone. Some have undergone extensive testing under clinical conditions and have been determined safe and effective by leading physicians and professional groups like the International Ozone Association and the International Scientific Committee of Ozone Therapy, while others have not. New methods are being introduced on a regular basis, including some that are considered highly experimental.

In most cases, tiny amounts of ozone are added to pure oxygen (consisting of 0.05 part of ozone to 99.95 parts of oxygen for internal use and 5 parts of ozone to 95 parts of oxygen for external applications). Doses are usually expressed in terms of micrograms of ozone per milliliter of oxygen ($\mu g/ml$). For example, if a physician were to require 1,200 micrograms of ozone, he or she would select a concentration of 12 $\mu g/ml$ and use a volume of 100 ml of oxygen. Because medical uses usually call for exact amounts of ozone, only ozone generators that allow measurements of precise concentrations should be used.

The exact amount of ozone to be used is determined on a case-by-case basis, after a careful medical diagnosis by a practitioner with extensive training in ozone therapy. That is the main reason why only representative ozone (and hydrogen peroxide) protocols are included in this book, the goal of which is to educate the reader about these therapies rather than promote self-treatment. In addition, protocols can change over time, and the medical needs of each patient must be determined on an individual basis before an oxidative therapy is used. For a current listing of specific medical protocols for ozone therapy, consult the latest edition of Viebahn-Haensler's *The Use of Ozone in Medicine,* chapter 9 ("The Clinical Applications of Ozone") in Bocci's *Ozone: A New Medical Drug,* and the latest edition of the *Madrid Declaration on Ozone Therapy.*

Over the years, some physicians have found that too much ozone can be immunosuppressive, while not enough can be ineffective. In an effort to discover the lowest possible dose of ozone needed to enhance immune activity, many researchers see microdosing as an important guideline in future therapeutic ozone applications.

Figure 5.1. Portable medical ozone generator. (Photograph courtesy of Kastner Praxisbedarf GmbH-Medizintechnik, Rastatt, Germany.)

OZONE DELIVERY

At the present time, there are numerous methods of ozone therapy that are used in medical practice. Some are designed for very specific health problems, while others have more generalized applications. Some methods are considered extremely safe; the safety of others is questionable.

According to *The Use of Ozone in Medicine,* the most common recommended applications include the following:

Systemic Applications

Major autohemotherapy

Minor autohemotherapy

Rectal/vaginal insufflation

Topical Applications

Intra-articular injection

Ozone bagging

Ozonated ointments

Ozonated water as sprays

Suction cup method[1]

Let's look at these and other applications in more detail.

Systemic Applications

Direct Intra-arterial Application

An oxygen-ozone mixture is slowly injected into an artery with a hypodermic syringe. This method has been used primarily for arterial circulatory disorders. However, this method has been abandoned by most physicians in favor of safer modalities. According to Gerard V. Sunnen, M.D., "Due to accidents produced by too rapid introduction of the gas mixture into the circulation, this technique is now rarely used."[2] It has been prohibited in Europe since 1984 to avoid the risk of gas embolism.

Rectal Insufflation

First pioneered by Payr and Aubourg in the 1930s, a mixture of ozone and oxygen is introduced through the rectum. In the past, it was believed that the ozone was absorbed into the body through the intestine. In fact, ozone reacts with the luminal content immediately and only some of the chemicals produced during the reaction are absorbed; this has been scientifically measured in both the portal and general circulation by Dr. Bocci and his colleagues.[3] Used for a wide variety of health problems, including arterial circulatory disorders, general immunoactivation, adjuvant cancer therapy, and hepatitis A, B, and C,[4] this method is considered one of the safest. Typically, between 100 and 800 ml of oxygen and ozone (for an average adult of normal body weight) is insufflated into the rectum, a process that takes between 1½ and 2 minutes.

Dr. Horst Kief believes that rectal insufflation is a valuable method of ozone-oxygen delivery due to several unique properties of the large intestine, especially its enormous surface of resorption, among these other properties:

- The intestinum of adults is approximately 12 meters long and, due to the multitude of intestinal villi and crypts, features a surface of 10 square meters.
- The lymphatic system of the intestinum (i.e., Peyer's patches) occupies more space within the human organism than is used by the spleen and the thymus together.
- The circulatory system of the intestinum is directly connected to the liver through the portal vein, where most of the biochemical, immunological, and metabolic processes take place.
- "Death lives in the intestines." This popular saying presumably is derived from the deeply rooted archaic knowledge that the intestinal flora—the pathological flora in particular—may trigger a number of diseases, which most frequently are misjudged or rather underestimated by traditional medicine.

Considering the anatomic, immunological, biochemical, and micro-biological particularities of the intestinum, the use of medical ozone may reasonably be expected to provide decisive therapeutic consequences in rectal application and to yield successful clinical results.

Dr. Kief adds that the use of medical ozone in rectal application should do the following:

- Provide for measurable resorption to be obtained upon insufflation of sufficient volumes
- Provide for a substantial immunological effect to be obtained due to direct contamination of the largest lymphatic system of the human organism
- Yield improvements relating to all oxidative processes taking place in the liver due to the increased flood of reactive oxygen metabolites supplied to this organ
- Provide for the microbiological milieu to be improved in cases of pathological changes of the intestinal flora due to old age and wrongful eating habits supported by our society[5]

Rectal insufflation is considered a safe and simple method of ozone delivery that is particularly suited to the elderly (who often have difficult access to veins), to babies and young children, and to others who don't like getting stuck with hypodermic syringes. While administered under medical supervision in Germany, Russia, and Cuba, a growing number of private individuals in the United States have used this method for self-treatment of cancer, HIV-related problems, heart and circulatory disorders, diabetes, and other degenerative diseases. It has also been found useful in treating localized health problems such as proctitis and colitis.

Whenever insufflation is used, the ozone-oxygen mixture must be humidified in order to prevent sensitive tissues from drying out.

Vaginal Insufflation/Urethral Insufflation

Vaginal insufflation is based on the wrong philosophy that ozone can be absorbed into the body through the vaginal wall, uterus, and fallopian tubes. In reality, oxygen and certain chemicals produced by the post-ozone reaction are absorbed. This method is considered safe and effective, and physicians have found not only that it can be useful for the same kinds of systemic diseases ordinarily treated by rectal insufflation, but also that the vaginal route can be used specifically to treat gynecological problems like yeast infections (such as candida) and uterine infections. This method is not recommended during pregnancy.

Using a silicone catheter, Cuban physicians apply oxygen-ozone to treat a variety of gynecological problems, including vulvovaginitis, vaginosis, and cervicitis. They report that the best results are obtained after the affected area is pretreated with ozonated water. Ozonated oil is also used after treatment to facilitate healing.[6]

Urethral insufflation is recommended primarily for treating bladder infections among men, but it may be useful in localized problems such as urethritis as well. In Cuban clinics a mixture of oxygen and ozone is administered via a fine-gauge silicone catheter. Treatment can be combined with ozonated water, which is also applied through a catheter.[7]

Ear Insufflation

Applying a mixture of oxygen and ozone through the ear is a recent but popular development in ozone therapy. This method is based on the idea that ozone is absorbed by the body through the tiny capillaries of the ear canal. Once again, this idea is wrong, and only some chemical compounds produced by a post-ozone reaction are absorbed into the ear canal.

Used only in a well-ventilated room (and preferably with a fan placed behind the patient to prevent inhalation of ozone), the generator is connected to a tube with a plastic catheter. The generator is turned on, and the catheter is placed gently into the ear. Some use a modified stethoscope to split the ozone flow so that both ears are treated at the same time. The gas is run at a slow flow rate through a glass humidifier, and it then interacts with the surface tissues of the eardrum. The chemical compounds produced by these interactions enter the middle ear and the inner ear and proceed down the eustachian tube into the sinuses, brain, and bloodstream. A typical treatment takes 1 to 2 minutes.

Typically, sick patients undergo three ear insufflation treatments a week, while others use it once or twice weekly for health maintenance. Although this method has not yet been clinically studied, doctors report that ear insufflation is helpful in treating ear infections, mastoiditis, tinnitus, sinusitis, head colds, hearing problems caused by candida, and more generalized symptoms of such conditions as Parkinson's disease, influenza, bronchitis, and asthma. However, some physicians question whether a prolonged and repeated course of treatment is safe considering the delicacy of and low levels of antioxidants in these auricular structures.

Intramuscular Injection

A small amount of an ozone and oxygen mixture (up to 10 ml) is injected into the patient (usually in the buttocks) like a normal injection would be. This method is commonly used to treat allergies and inflammatory diseases, and it is sometimes used as an adjunct to traditional cancer therapies in Europe. However, it has been reported that ozone concentrations over 20 µg/ml in volumes exceeding 10 ml can be very painful and may produce feelings of faintness in some patients.

Minor Autohemotherapy

Used since the 1960s, minor autohemotherapy involves removing a small amount (usually 10 ml) of the patient's blood from a vein with a hypodermic syringe. The blood is treated with ozone and oxygen and then returned to the patient via intramuscular injection. Thus the blood and ozone mixture becomes a type of autovaccine given to the patient that is derived from his or her own cells and can be very specific and effective in treating the patient's health problem. This method is primarily used to treat acne, allergies, and furunculosis and as an adjunct to traditional cancer therapy.[8]

Major Autohemotherapy (MAHT)

Major autohemotherapy is perhaps the most popular form of generalized ozone therapy. A type of extracorporeal blood treatment (in which blood is taken from the body, treated, and reinfused), MAHT has been analyzed and evaluated under a wide variety of clinical conditions.

Major autohemotherapy typically calls for the removal of up to 250 ml of the patient's blood. Ozone and oxygen are carefully added to the blood for several minutes, and then the ozonated blood is reintroduced into the vein in the form of an intravenous (IV) drip. Care must be taken on the introduction of the ozone-oxygen mixture to prevent bubbling, which causes foaming that damages blood cells and must be avoided.

Like rectal insufflation, MAHT has been found to activate red blood cell metabolism, increase ATP production and oxygen release, activate the immune system with the release of cytokines (such as interferon and interleukins), aid in immune system modulation, and increase the body's antioxidant capacity.[9] For these reasons, it has been used successfully to treat a wide variety of health problems, including herpes, arthritis, cancer, circulatory disorders, and HIV infection. It is probably the most commonly used type of ozone therapy today.

MAHT involves the following steps (see figure 5.2):

1. One-half pint of blood is removed from the patient.
2. Ozone is taken from the medical ozone generator.
3. The ozone is allowed to mix with the blood. (This is done by simply rotating the bottle gently for a few minutes to mix the blood and gas phases.)
4. The blood is then infused into the patient.

Body Ozone Exposure (BOEX): The Sauna Bag

Ozone pumped into a "sauna bag" is now being used to treat more generalized health problems, such as HIV infection, circulatory problems, and diabetes. Typically the patient takes a warm shower and gets into the bag, which covers the entire body except the head. A special closure

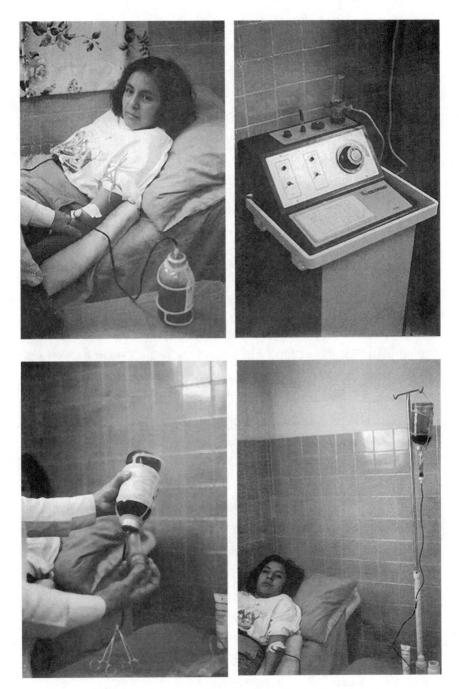

Figure 5.2. Major autohemotherapy, Cira Garcia Hospital, Havana. (Photographs by Nathaniel Altman.)

is used to prevent the patient from breathing in the oxygen-ozone mixture. Pure oxygen mixed with small amounts of ozone is then pumped into the bag for a period of 20 to 30 minutes, making contact with all skin surfaces. The skin interacts with the ozone, and only the oxygen and ozone-reactive products are absorbed. According to Dr. Sunnen: "Surprisingly, the mixture is able to penetrate far enough into the capillary networks to raise blood oxygen pressure. Presumably, then, ozone is able to exert its biochemical influence."[10]

Body Ozone Exposure: The Steam Cabinet Method

Another BOEX delivery system calls for the patient to sit in a steam cabinet (see figure 5.3). In addition to steam, a mixture of oxygen and ozone is pumped into the cabinet through a tube from an ozone generator. Wet towels are placed around the patient's neck and a ventilating fan is placed behind the head so that ozone is not breathed into the lungs. A session will normally last from 10 to 20 minutes, or until the patient feels uncomfortable from the heat. Like the sauna bag technique described above, the theory behind this method is that the ozone will react with the surface of the skin, and the oxygen and ozone-reactive products will be absorbed and eventually find their way into the bloodstream.

BOEX with a steam cabinet can easily be done at home with a minimum of technical skill, and many enjoy it as a spa treatment or in health maintenance programs. A growing number of physicians and patients have expressed enthusiasm for the steam cabinet method for treating a wide variety of health complaints, although more scientific research needs to be done. In addition, standardized protocols need to be developed for this relatively new form of ozone application.

While the method itself is considered very safe, ozone must not be inhaled, even in small amounts. For this reason, the steam cabinet must be sealed to prevent ozone leakage and the room in which treatment takes place must be adequately ventilated.

One of the few researchers to document the effects of BOEX is Dr. Velio Bocci, in his book *Oxygen-Ozone Therapy: A Critical*

Evaluation. While acknowledging the problems mentioned above, Dr. Bocci cites several advantages of BOEX over other methods like MAHT: it is simple to perform, fairly inexpensive, and noninvasive (no puncturing of veins) and does not involve the handling of blood. He points out that BOEX can be potentially useful in treating a variety of health problems, such as viral diseases (including HIV and herpes), chronic fatigue syndrome, certain circulatory diseases at low temperature levels (such as hind limb ischemia due to atherosclerosis, Buerger's disease, and diabetes), moderate burns, skin diseases, scleroderma, certain types of musculotendinous lesions in athletes, and advanced lipodystrophies, such as Madelung disease.

Figure 5.3. Steam cabinet for BOEX.
(Photograph courtesy of Ozone Services.)

As with other ozone therapies, Dr. Bocci recommends the "start low, go slow" protocols, with low initial concentrations of ozone to help the body adapt to chronic oxidative stress. He recommends a course of therapy every other day for several weeks at temperatures from 70 to 90°C for periods of 10 to 25 minutes for each treatment.[11]

Direct Intravenous Injection

This controversial method involves injecting a mixture of oxygen and ozone directly into a vein. This method has long been promoted by Ed "Mr. Oxygen™" McCabe in his publications and lectures, and he includes a protocol for the treatment in his popular book *Flood Your Body with Oxygen*. When determining how much ozone to use, McCabe writes:

> I have always used the analogy of filling up the gas tank in your car. You pump the gas in and when it's full, if you keep pumping it in the gas runs down the side of the car. The lungs are the oxygen overflow mechanism for the blood. When the bloodstream is full, the blood out-gasses into the lungs, and the oxygen-ozone sub species "run down" the inside of the lungs, causing rapid lung pollution detoxification, heat, and possible slight temporary edema. All the patient knows is that he or she can't stop coughing if you do not quickly stop the procedure at the first sign of this.[12]

Although a number of health practitioners in the United States and Canada claim that this method is safe and effective, many physicians (especially those trained in Europe and Cuba) consider it dangerous and without clinical advantages over other ozone delivery methods.

In my own work as a journalist covering the subject of ozone therapy, I've come across stories of embolism, including one of a patient becoming comatose and another patient suffering respiratory arrest after direct IV treatment. Dr. Robert Atkins's medical license was temporarily revoked after a patient went to the hospital complaining of adverse side effects from direct IV injection, which led the doctor to abandon it permanently.

Dr. Frank Shallenberger, perhaps the most respected ozone practitioner in the United States today, has treated thousands of patients with therapeutic ozone since 1985. After several negative experiences with direct IV injection early in his practice, he stopped using the method completely in favor of autohemotherapy. In his training manual for physicians who attend his workshops, Dr. Shallenberger offered six reasons why direct IV injection should not be used:

1. Precise dosing is impossible, because the induction effects of ozone vary according to the volume amount of blood being treated. Since it is impossible to know with any precision what volume of blood is being treated in a direct IV application, it is impossible to maximize the treatment effect.
2. Autopsy studies of dogs treated with the direct IV method have consistently demonstrated that the technique causes pulmonary embolisms. These embolisms are caused by the oxygen in the gas mixture, not the ozone.
3. The embolisms associated with direct IV injection will induce bronchospasm, which in the case of patients with a history of either asthma or chronic lung disease may result in fatal acute respiratory failure.
4. The treatment of many clinical conditions requires fairly large doses of ozone. While these doses are readily achieved using MAH [major autohemotherapy], they are extremely time-consuming using the direct IV method.
5. The direct IV method is very uncomfortable to patients. The embolisms cause chest pain, coughing spasms, and tachycardia.
6. Phlebitis at the injection site is a common side effect of this modality.[13]

Dr. Bocci has also spoken out strongly against direct IV injection. In a 1995 speech on the future of ozone therapy presented at the

Twelfth World Congress of the International Ozone Association in Lille, France, he cautioned: "[The] use of the intravenous administration route is extremely dangerous, because even if the gaseous mixture of oxygen-ozone is administered very slowly with a pump, it frequently procures lung embolization and serious side effects, particularly when daily dosing is up to 120 ml."[14]

In a 2005 communication, Dr. Bocci cited a number of fatalities in Italy resulting from subcutaneous (under the skin) ozone injections to treat lipodystrophy, commonly known as cellulite. Three deaths, from March 1998 to December 2002, caused the Italian Ministry of Health to prohibit the use of ozone therapy not only in all cosmetic and beauty centers but also in public hospitals.

Bocci adds bluntly:

> I am always very emphatic in proscribing direct IV injection of the gas [oxygen-ozone] mixture: Unfortunately charlatans and technicians without medical qualification do this because they either are stupid or because they cannot do major AHT [autohemotherapy]. It has been well defined that a gas injection with a volume above 20 ml can produce a deadly embolism. Thus why risk harming the patient? Moreover, it does not matter that it is not ozone, but actually oxygen [that] kills the patients. Indeed the minute volume of ozone is immediately dissolved and disappears because of extreme reactive capacity.[15]

Dr. Bocci also points out that in the often-cited 1983 German survey on the safety of ozone applications (see chapter 2, note 3), the only adverse side effects were attributed to direct IV injection. Administering ozone through this method is considered medical malpractice in Europe and has been outlawed there since 1984.[16]

The International Scientific Committee of Ozone Therapy's position on direct IV injection of ozone and oxygen was stated clearly in the *Madrid Declaration on Ozone Therapy* in 2015:

Its application is strongly discouraged due to the risk of air embolism which can occur even in the case of using a slow infusion pump and volumes of 20 ml. The complications of stroke range from a simple axillary bubbling sensation, then cough, a feeling of retrosternal weight, dizziness, to changes in vision (ambioplia), hypotensive crisis, with signs of cerebral ischemia (paresis of the members) and death. It is important to note that five patients died as a result of gas embolism after administration of ozone by direct intravenous injection. Furthermore, there is no justification to put the patient and the therapy at risk when there are methods that are safe, have been tested and are effective such as the major autohemotherapy, minor autohemotherapy and rectal insufflation.[17]

Ozone IV and Saline

First developed by researchers affiliated with the Russian Association of Ozonetherapy in Nizhny Novgorod, the intravenous IV method of using a liquid oxygen-ozone saline drip (as opposed to direct IV injection of ozone and oxygen) appears to be free of the dangers of embolism.[18]

Using an ozone generator, fill spout, and ozone destructor unit, oxygen and ozone are bubbled into a prescribed amount of saline (the Russians use 200 or 400 ml of sterile physiological 0.9 percent sodium chloride solution), the kind usually used in IV drips. The ozonated saline is then infused slowly into the patient through a vein, as a normal intravenous saline drip would be.

While Russian studies have found this method to be both safe and effective,[19] similar research has not been done in the West. However, physicians who have used this method have reported good results with minimal adverse reactions. Some possible clinical applications for this ozone delivery method could include treating disease-causing microorganisms in the blood, as well as rheumatic diseases, inflammatory conditions, and degenerative diseases such as arteriosclerosis, diabetes, and cancer. According to Natalia Bernikova of Medozons Ltd. (a company formed by the Russian Association of Ozonetherapy and the Russian Federal Nuclear Center Arzamas-16):

> Intravenous infusion of ozonated saline is still procedure No. 1 in Russia, being a priority of the Russian technology of ozone therapy and considered as a better systemic alternative to major autohaemo- therapy and rectal insufflations. Nevertheless, the latter methods have been used in Russia as well, depending on the indication.[20]

However, this method is not without its critics. Dr. Bocci, who is one of them, writes, "Unless very low levels of ozonation are adopted, some formation of hypochloric acid, with time, will cause venous damage, pos- sibly phlebitis" and could "possibly induce intravascular coagulation." He also dismisses this method as more a placebo than a real treatment.[21]

Figure 5.4. IV delivery system for ozonated saline.
(Graphic courtesy of Ven-Mar Scientific.)

I also asked Dr. Renate Viebahn-Haensler her views on this subject. She replied:

> As to the ozonization of saline I am of the same opinion as Prof. Bocci: we have measured the reaction products under different conditions and approaches. The results are not promising: we always got NaOCl [hypochloric acid] which is toxic to blood and blood vessels. So, there is no recommendation to treat saline or another solution containing physiological NaCl solution. I know there are Russian groups treating patients that way but with very, very low ozone concentrations.[22]

Extracorporeal Blood Circulation (EBOO)

EBOO is an experimental procedure developed by Velio Bocci and others in Italy. Its goal is to ozonate large amounts of blood in a single session (5 liters over a period of 30 to 45 minutes) using a method similar to kidney dialysis. However, Bocci is critical of the use of dialysis filters:

> I condemn the use of dialysis filters because they are ineffective and toxic, and unfortunately Russians and other charlatans in Kenya, Malaysia, etc. use them. We need only to exchange gas and therefore we can use only appropriate hydrophobic gas exchangers coated with biocompatible compounds to prevent platelet activation. The system operates quite differently from dialysis because blood runs outside the ozone-resistant hollow-fiber tubings.[23]

By 2006, EBOO had been used on several dozen volunteers, mostly patients suffering from serious coronary disease. Most received fourteen treatments over a period of several weeks, with periodic follow-up treatments. Improvements were noted in all patients.

Dr. Bocci believes that EBOO can be potentially useful in patients with chronic, inoperable ischemic limbs (where amputation is the only alternative); severe coronary angiostenosis (narrowing of the blood vessels); chronic hepatitis C; acute cardiac ischemia; inoperative metastatic cancer; and severe lipodystrophies that are characterized by abnormalities in fatty tissue (which can be associated with total or partial loss of body fat), abnormalities of carbohydrate and lipid metabolism, severe resistance to insulin, and immune system dysfunction.

However, disadvantages include the high costs of a disposable oxygenator and of training a highly qualified technician, possible deterioration of access to veins, and complications associated with the occasional need to insert a catheter into a central vein.[24]

In an article published in *Redox Report: Communications in Free Radical Research,* a team of researchers from the Nephrology and Dialysis Department at the University Hospital in Siena, Italy, praised EBOO for its ability to treat large amounts of blood more efficiently than major autohemotherapy: in one hour of extracorporeal circulation, up to 4,800 ml of heparinized blood can be treated without technical or clinical problems, whereas only 250 ml of blood can be treated with ozone by major autohemotherapy.

In addition to a configuring this method for use in hemodialysis, researchers saw great potential for EBOO in treating patients with severe peripheral arterial disease, coronary disease, cholesterol embolism, severe dyslipidemia (an abnormal amount of lipids—such as cholesterol and/or fat—in the blood), sudden deafness of vascular origin, and Madelung disease, a rare condition involving the presence of multiple symmetric, nonencapsulated masses of fatty tissue, usually in the neck and upper part of the trunk.[25]

By 2015, the International Scientific Committeee of Ozone Therapy considered EBOO to be an advanced variant of autohemotherapy. It is currently being used to treat a variety of serious health problems, including severe peripheral artery disease, coronary disease, cholesterol embolism, severe dyslipidemia, Madelung disease, ischemic stroke, chronic heart failure, and hepatitis C.[26]

Intraperitoneal Ozone

Another highly experimental yet promising method is administering oxygen and ozone into the peritoneum, a thin membrane that lines the abdominal and pelvic cavities and covers most abdominal viscera. Russian physicians have been washing out purulent material with ozonized water in treating peritonitis and pleural empyema for years with good results, and Dr. Bocci has explored the possibility of using this method to treat chronic viral hepatitis.[27]

Administering medication through the peritoneum is rare, but not unknown. A 2006 article in the *New York Times* highlighted how this method can help prolong the lives of ovarian cancer patients and reported that the National Cancer Institute took the unusual step of encouraging doctors to adopt this previously little-used abdominal treatment.[28]

In Cuba, intraperitoneal ozone is used primarily in patients suffering from peritonitis. Oxygen and ozone are applied as autohemotherapy via a catheter implanted into the peritoneal cavity. In addition, Cuban physicians deliver ozonated water via a catheter to cleanse the affected area. They consider this method to be safe because it avoids risk of embolism.[29]

A technique to administer intraperitoneal ozone was developed by Dr. Siegfried Schulz and others from various institutes and departments (Veterinary Services and Laboratory Animal Medicine; the Department of Otorhinolaryngology, Head and Neck Surgery; the Department of Pathology; the Institute of Anatomy and Cell Biology; and the Department of Pediatrics) at the Philipps-Universität of Marburg, Germany. Dr. Schulz and his colleagues believe that intraperitoneal ozone application can yield great benefits for patients suffering from cancer and severe bacterial diseases like sepsis and enterocolitis.[30] By 2016, the use of intraperitoneal ozone was still in the experimental phase with animals, although washing of the abdominal cavity with ozonated saline solution during surgery for peritonitis has been successfully used on humans. Details of their research will be discussed in chapters 11 and 23.

Intratonsilar

In Cuba, oxygen-ozone injections are administered to patients diagnosed with tonsillitis. Between 1 and 5 ml of oxygen-ozone at a concentration of between 40 and 45 mg/L is injected into each tonsil. Four or five applications is the norm.[31]

Topical Applications

Ozonated Water

This method calls for ozone gas to be bubbled through water, which is then used externally to bathe wounds, burns, and slow-healing skin infections. It is also used as a disinfectant by dentists who perform dental surgery. In Russia, physicians are using ozonated water to irrigate body cavities during surgery. In both Russia and Cuba, ozonated water is used to treat a wide variety of intestinal and gynecological problems, including ulcerative colitis, duodenal ulcers, gastritis, diarrhea, and vulvovaginitis. Ozonated water can also be used for colonics or enemas.

Intra-articular Injection

In this method ozone gas is bubbled through water and the mixture is injected directly between the joints, primarily those of the knee and shoulder. Some feel that using water is not necessary because synovial fluid (a transparent viscid lubricating fluid secreted by a membrane of an articulation, bursa, or tendon sheath) contains plenty of water. And unless the water and the delivery system are sterile, they may also contaminate the gas.

Intra-articular injection is used primarily by physicians in Europe and Cuba to treat rheumatoid arthritis, knee arthrosis, rheumatism, traumatic knee disorders, and other joint diseases. A variation of this method, known as Prolozone therapy, was developed by Dr. Shallenberger. We'll discuss this unique therapy in detail in chapter 14.

Ozone Bagging

This noninvasive method uses a special ozone-resistant plastic bag containing some water that is placed around the area to be treated. An ozone-oxygen mixture is pumped into the bag, and the oxygen and ozone-reactive products that result are absorbed into the body through the skin. Ozone bagging is primarily recommended for treating leg ulcers, gangrene, fungal infections, burns, and slow-healing wounds. Without water in the bag, ozone is practically ineffective. A normal treatment takes 10 to 20 minutes using approximately 80 to 100 microns of ozone. A photo of a patient receiving an ozone treatment with this method is found in figure 5.5.

Ozone Glass Cupping Funnel

Another form of transdermal ozone application is ozone cupping, which utilizes a small glass cup with a funnel attached to administer ozone to specific areas of the skin (see figure 5.6 on page 78). The cupping funnel has an ozone destruct and an ozone line to introduce ozone into the funnel. The physician first applies a small amount of water to the skin, and then the glass cup is applied firmly to the area being treated. A mixture of oxygen and ozone is pumped into the cup, and the oxygen and ozone-reactive products penetrate the skin. This method has been

Figure 5.5. The "ozone bagging" method.
(Photograph by Nathaniel Altman.)

Figure 5.6. Ozone
cupping funnel.
(Photograph by
Nathaniel Altman.)

found to be especially effective in treating poorly healing wounds, abrasions, skin infections, herpes, decubitus ulcers, fungal skin infections, burns, and radiodermatitis. A typical treatment involves a low flow of ozone administered for 10 to 15 minutes.

Ozonated Oils

Ozonated oil has been used to treat skin problems for over a century. Although not yet widely available in pharmacies, it became quite popular in Europe during the 1950s and is marketed by mail through a number of ozone suppliers in the United States and Canada (see the resources—appendix 2). Ozone gas is added to olive oil and applied as a balm or salve for long-term, low-dose exposure. Other bases (such as sunflower oil) for salves and creams have been developed in Cuba, where their effects have been extensively documented in hospitals and clinics.

Ozonated oil has been found to be useful in treating a wide variety of skin problems, including dermatitis, bacterial infections of the skin (including staphylococcal diseases such as cellulitis, impetigo, ecthyma, and scalded skin syndrome), fungal infections (including infections of the nail bed and athlete's foot), fistulas, leg ulcers, bedsores, gingivitis, herpes simplex, hemorrhoids, vulvovaginitis, bee stings and insect bites, acne, furuncles and carbuncles, infections of the sweat glands (hidradenitis suppurativa), and yeast infections of the skin including candidiasis (caused by *Candida albicans*). It is also useful in the postsurgical treatment of wounds, and Cuban physicians are using capsules filled with ozonated oil to treat gastroduodenal ulcers, gastritis, giardiasis, and peptic ulcers.

Inhalation of Ozone?

Physicians who use medical ozone warn that inhaling ozone into the lungs can bring about alterations in the density of the lung tissue, damage delicate lung membranes, irritate the epithelium (the surface layer of mucus) in the trachea and bronchi, and lead to emphysema. They caution users that no ozone should escape into the room in which it is being used; properly designed medical ozone generators that avoid the accidental escape of ozone gas are becoming available for use. Dr. Stephen A. Levine, the coauthor of *Antioxidant Adaptation,* cautions people against using commercial air purifiers that generate small amounts of ozone to clean the air, since ozone should not be inhaled.

Having said this, it is important to point out that in Russia, tiny amounts of ozone are being added to oxygen for therapeutic inhalation in certain cases. This has been done with patients suffering from carbon monoxide poisoning, and doctors have been impressed with the results. No adverse side effects were observed.[32]

Here in the United States, some physicians have begun to experiment with inhalation of ozone filtered through olive oil, because bubbling ozone and oxygen into olive oil produces a different gas ($C_{10}H_{18}O_3$) that can be safely inhaled through the nostrils. We will see how this method is used in veterinary medicine in chapter 26.

Pure oxygen is used as the feed gas through a medical ozone generator. A low concentration of ozone is used at a flow rate of 0.25 to

0.5 liter per minute. A humidifier or nebulizer is filled half-full with extra-virgin, cold-pressed olive oil, and the oxygen-ozone gas is bubbled through the olive oil. The patient either inhales the vapors directly from the olive oil or inhales it through an oxygen mask or nasal cannula. A typical treatment takes approximately 20 minutes. Practitioners in both Europe and the United States report that this delivery system is both safe and effective for treating allergies, asthma, and other respiratory diseases. However, they warn that this method is *never to be used without olive oil or at high ozone concentrations.*

Autohomologous Immunotherapy (AHIT)

This controversial method of ozone therapy was developed by the German physician Horst Kief in the early 1980s. It is a patented new form of autohemotherapy currently used by a small number of physicians in Europe. AHIT is not approved for treatment in the United States.

In AHIT, the patient's own blood and urine are taken to a laboratory and are broken down into their different cellular and fluid parts, known as *fractions*. Each fraction undergoes more than a dozen special biochemical and processing steps, including ozonation. These different fractions are then recombined according to the patient's diagnosis and are administered as drops, injections, or inhalation fluids over a period of several months.

Dr. Kief and others have found AHIT to have a strong influence on the immune system. It causes a change in the immunological cell systems that aid in stimulating the body's natural defense mechanisms. Unlike antibiotics and other medications, AHIT has produced no adverse side effects in literally thousands of applications. AHIT has been clinically shown to have a potent effect on a wide variety of diseases, including cancer, eczema, bronchial asthma, allergies, rheumatic joint diseases, chronic infections, and premature aging. It also holds promise for the treatment of other diseases like hepatitis, HIV-related problems, cirrhosis, and ulcerative colitis.[33]

Dr. Kief's method is not without its critics, even within the ozone community. In *Oxygen-Ozone Therapy: A Critical Evaluation,* Dr. Bocci questions the claims that AHIT can cure cancer and notes that the three cases he followed showed no improvement. Knowing that many cancer patients visit Dr. Kief when all other therapeutic methods have failed, Bocci writes, "My feeling is that once the disease has reached the point of no return, any therapy becomes practically useless."[34] He is also skeptical of findings that have never been reported in a peer-reviewed medical journal. However, in chapter 11, we will review some of Dr. Kief's clinical evidence showing that AHIT can help fight cancer, even at late stages of progression.

OZONE: EXACT MEASURE

Different therapies require very specific concentrations of ozone, and the ozone must be given in exact amounts. According to Dr. Bocci, "The ozone therapist must be aware of the dilemma that either too low or too high ozone doses can be either ineffective or toxic, respectively."[35]

Figure 5.7. Different applications of ozone; *gamma* stands for micrograms/ml. (Reproduced courtesy of Ozone Services.)

Some generators, like the German, Canadian, and Cuban machines referred to earlier in this chapter, are capable of generating ozone for all therapeutic applications, while others (especially inexpensive models designed primarily for treating tap water in the home) are not. This is why it is important to verify a generator's capacity before purchase and to determine the exact ozone concentration produced by the generator for a specific therapeutic use. Figure 5.7 on page 81 illustrates the typical concentrations of ozone required for different therapeutic applications.

In part 2, we will examine how these different forms of ozone therapy (as well as therapeutic applications of hydrogen peroxide) have been used to successfully treat a wide range of specific health problems, both alone and as adjuncts to other forms of medical treatment.

6
Hydrogen Peroxide

Hydrogen peroxide is a clear, colorless liquid that easily mixes with water. Made up of two hydrogen atoms and two oxygen atoms, it is known chemically as H_2O_2. Hydrogen peroxide is created in the atmosphere when ultraviolet light strikes oxygen in the presence of moisture. Ozone (O_3) is free oxygen (O_2) plus an extra atom of oxygen. When it comes into contact with water, this extra atom of oxygen splits off very easily. Water (H_2O) combines with the extra atom of oxygen and becomes hydrogen peroxide (H_2O_2).

We can call hydrogen peroxide a close relative of ozone. Aside from being known as a powerful oxygenator and oxidizer, hydrogen peroxide readily decomposes into water and oxygen. Like ozone, hydrogen peroxide reacts easily with other substances and is able to kill bacteria, fungi, parasites, viruses, and some types of tumor cells.

Hydrogen peroxide occurs naturally within the earth's biosphere; traces of it are found in rain and snow. It has also been found in many of the healing springs of the world, including Fatima in Portugal, Lourdes in France, and the Shrine of St. Anne in Canada. Hydrogen peroxide is an important component of plant life, and small amounts are found in many vegetables and fruits, including fresh cabbage, tomatoes, asparagus, green peppers, watercress, oranges, apples, and watermelons.[1]

Hydrogen peroxide is also found in the animal kingdom and is involved in many of our body's natural processes. As an oxygenator, it is able to deliver small quantities of oxygen to the blood and other vital systems throughout the body. However, hydrogen peroxide does not oxygenate the body merely by producing modest amounts of oxygen; it has an extraordinary capacity to stimulate oxidative enzymes, which have the ability to change the chemical components of other substances (like viruses and bacteria) without being changed themselves. Rather than providing more oxygen to the cells, hydrogen peroxide *enhances* natural cellular oxidative processes, which increases the body's ability to use what oxygen is available. According to the late Charles H. Farr, M.D., Ph.D., one of the world's leading authorities on the chemical properties and therapeutic applications of hydrogen peroxide:

> It functions to aid [cell] membrane transport, acts as a hormonal messenger, regulates thermogenesis (heat production), stimulates and regulates immune functions, regulates energy production [similar to insulin] and has many other important metabolic functions. It is purposely used by the body to produce hydroxyl radicals to kill bacteria, virus, fungi, yeast, and a number of parasites. This natural killing or protective system has nothing to do with increasing the amount of available oxygen.[2]

Hydrogen peroxide must be present for our immune system to function properly. The cells in the body that fight infection (the class of white blood cells known as granulocytes) produce hydrogen peroxide as a first line of defense against harmful parasites, bacteria, viruses, and fungi. Hydrogen peroxide is also needed for the metabolism of protein, carbohydrates, fats, vitamins, and minerals. It is also a by-product of cell metabolism (that is actively broken down by peroxidase) and a hormonal regulator that is necessary for the body's production of estrogen, progesterone, and thyroxine. If that weren't enough, hydrogen peroxide is involved in the regulation of blood sugar and the production of energy in body cells.[3]

HISTORY AND CHARACTERISTICS

Hydrogen peroxide was first discovered in 1818 by the French chemist Louis-Jacques Thenard, who named it *eau oxygénée,* or "oxygenated water." It has been used commercially since the mid-1800s as a nonpolluting bleaching agent, oxidizing agent, and disinfectant.

Although it is found in nature, small quantities of hydrogen peroxide can be made in the laboratory by reacting barium peroxide with cold diluted sulfuric acid. Larger amounts are produced by electrolyzing chilled concentrated sulfuric acid. This process causes a series of chemical reactions to occur and make a substance called peroxydisulfuric acid. When the solution is warmed to room temperature, it becomes hydrogen peroxide.[4]

Hydrogen peroxide is found in a variety of different grades:

- *3 percent grade hydrogen peroxide* is the type we find in pharmacies and grocery stores. Made primarily of 50 percent "super D peroxide" and diluted, it contains a variety of stabilizers like phenol, acetanilide, and sodium stannate. It is used mostly to disinfect wounds and treat skin rashes and as an effective, inexpensive (though unpleasant-tasting to some) mouthwash. This grade of hydrogen peroxide is also used around the house to freshen the bathroom and to wash fresh fruits and vegetables. While safe for these applications, 3 percent grade H_2O_2 should not be ingested.
- *6 percent grade hydrogen peroxide* contains an activator that makes it an effective bleaching agent. For this reason, it is used primarily by hairdressers, surfers, and teenagers for coloring their hair.
- *30 percent reagent-grade hydrogen peroxide,* like other grades, looks like harmless water. However, it is a highly concentrated chemical compound that is very corrosive. Strict precautions must be taken by those who plan to use it. When it makes contact with skin, burns can result. Breathing the vapor or ingesting

it full-strength can be hazardous and even fatal. Yet when used properly, reagent-grade hydrogen peroxide is safe. Because it is relatively free of heavy metals and other trace elements, it is used primarily in medical research. It is also highly recommended for use (in diluted form) in oxidative therapy. Reagent-grade hydrogen peroxide can be found in chemical and farm supply stores.

- *35 percent food-grade hydrogen peroxide* has traditionally been used by the food industry as a nontoxic disinfectant. Added to water, it is sprayed on cheese, eggs, vegetables, fruits, and whey products to keep them free of unwanted bacteria. It is also used to disinfect metal and foil-lined food containers. In addition, food-grade hydrogen peroxide is used in the dairy industry as a disinfectant and bactericide. While considered less desirable than reagent-grade for use in oxidative therapy, food-grade hydrogen peroxide is easily obtainable in any large natural foods store. It is also easily found on the Internet, although it must be shipped as a "hazardous material" involving extra packaging and additional shipping fees.

- *90 percent hydrogen peroxide* is used by the military and in space exploration as a propulsion source for rocket fuel. A highly unstable compound that can explode unless handled very carefully, it is *not* recommended for use in oxidative therapy.

MAJOR USES

Like ozone, hydrogen peroxide is used in a wide variety of ways.

Bleaching

One of the major industrial uses of hydrogen peroxide is in the bleaching of cotton textiles and, to a lesser extent, wool, silk, and certain vegetable fibers. It is also used to bleach chemical pulps, groundwood, and linoleum and to improve the color of certain waxes and oils. In addition, hydrogen peroxide is used to de-ink waste paper in the recycling process. These industries like using hydrogen peroxide because it is environmentally friendly. When hydrogen peroxide decomposes, it yields only water and oxygen.

Pollution Control

Like ozone, hydrogen peroxide is a powerful oxidizer, bactericide, and virucide. When added to industrial and residential sewage and waste-waters, it is able to kill harmful pathogens, making effluents safe for the environment. Hydrogen peroxide removes toxic and foul-smelling pollutants from industrial gas streams and can also limit chlorine concentration in water supplies. When 3 to 10 percent hydrogen peroxide is added to water, it can be used to disinfect bathrooms and kitchens without the use of harmful chemicals.

Hydrogen peroxide is one of the materials approved by the U.S. Environmental Protection Agency (EPA) for use in anthrax decontamination efforts to reduce spore populations.[5]

Chemicals, Pharmaceuticals, and Mining

Hydrogen peroxide is used by the chemical industry in the production of a wide variety of organic and inorganic chemicals, as well as in the manufacture of household bleaches. It is also an ingredient in contact lens cleaners, eye drops, aloe vera extracts, mouthwashes, and tooth-whitening products. Hydrogen peroxide is also an oxidizing agent in the mining industry.

Propellant

High-grade (90 percent) hydrogen peroxide has been used as a propellant by the military in both the U.S. and British military for over fifty years, primarily in torpedoes and missiles. It was also used by the National Aeronautics and Space Administration (NASA) in Mercury spacecraft and other programs.

At the present time, scientists at the U.S. Naval Air Warfare Center (Weapons Division) at China Lake, California, are developing self-contained power sources based on novel heterogeneous catalysts that provide more effective decomposition of high-strength hydrogen peroxide. They are developing lighter, more efficient, and lower-cost technologies for releasing the chemical energy of hydrogen peroxide to be suitable for use in a variety of power sources. Applications include lightweight power generators for recreational or emergency uses and power sources for surface and submersible watercraft.

Because water and oxygen are the only decomposition products of hydrogen peroxide, the scientists at China Lake are studying other applications that require an environmentally clean power source, such as projectile propulsion, electrical power generation, and small-vehicle propulsion (using either turbine systems or direct thrust).[6] Perhaps the most exciting possibility of this research is the development of motor vehicles that are run on cheap, renewable, efficient, and nonpolluting hydrogen peroxide!

Agriculture

As an inexpensive way for farmers to purify drinking water, one pint of 35 percent food-grade hydrogen peroxide can be added to one thousand gallons of drinking water for farm animals. In addition to serving as a catalyst for promoting oxygenation of the blood and killing harmful viruses and bacteria, hydrogen peroxide added to drinking water helps eliminate worms and other parasites from the intestine. When given to dairy cows, it can increase both the milk production and its butterfat content.

One farmer relates his experience with hydrogen peroxide:

In 1990, I was administering 35% H_2O_2 orally to bovines (a dairy herd), at 30 ppm, added to their drinking water. All the water on the farm was treated, so it was also in all cleanup water, etc. The cows became extremely healthy. Bacteria counts dropped and butterfat went up. Those two criteria convert immediately to money for the farmer. He is paid more for his milk the very next pickup. So, I started taking it myself.[7]

Food-grade hydrogen peroxide is also used to rinse milk cans and bulk tanks to destroy bacteria and other pathogens. It is diluted with water and used as a spray to clean barn walls and floors. Hydrogen peroxide mixtures are used to clean wounds and wash the udders of cows, which results in a lower bacteria content in their milk.

Because oxygen is essential for both plant life and animals, hydrogen peroxide is being used in various ways to increase the growth rate and productivity of plants. Mushroom farmers find hydrogen peroxide a cheap and efficient way to promote mushroom growth and protect mushrooms from harmful spores. Farmgard Products of Minnesota reports that nonbearing fruit trees are able to grow fruit when given water containing hydrogen peroxide, and that nonproductive rice paddies in Japan were able to bear crops after being irrigated with water mixed with hydrogen peroxide. Hydrogen peroxide is also used by farmers to make an effective nonpolluting insecticide in the field, and it can be used by home garden enthusiasts as a spray for home and garden plants.[8]

Sterilization of Medical Devices

Like ozone, hydrogen peroxide has also been used to sterilize medical instruments for years, although new technologies are being developed to maximize its use and effectiveness. One is vaporized hydrogen peroxide (VHP). The VHP sterilizer is first filled with the objects to be sterilized. The basic VHP sterilization cycle consists of three stages (conditioning, including vacuum generation; H_2O_2 injection; and aeration) and takes approximately 90 minutes. Another method is hydrogen peroxide plasma sterilization. The sterilizer is first filled with the objects to be sterilized, followed by a cycle consisting of four stages (vacuum generation, H_2O_2 injection, diffusion, and plasma discharge). The process takes approximately one to three hours.[9]

Perhaps the most revolutionary development in the field of sterilization of medical instruments is the Sterizone VP4 sterilizer, which utilizes both vaporized hydrogen peroxide and ozone. Considered a model of both efficiency and cost-effectiveness in killing viruses, spores, and harmful microorganisms—including superbugs—the VP4 uses a patented multistep process to achieve 100 percent sterilization of heat- and moisture-sensitive metal and nonmetal reusable medical devices. It was cleared for commercial use in the United States in 2014 and in Canada the following year, and its single preprogrammed cycle can effectively sterilize up to 75 pounds (34 kilograms) of medical instruments per load. In 2016, the VP4 became the only sterilizer validated by the FDA to completely sterilize large, complex, and hard-to-clean medical instruments like colonoscopes, gastroscopes, and other multichannel flexible endoscopes.[10]

7
Hydrogen Peroxide
in Medicine

The first medical use of hydrogen peroxide was reported by I. N. Love, M.D., a consulting physician to City Hospital in St. Louis, Missouri, in the March 3, 1888, issue of the *Journal of the American Medical Association* under the title "Peroxide of Hydrogen as a Remedial Agent." The article, based on a talk given to the St. Louis Medical Society the previous month, related Dr. Love's success in treating patients with a variety of diseases, including scarlet fever, diphtheria, nasal catarrh, acute coryza (head catarrh), whooping cough, asthma, hay fever, and tonsillitis. In these cases, treatment primarily involved administering a diluted solution of hydrogen peroxide into the nostrils with a syringe. Dr. Love commented: "From its very nature this agent should be a powerful antiseptic and a destroyer of microbes; anything which accomplishes oxidation as rapidly, if it can be applied safely, must be an excellent application to purulent surfaces for its cleansing effect." The author also mentioned its use (unsuccessfully) in treating diabetes and addressed possible clinical applications in treating some forms of atonic dyspepsia and gonorrhea. Dr. Love observed: "The beneficial effect of the application was apparent, all the distressing symptoms were much abated, and within three or four days they had passed away." Dr. Love also documented the use of hydrogen peroxide in treating uterine cancer as a "cleanser, deodorizer and stimulator of healing."[1]

Later that year, P. R. Cortelyou, M.D., reported his clinical experience with hydrogen peroxide to treat disorders of the throat and nose at the annual meeting of the Medical Society of Georgia. Dr. Cortelyou diluted hydrogen peroxide and used the fluid as a fine spray to treat people with chronic pharyngitis, rhinitis, cough, sore throat, tonsillitis, and diphtheria. In some cases, Dr. Cortelyou used hydrogen peroxide in combination with other medicines of the time, including "muriate of cocaine" and a solution made with iodine, potash, and glycerin. After treating a woman suffering from severe cough and high fever with this combination for four weeks, the doctor reported: "The throat was feeling so much better that the treatment was only given twice a week, and patient has kept in good condition all winter."[2]

The first known use of intravenous hydrogen peroxide was reported by British physician T. H. Oliver in 1920. In India the previous year, he had treated twenty-five patients who were critically ill with influenzal pneumonia by injecting hydrogen peroxide directly into their veins. Compared with a death rate of over 80 percent with this disease, Oliver's patients had a mortality rate of only 48 percent.[3] Although this method of hydrogen peroxide delivery can cause gas embolism, a condition that can obstruct blood vessels and may lead to a stroke, this apparently did not occur in any of the patients treated, probably because he performed a very slow infusion.

In the United States, studies with hydrogen peroxide were conducted by noted German chemist and physician William Frederick Koch in the 1920s with cancer patients. Dr. Koch used a substance he called glyoxylide, which is believed to be the same oxygen found in hydrogen peroxide. Rather than using intravenous administration like Dr. Oliver, he preferred giving the substance intramuscularly.

Although his treatments were successful, Dr. Koch was later sued by the U.S. Food and Drug Administration. He was acquitted, but he decided to leave the United States and continue his research in Brazil. He died there in 1967.[4]

In the early 1960s, major studies in the medical uses of hydrogen peroxide were conducted at Baylor University Medical Center in Texas.

In an early study involving cancer, researchers found that cells containing a high amount of oxygen responded more favorably to radiation therapy than ordinary cells. Before that study, hyperbaric oxygen was often used by physicians to oxygenate the cells; in a rather cumbersome and expensive method using a specially built oxygen chamber, oxygen was delivered under a pressure greater than the normal atmospheric pressure. However, the doctors at Baylor found that small amounts of hydrogen peroxide injected into a vein could achieve the same effect as hyperbaric oxygen at a much lower cost and with fewer adverse side effects.

The Baylor researchers also discovered that hydrogen peroxide has an energizing effect on the heart muscle that could be of great benefit to patients suffering heart attacks. Myocardial ischemia, or lack of oxygen to the heart muscle, was relieved with hydrogen peroxide.[5] Writing in the journal *Circulation,* Dr. H. C. Urschel Jr. reported that ventricular fibrillation—a life-threatening condition involving extremely rapid, incomplete contractions of the ventricle area of the heart—was completely relieved through the intravenous administration of hydrogen peroxide.[6]

Researchers at Baylor also studied the effect of intravenous hydrogen peroxide on the accumulation of plaque in the arteries. They found that not only could hydrogen peroxide remove plaque buildup efficiently, but its effects were long-term.[7] While these findings offered hope to individuals destined for expensive, dangerous, and often ineffective heart bypass operations, the Baylor studies were largely ignored by the medical establishment. They will be presented in more detail in part 2 of this book.

Perhaps the most important medical research in hydrogen peroxide therapy during the 1990s can be credited to Charles H. Farr of Oklahoma, who held doctorate degrees in both pharmacology and medicine. Dr. Farr was among the first to suggest the clinical benefits of treating illnesses with hydrogen peroxide injected intravenously, and he conducted more clinical research in the fields of chelation therapy and hydrogen peroxide therapy than anyone else. In addition to having written over thirty-five scientific and medical articles and books, he was the founder of the International Oxidative Medicine Association.

Dr. Farr's work in hydrogen peroxide, like that of many pioneers who have researched the value of the medical applications of ozone, has been largely ignored by the scientific and medical establishment in the United States and Canada. However, his work has been carefully evaluated by eminent scientists abroad. He wrote:

> When hydrogen peroxide and/or ozone are used as therapeutic agents, it soon becomes obvious that they are useful in treating a wide variety of seemingly unrelated conditions. Since most of us have come to think in terms of "one cause, one disease, one cure," we have difficulty accepting the idea that a broad-scope panacea may have been discovered. Yet the concept that hydrogen peroxide, for example, may indeed be a panacea is not so far-fetched when we begin exploring the role of the substance in body metabolism.[8]

HOW DOES IT WORK?

We mentioned before that hydrogen peroxide is both an effective oxygenator and a powerful oxidizer. Numerous physiological effects of hydrogen peroxide have been described in medical and scientific literature for over sixty years.

On the Lungs

Hydrogen peroxide helps stimulate the process of oxygenation in the lungs by increasing blood flow so that blood has more contact with air; it also helps red blood cells and hemoglobin carry oxygen to the cells of the lungs. This helps remove foreign material, including dead and damaged tissue, from the *alveoli,* the tiny air sacs in the lungs where oxygen is taken into the bloodstream.

On Metabolism

A number of hormonal effects are regulated by the actions of hydrogen peroxide, including the production of progesterone and thyroxine as well as the inhibition of bioamines, dopamine, noradrenaline, and serotonin. Hydrogen peroxide also stimulates (either directly or indirectly) certain oxidative enzyme systems. Enzymes are complex proteins that are able to bring about chemical changes in other substances; digestive enzymes, for example, are able to break down foods into simpler compounds that the body can use for nourishment.

On the Heart and Circulatory System

Hydrogen peroxide can dilate (expand) blood vessels in the heart, the extremities, the brain, and the lungs. It is also able to decrease heart rate, increase stroke volume (the amount of blood pumped by the left ventricle of the heart at each beat), and decrease vascular resistance (which makes it easier for blood to move through the blood vessels). As a result, it can increase total cardiac output.

On Sugar (Glucose) Utilization

Hydrogen peroxide is said to mimic the effects of insulin and has been able to stabilize cases of diabetes mellitus type 2.

On Immune Response

As previously mentioned, granulocytes are a type of white blood cell that the body uses to fight infections. When the body is infused with hydrogen peroxide, the number of granulocytes in the body first goes down but then increases beyond the original number.

Intravenous treatment with hydrogen peroxide has also been found to stimulate the formation of *monocytes,* a type of white blood cell that scavenges, hunts, and kills bacteria; stimulate *helper T cells* (white blood cells that orchestrate the immune response and signal other cells in the immune system to perform their special functions); and help increase the production of *gamma interferon,* a protein found when cells are exposed to viruses, as well as *cytokines* (cellular messengers) that promote healing. Noninfected cells that are exposed to interferon become protected against viral infection.[9]

According to Dr. Farr:

> Hydrogen peroxide is manufactured by the body and is maintained at a constant level throughout our life. It is part of a system that helps the body regulate living cell membranes. It is a hormonal regulator, necessary for the body to produce several hormonal substances such as estrogen, progesterone, and thyroxine. It is vital for the regulation of blood sugar and the production of energy in all body cells.
>
> Hydrogen peroxide helps regulate certain chemicals to operate the brain and nervous system. It has a stimulatory and regulatory effect on the immune system and may either directly or indirectly kill viruses, bacteria, parasites, yeast, fungi, and a variety of harmful organisms. Our studies demonstrate a positive metabolic effect of an intravenous infusion of hydrogen peroxide. Its ability to oxidize almost any physiological and pathological substance, in addition to producing increased tissue and cellular oxygen tensions, has proved to have therapeutic value.[10]

WHAT DISEASES CAN HYDROGEN PEROXIDE TREAT?

Low-grade (3 percent) hydrogen peroxide is well known to most of us. When we apply it externally to an open wound, hydrogen peroxide produces a bubbling sensation, which is just the oxygen coming out of solution. However, few people know about the wide range of therapeutic possibilities of 30 percent reagent-grade or 35 percent food-grade hydrogen peroxide when diluted and taken internally as oxidative therapy.

Like ozone, hydrogen peroxide can treat a broad spectrum of diseases because it kills bacteria, fungi, parasites, and viruses. It can also destroy certain tumor cells. According to Dr. Farr, the following diseases have been clinically treated with intravenous hydrogen peroxide with varying degrees of success.

acute and chronic viral
   infections
allergies
Alzheimer's disease
angina
asthma
cardiac arrhythmias
   (irregular heartbeat)
cardioconversion
   (heart stoppage)
cardiovascular disease
   (heart disease)
cerebral vascular disease
   (stroke and memory loss)
chronic obstructive
   pulmonary disease
chronic pain syndromes
   (from various causes)
chronic recurrent
   Epstein-Barr infection
chronic unresponsive
   bacterial infections
cluster headaches

diabetes mellitus type 2
emphysema
herpes simplex
   (fever blister)
herpes zoster
   (shingles)
HIV-related infections
influenza
metastatic carcinoma
   (cancer)
migraine headaches
multiple sclerosis
parasitic infections
Parkinson's disease
peripheral vascular disease
   (poor circulation)
rheumatoid arthritis
systemic chronic candidiasis
   (yeast infections)
temporal arteritis
   (inflammation of the
   temporal artery)
vascular headaches[11]

Hydrogen peroxide is the reactive oxygen species most damaging to human spermatozoa. This has led Indian researchers at the Department of Reproductive Biomedicine at the National Institute of Health and Family Welfare in New Delhi to explore the possible use of hydrogen peroxide as an active ingredient in a water-based contraceptive gel. In a study with rats carried out in 2002, they found that 2 percent hydrogen peroxide in a 0.9 percent solution of sodium chloride showed 100 percent efficiency in mating studies two hours after vaginal application.[12] Though the results are promising, one should not attempt to duplicate these findings at home.

H$_2$O$_2$ AND HONEY

The use of honey in healing goes back thousands of years. It is used to treat a broad range of health problems such as wounds, ulcers, diabetes, and infections, including those resistant to antibiotics. Several of these infections even include "superbugs" like MRSA (methicillin-resistant *Staphylococcus aureus*) and *Pseudomonas aeruginosa*. As mentioned in my book *The Honey Prescription* (Healing Arts Press, 2010), there has been an explosion in scientific research on the medicinal uses of honey at universities, research centers, and medical clinics around the world.

Although honey's ability to draw fluids out of wounds through osmosis and its low Ph (which kills bacteria) are factors in its healing abilities, honey also contains hydrogen peroxide. Bees secrete an enzyme, called *glucose oxidase,* from their hypopharyngeal gland into the nectar, where it catalyzes glucose into gluconic acid and hydrogen peroxide. It is believed that the hydrogen peroxide is used as a sterilizing agent during the honey's ripening process.

It's interesting to note that full-strength honey has a negligible level of hydrogen peroxide because this substance is short-lived in the presence of the transition metal ions and ascorbic acid found in honey, which cause the hydrogen peroxide to decompose to oxygen and water. Glucose oxydase has been found to be practically inactive in full-strength honey, giving rise to hydrogen peroxide only when the honey is diluted. This often takes place when honey is applied to the skin or to other parts of the body where moisture—even in tiny amounts—is present.

Dr. Katrina Brudzynski of the Department of Biological Sciences at Brock University in Ontario studied forty-two samples of Canadian honey to determine their antibacterial potential against strains of *Escherichia coli* and *Bacillus subtilis.* After tabulating the results, she concluded: "These data indicate that all Canadian honeys exhibited antibacterial activity, with higher selectivity against *E. coli* than *B. subtilis,* and that these antibacterial activities were correlated with hydrogen peroxide production in honeys. The hydrogen peroxide level in honey, therefore, is a strong predictor of the honey's antibacterial activity."[13]

When it comes to clearing infections, honey supplies low levels of hydrogen peroxide to wounds continuously over time as opposed to a large amount at the moment of treatment. In essence, it becomes a powerful yet effective slow-release antiseptic at a level that is antibacterial but does not damage tissue. In an article published in *Archives of Medical Research* on the activity of honey against medically significant bacteria by members of the School of Biomedical Sciences at Charles Sturt University in Australia, the authors note: "The mild acidity and low-level hydrogen peroxide release assists both tissue repair and contributes to the antibacterial activity of honey. The antibacterial activity is a major factor in promoting wound healing where infection is present."[14]

Dilution with water has not been found to seriously inhibit hydrogen peroxide production in honey, an important factor to consider when treating exuding wounds. In a study carried out at the Honey Research Unit at the University of Waikato in New Zealand, eight honey samples from six different floral sources were tested. The maximum levels of accumulated hydrogen peroxide occurred in solutions diluted to concentrations of between 30 percent and 50 percent. The authors concluded: "Significant antibacterial activity can be maintained easily when using honey as a wound dressing, even on a heavily exuding wound."[15]

Pasteurization destroys the enzymes that produce hydrogen peroxide, so any honey used therapeutically should be raw and unpasteurized. The honey should be stored in a cool place and away from light. If it is necessary to liquefy honey, it should be heated at a temperature no higher than 37°C (98.6°F).

We will see later on that hydrogen peroxide is playing an increasing role in dentistry and oral hygiene, as well in treating skin and gynecological problems. Treatment protocols are under investigation for many other health problems, including Legionnaire's disease, candidiasis, salmonella poisoning, *Pneumocystis jiroveci* (AIDS-related pneumonia), *Toxoplasma gondii*, malaria, cytomegalovirus, HIV infection, and Ehrlich ascites carcinoma.

8

How Is Hydrogen Peroxide Administered?

Hydrogen peroxide can be introduced into the body in a number of different ways.

INTRAVENOUS INFUSION

An intravenous infusion is prepared by diluting 30 percent reagent-grade hydrogen peroxide with equal amounts of sterile distilled water to make a 15 percent "stock solution." This is then passed through a Millipore 0.22-micrometer medium-flow filter both to sterilize the solution and to remove any particulate matter from it. The stock solution is refrigerated in 100 ml sterile containers until needed.

At the time of application, physicians use 5 percent dextrose in water or normal saline solution as the carrier. Adding 0.4 ml of the stock solution to 200 ml of dextrose in water yields a 0.03 percent concentration, which is the recommended strength for most intravenous infusions. Because of its tremendous oxidizing power, Dr. Farr cautions that "vitamins, minerals, peptides, enzymes, amino acids, heparin, EDTA or other injectable materials should never be mixed with the H_2O_2 solution."[1] The mixture is then slowly infused into a vein over a period of one to three hours, depending on the patient's situation. According to the International Oxidative Medicine Association, "Treatments are usually given about once a week in chronic illness but can be given daily in patients with acute illness such as pneumonia or flu. Physicians may recommend 1 to 20 treatments, depending on the condition of the patient and the illness being treated."[2]

Follow-up treatments are sometimes necessary. Although adverse side effects are rare (some people experience irritation in the vein or slight temporary pressure in the chest), the patient is often monitored by a doctor or nurse during and shortly after the infusion.

Because the hydrogen peroxide solution is administered in exact amounts, this is the method most preferred by physicians. It is also considered the most efficient way to introduce hydrogen peroxide into the body.

INTRAVENOUS HYDROGEN PEROXIDE OR OXYGEN-OZONE AUTOHEMOTHERAPY?

There are always disagreements about whether intravenous hydrogen peroxide is more or less effective than autohemotherapy with ozone. As we'll see later on, both methods have been used to effectively treat similar health problems. Ozone is used more widely in Europe, partly because it was first developed there.

Dr. Bocci believes that comparative studies could be useful, because hydrogen peroxide is one of the early ozone messengers. These ozone messengers are the Reactive Oxygen Species (ROS) and Lipid Oxidation Products (LOPs) that are created after ozone biochemically reacts with blood plasma. These messengers are responsible for the biological therapeutic effects of ozone. Yet he believes that "late products, like LOPs [lipid oxidation products] may not be generated in vivo owing to the rapid reduction of H_2O_2,"[3] which would possibly render hydrogen peroxide less effective than ozone.

However, Bocci and others have pointed to several advantages of therapeutic hydrogen peroxide over ozone therapy, especially in poor countries where health facilities are either primitive or nonexistent, and where electricity may be difficult to come by. In order to produce ozone, an ozone generator, which can cost several thousand dollars, is needed. And because generators run on electricity, a suitable energy source must be available. By contrast, hydrogen peroxide is comparatively very inexpensive to buy, and preparing the standardized solution is simple and reliable. Hydrogen peroxide can also be stored for a longer length of time. It can be taken anywhere and easily administered, either at a patient's home or at a field hospital or clinic. This would make hydrogen peroxide especially useful in isolated communities in rural Latin America, Africa, and Asia.

ORAL INGESTION

The oral method calls for drops of 35 percent hydrogen peroxide to be added to a glass of water and then ingested two or three times daily. One of the more prominent advocates of this method was renowned heart surgeon Dr. Christiaan Barnard. In a letter dated March 10, 1986, he wrote: "It is true that I have found relief from the arthritis and I attribute it to taking hydrogen peroxide orally several times a day."[4]

Dr. Kurt Donsbach, a noted holistic practitioner and writer, uses hydrogen peroxide and other natural substances to treat patients with cancer, heart disease, and other illnesses at his Hospital Santa Monica in Mexico. Although Dr. Donsbach prefers the intravenous method at the hospital (and estimates that he and his staff have administered over 120,000 hydrogen peroxide infusions without significant side effects), he recommends oral administration for outpatient use. He created a product for this purpose known as Superoxy Plus, made from aloe vera saturated with magnesium peroxide. Each ounce is said to be equivalent to twenty drops of hydrogen peroxide.[5] Well-known lay researcher Conrad LeBeau suggests that adults take ten drops of food-grade hydrogen peroxide in an eight-ounce glass of distilled water two or three times a day on an empty stomach 30 minutes before eating or three hours after eating.[6] Some people find the taste of hydrogen peroxide unpleasant. To help disguise the taste, several drops of olive oil can be added to the water.

One can also begin taking one drop of hydrogen peroxide in a glass of water on the first day and add a drop per glass each day until ten drops per day are achieved. Dr. Donsbach cautions against taking hydrogen peroxide with juice, milk, or other flavorings because it will "create oxidation, robbing the oxygen which is what you are trying to get into the bloodstream,"[7] while Dr. Farr notes that "almost without exception, hydrogen peroxide, added to anything besides oil and/or water will cause dismutation and destruction of the hydrogen peroxide."[8]

Physicians also caution against adding hydrogen peroxide to water containing iron, because the combination of hydrogen peroxide and iron produces a very high number of free radicals and can promote stomach upset, possibly leading to cancer over the long term. If one's water contains iron, distilled water is recommended instead. It is also suggested that iron supplements not be taken within an hour of ingesting hydrogen peroxide.

Not all physicians who advocate the use of hydrogen peroxide are in favor of taking it orally. One of these critics is Dr. Farr. He believes that, in addition to the presence of iron in the stomach, combinations of fatty acids may reduce hydrogen peroxide to a number of free radicals, thus causing negative effects upon the gastric and duodenal mucosa, the delicate membrane lining the stomach and the first part of the small intestine. This may lead to an increase of glandular stomach erosion, an abnormal increase in the number of cells in the duodenum, and the possible formation of cancerous and noncancerous tumors in the stomach and duodenum.[9]

Dr. Farr's views are supported by Dr. Bocci, who writes: "Hydrogen peroxide coming into contact with the acidic gastric juice will decompose immediately. Very little—if any—oxygen will reach the bloodstream and the effect on the gastric mucosa remains totally uncertain."[10] Hugo Vietz, M.D., a Pennsylvania practitioner who has had extensive experience using hydrogen peroxide therapeutically, agrees as well. In an article published in *East West* magazine, he strongly discourages the oral self-administration of hydrogen peroxide:

> You're putting a fairly caustic substance into the intestinal tract, which, from the mouth to the rectum, is lined with highly sensitive, delicate, multi-purpose mucous membrane. This membrane has some extremely important functions to perform. Introduce a caustic substance like hydrogen peroxide even in the dilute concentrations

that they are using, and it scares me. A lot of people who are doing it are going to get away with it. But there are going to be some who will wind up with damaged intestinal tracts. If you cause permanent damage to an organ like this, I think you're in for real trouble.[11]

This subject of oral self-administration of hydrogen peroxide remains a controversial one, since many long-term users of oral hydrogen peroxide have not become sick, and clinical studies are lacking. Until such studies are done, many feel that oral hydrogen peroxide should be avoided in favor of less risky applications.

IN BATHING

A much safer (and less controversial method) involves adding one pint of 35 percent food-grade hydrogen peroxide to a bathtub of warm water and soaking in the water for a minimum of 20 minutes. The rationale for this treatment is that hydrogen peroxide is absorbed through the skin, and the reactive oxygen species that result are absorbed into the bloodstream. People have reported relief from stiff joints, rashes, psoriasis, and fungal infections from using this method one to three times a week. There is little clinical evidence attesting to the effectiveness of this method in treating serious diseases (some critics believe that the warm bath alone may produce a placebo effect). However, there is anecdotal evidence that it can be very helpful to people dealing with HIV infection and related health problems. Hydrogen peroxide in bathwater is often recommended as an adjunct to traditional medical therapies.

Another safe way to enjoy a hydrogen peroxide bath is to spray the body with a 3 percent solution of hydrogen peroxide (either diluted from food-grade hydrogen peroxide, or the common drugstore variety). The hydrogen peroxide is placed in a small spray bottle and applied to the entire body after a shower. The peroxide can then be massaged lightly into the skin. Care should be taken to avoid contact with eyes. The primary disadvantage to this method may affect men with abundant body hair, which may turn reddish blond. Those who utilize this method claim that the spray offers the same benefits of a hydrogen peroxide bath; some have reported that it clears up skin blemishes very effectively.

INJECTION IN JOINTS AND SOFT TISSUE TRIGGER POINTS

Dr. Farr discovered and reported the use of 0.03 percent hydrogen peroxide injected into joints and soft tissues. He found that the swelling and inflammation of rheumatoid arthritis and other types of inflammatory arthritis responded quickly to intra-articular injections of hydrogen peroxide. He also found that it was especially effective when injected into osteoarthritic joints such as fingers and knees. Trigger points in muscles and tendons are rapidly relieved with the same type of injection. Some physicians have reported good results in reconstruction of joint surfaces and spaces using hydrogen peroxide injections.[12]

FREE RADICALS AND HYDROGEN PEROXIDE

In chapter 1 we discussed the issue of free radicals in detail. Hydrogen peroxide is an activated oxygen species that can break down and liberate free radicals and may sometimes act as a free radical itself. However, it is more often an "intermediate" for the formation of other free radicals, such as hydroxyl. While hydroxyl is essential for fighting off disease, excessive amounts in the body have been linked to genetic mutations and the destruction of cell membranes. Many physicians believe that hydrogen peroxide is harmful to use in medical therapy because it can lead to the uncontrolled production of free radicals like hydroxyl in the body. However, this is very unlikely because hydrogen peroxide is reduced in blood within seconds. A closer look at recent findings in the field of free radical production is needed before reaching such a conclusion.

It has already been mentioned that small amounts of hydrogen peroxide are vital for the proper functioning of our immune system, as well as the metabolism of protein, fats, carbohydrates, vitamins, and minerals; the production of hormones; and the regulation of blood sugar. Yet hydrogen peroxide is also a powerful agent in oxidizing harmful bacteria, viruses, and fungi while providing vital oxygen to the body's cells.

Dr. Farr found that hydrogen peroxide leads to the formation of hydroxyl radicals only under special circumstances, primarily when ferrous oxide is present. This is why physicians suggest that iron supplements not be taken when hydrogen peroxide is given intravenously or orally and that tap water containing iron should not be used to take hydrogen peroxide orally.

When ferrous oxide is not present—which is true most of the time—Dr. Farr discovered that hydrogen peroxide is normally dealt with by the enzyme catalase, which renders the hydrogen peroxide beneficial to the body:

> The action of catalase on hydrogen peroxide is to add an electron in the presence of hydrogen to pure water and diatomic oxygen. The oxygen is again reduced to superoxide and then to hydrogen peroxide and around the reaction continues. . . . One molecule of catalase can convert millions of molecules of hydrogen peroxide into oxygen and water within seconds and is the body's first line of defense against hydroxyl radical formation.[13]

When taken into the body in small amounts, hydrogen peroxide oxidizes sick, weak, and devitalized cells while making healthy cells (such as T cells) stronger and more resistant to oxidation. It also permits the formation of new, healthy cells that are better able to resist disease. This process is essential for healing. In chapters 28 and 29, we will discuss the importance of antioxidants (which can be easily found in a number of popular vegetables and fruits and nutritional supplements) as important adjuncts to oxidative therapy, because they help keep the body's production of free radicals in check.

As with ozone, there is a wealth of documented evidence that attests to the value of hydrogen peroxide in medical therapy. Part 2 of this book will explore the latest laboratory and clinical findings that evaluate the use of oxidative therapies to treat many of our most serious health problems.

9

Hyperbaric Oxygen Therapy and Oxygen Multistep Therapy

Although hyperbaric oxygen (HBO) therapy (also referred to as HBOT) has been around for centuries, it received widespread press attention as an adjunct modality to treat the only survivor of the Sago Mine disaster of January 2006. Suffering from severe carbon monoxide poisoning and oxygen deprivation to the heart, brain, and other organs, Randal McCloy Jr. received several hyperbaric oxygen treatments at Allegheny General Hospital in Pittsburgh, Pennsylvania, with good results.[1]

In hyperbaric oxygen therapy, 100 percent pure oxygen is administered at two to three times normal atmospheric pressure. To begin, the patient is placed in a specially designed chamber. The pressure in the chamber is gradually increased, which causes a rise in the body's blood plasma oxygen content. This results in enhanced oxygen delivery to compromised tissues. With HBO therapy, oxygen can be dissolved in the blood plasma and go directly into tissues. The technique also has an important systemic effect on bacterial growth and enhances the body's overall inflammatory response. Hyperbaric oxygen reduces swelling or edema in body tissues, produces antioxidant effects, and promotes new blood vessel formation in areas of the body where blood supply is limited.

Hyperbaric oxygen has been used to treat a wide range of health problems. It is best known as a primary therapy in treating carbon monoxide poisoning, gas gangrene, and tissue decompression, known in scuba diving as "the bends." However, hyperbaric oxygen therapy is now increasingly being used as an adjunct to standard medical and surgical care, including the treatment of problem wounds, anaerobic infections, chronic bone infections, gas embolism, crush injuries, soft tissue injuries, thermal burns, compromised skin grafts, and radiation injuries. It has been found to be useful in treating patients suffering from impaired healing or compromised blood circulation where oxygen cannot reach important tissues.

HBO therapy has also been found useful in treating people with diabetes and vascular disease, as well as amputees, cancer patients undergoing radiation therapy, and patients recovering from plastic, cosmetic, or laser surgery. Research is now under way to study the effects of HBO therapy on patients suffering from stroke and chronic fatigue syndrome.[2]

HBO therapy has also been studied in treating HIV and AIDS. In 1990, Michelle R. Reillo, R.N., began research on three hundred patients with late-stage AIDS who underwent HBO treatment for diverse AIDS-related complications. Results were reported in her book *AIDS under Pressure* (see the resources—appendix 2, page 442). Although the patients' life expectancy was just two years at the time the study was begun, more than half of the patients were still alive six years later, even though they did not take antiviral drugs. Reillo investigated how HBO therapy works in the manifestation of peripheral vascular insufficiency, pulmonary complications, neurological manifestations, dermatological manifestations, metabolic disorders, and liver problems and found the therapy—whether used alone or as an adjunct to traditional medical therapy—safe, clinically beneficial, and cost effective. In some cases, HBO therapy enhanced drug effectiveness.[3]

Hyperbaric oxygen therapy is finding greater acceptance in treating sports injuries and is believed to enhance performance in competitive athletics. Hyperbaric chambers have been widely used in Russia, East Germany, and other socialist countries. In the West, some professional sports teams have hyperbaric chambers in their training rooms, including the Vancouver Canucks hockey team. However, large-scale scientific studies on the ability of HBO therapy to enhance athletic performance have yet to be carried out.

A typical HBO treatment lasts between 60 and ninety minutes, and the number of treatments given depends on the patient's medical condition. For example, divers suffering from the bends would normally receive one or two treatments, while an individual with a severe or infected wound may require daily HBO treatments for several weeks.

Hyperbaric oxygen therapy has several general health benefits:

- It reduces gas embolism. Any free gas trapped in the body will decrease in volume as pressure exerted on it increases. This may allow it to pass through into general blood. This makes HBO therapy especially useful in management of gas embolism and decompression illness among divers.
- Hyperbaric oxygen causes the blood vessels to contract. This can result in the reduction of healing time for burn or crush injuries. At the same time, HBO therapy provides extra oxygen to the blood plasma, so that a net increase in tissue oxygen occurs. This, in turn, promotes healing.
- HBO has an anti-ischemic effect on body tissues. Ischemia occurs when the flow of blood is reduced to a part of the body, which slows the healing process. Hyperbaric oxygen physically dissolves oxygen into plasma. This allows an increase in the quantity of oxygen transferred to the ischemic tissue by the blood, thus promoting healing.
- Oxygen is a powerful antimicrobial. Anaerobic bacteria (or bacteria that thrive in a low-oxygen environment) do not contain natural defenses to protect them from superoxides, peroxides, and other compounds formed in the presence of high oxygen tension.

Many of the body's defense mechanisms are dependent on oxygen, and when tissue pO_2 [oxygen partial pressure] drops too low, effective infection-fighting mechanisms are retarded. By reoxygenating those body tissues, we allow the body's defense mechanisms to function at an optimal level once more.

- Oxygen promotes the formation of new blood cells. Our body's defense mechanisms (such as the "oxidative burst") are necessary for the formation of white blood cells, which kill bacteria and produce collagen, a protein that helps heal wounds. When hypoxia (or oxygen starvation) is reversed by HBO therapy, these body processes are enhanced.[4]

HBO AND OXIDATIVE THERAPIES

Because side-by-side clinical comparisons between oxidative and HBO therapies are difficult to come by, Dr. Bocci has attempted to compare the effectiveness of both hyperbaric oxygen therapy and ozone therapy in treating specific health problems. Based on his personal experience, he believes that HBO therapies excel in treating arterial gas embolism, decompression sickness, severe carbon monoxide poisoning, severe anemia due to blood loss, and clostridial myonecrosis (gas gangrene). Ozone therapy is not effective or its effectiveness has not been determined regarding these health problems.

By contrast, Bocci believes that ozone therapy has "good activity" in treating compromised skin grafts and flaps, radiation damage, refractory osteomyelitis, necrotizing fasciitis, traumatic ischemic injury, thermal burns, chronic ulcers, and failures in wound healing; it is also helpful in preventing osteoradionecrosis. The effectiveness of HBO therapy with these diseases is considered minimal. Dr. Bocci also believes that ozone therapy is more effective in treating senility and chronic fatigue syndrome than is hyperbaric oxygen therapy.[5]

Although HBO therapy is worthy of deeper consideration, it will not be included in the scope of our discussion in this book. For a comprehensive book on the subject, consult *Hyperbaric Oxygen Therapy* by Richard A. Neubauer, M.D., and Morton Walker, D.P.M. (see the resources—appendix 2, page 442).

During their groundbreaking research at Baylor University in Texas during the 1960s, scientists discovered that many of the positive effects of HBO therapy could be reproduced or enhanced through the therapeutic use of hydrogen peroxide, resulting in much lower treatment cost. Similar findings have been discovered with ozone therapy; both therapies are easily available in a traditional medical setting and to patients living in developing countries or in other areas where expensive hyperbaric oxygen chambers are rarely found.

OXYGEN MULTISTEP THERAPY

Oxygen multistep therapy (O_2MT) was developed by Dr. Manfred von Ardenne (1907–1997), a German researcher and inventor known for his pioneering work in the development of television technology, electron microscopy, scanning microscopy, and isotope separation.

In the 1960s, von Ardenne met the Nobel Prize winner Otto Warburg several times. As mentioned earlier in this book, Dr. Warburg believed that the key precondition for the development of cancer was a lack of oxygen at the cellular level. Inspired by Warburg's research, von Ardenne decided to explore how oxygen and other natural modalities could be used in cancer therapy. He developed a treatment he called "systemic cancer multistep therapy" or sCMT. His protocol utilized whole-body hypothermia, induced hyperglycemia, and oxygen enrichment of the blood in addition to traditional cancer treatment.

During the 1970s von Ardenne began suffering from extreme fatigue. Although his doctors could not provide a clear diagnosis or effective treatment, von Ardenne decided to inhale pure oxygen several times a day. Within a week he reportedly regained his health and energy. This resulted in the development of oxygen multistep therapy, popularly known as exercising with oxygen therapy or EWOT. He explored this therapy in great detail in his textbook *Oxygen Multistep Therapy: Physiological and Technical Foundations* (Thieme, 1990). Dr. von Ardenne's clinic, which closed in 2000, claimed that some hundred thousand people utilized this therapy in German-speaking countries alone.[6]

Proponents of EWOT point out that during periods of strenuous exercise—such as long-distance running or competitive cycling—the body utilizes more oxygen than it receives from the air.[7] EWOT is designed to reverse this imbalance. While EWOT is viewed as a medical therapy in Germany, it is not approved as such in the United States, Canada, or Australia. Because medical claims cannot be made for EWOT in these countries, it is considered primarily an exercise modality.

The most important feature of EWOT is the targeted, time-restricted, and controlled oxygen supply that is inhaled, often during exercise at home, at a gym, or at a clinic with a stationary bike, elliptical machine, or treadmill. Oxygen is provided by a special oxygen concentrator that removes nitrogen from the ambient air, providing between 92 percent and 97 percent pure oxygen to the user. As a result, the body is believed to increase its intake of oxygen, resulting in higher amounts of oxygen dissolved in blood (pO_2 levels). This is believed to result in improved mental clarity, increased energy, and a strengthened immune system. A total EWOT package, which includes an oxygen concentrator, face mask with nasal cannula, bubble humidifier, and tubing, begins at $1,000 and is available from a wide number of online companies that sell EWOT equipment.

PART TWO

Oxidative
Therapies
in Medicine

Although some of the studies presented in this section are the result of double-blind research (in which neither the patient nor the investigator knows what treatment the patient is receiving), most are objective and subjective clinical findings based on empirical knowledge or practical experience.

Double-blind trials have become the "gold standard" of scientific research, especially in the United States. The main advantage of this type of research is that complete objectivity is achieved and measurable results are easier to obtain and evaluate. It also prevents the physician from giving any preferential treatment to the patient. Much of the newer scientific research presented in this section is based on double-blind studies. Ozone researchers like Dr. Bocci believe that randomized, double-blind studies will open the door to greater acceptance of these therapies by the scientific community. He writes: "We must perform RCTs [randomized clinical trials] in selected diseases, for which we have good evidence of ozone's activity. In order to convince skeptics, the results must be more than adequate and be published in peer-reviewed journals."[1]

The primary drawback to double-blind trials is that people who may be in need of a valuable treatment do not receive it. In some cases, patients are not permitted to take any other experimental medications (some of which may be lifesaving) during the trials because the findings of the study might be compromised.

Most German physicians who have done research with medical ozone therapy believe that double-blind studies are immoral. They maintain that ozone is not an experimental drug; it has been used since World War I and has been proven to be safe and effective on millions of patients. They believe that to deny a sick patient a treatment that is likely to relieve suffering or save his or her life is a violation of the

Hippocratic oath and an affront to the people who go to them for care. Dr. Joachim Varro, a physician from Dusseldorf, Germany, who worked primarily with cancer patients, shared his views on double-blind studies at the 1983 World Ozone Conference in Washington, D.C.:

> For ethical reasons, and as a practicing physician facing the threat of life in advanced cases, I cannot do a so-called random study or double-blind study. I leave that to science and research with responsibility for such methods. Largely, I adhere to research findings and clinical experiences, and I try to adapt these so that they can be practically applied in my range of activities. As a result, I am able to constructively bring my empirical long-term observations into the medical discussion.[2]

Another problem with double-blind studies is that although they may be a good idea in theory, they do not always work in actual practice. Participants in double-blind trials are known to cheat, especially when their lives are on the line. Several such cases were reported by Paul A. Sergios in *One Boy at War: My Life in the AIDS Underground*. In one instance, he spoke of a double-blind trial for a promising AIDS drug. Some participants received an inert sugar pill while others were given the experimental drug. He wrote, "Numerous patients who were admitted to the trial between February and April 1986 opened their capsules to taste the contents. If the powder tasted bitter, they continued the treatment. If it tasted sweet, they threw the bottle away and rushed to catch a plane to try their luck at getting an actual drug at another site."[3]

Sergios also wrote of his own experience as a participant in another trial for a promising AIDS drug in which he shared half of his pills with another participant in order to increase their chances of survival in the event that one of them was receiving the experimental medication. When first offered the option of sharing the pills, he said that he felt it was immoral because it could disrupt the trial. His friend replied: "Immoral? . . . What about their twisted morality in giving half of us a sugar pill for a year or two in order to see how fast we go to our deaths while others get a drug that could potentially save their lives? Not only that—this study prohibits us from taking certain drugs to prevent opportunistic infections. The odds are stacked against *us*."[4]

An unlikely mainstream criticism of double-blind studies was reported on the front page of the September 18, 1997, edition of the *New York Times*. The article highlighted objection by U.S. government scientists and others over sponsorship by the National Institutes of Health and Centers for Disease Control and Prevention of overseas AIDS studies where half of 11,211 pregnant women in seven third-world countries were given AZT to determine minimal doses of the drug to prevent HIV infection, while the other half were given dummy pills. It is believed that as a result of this study, more than one thousand infants would contract HIV. The article quotes Dr. Peter Lurie of Public Citizen, an advocacy group, as saying, "We have turned our backs on these mothers and their babies," and cited the government's own scientists as questioning whether these double-blind studies are ethical.[5]

The decision to use double-blind or random clinical trials involves a number of difficult moral issues that will likely be debated among scientists, physicians, and their patients for years to come. One of my primary goals in this book is to present the evidence, whether it be preliminary, empirical, or the result of double-blind studies. After readers see the evidence, it is their task to either come to their own conclusions or do additional research on their own.

10
Cardiovascular Diseases

Physicians have utilized oxidative therapies to treat heart disease and related circulatory problems for over forty years. Ozone therapy (administered as autohemotherapy, intramuscular injection, intra-arterial injection, or rectal insufflation) and hydrogen peroxide (primarily in the form of intravenous or intra-arterial injection) have been used to treat heart attack, stroke, high blood pressure, cardiac insufficiency, high cholesterol levels, angina, atherosclerosis, and a wide variety of other problems relating to poor circulation.

Because ozone has been found to improve blood flow and enhance oxygen release from cells, Dr. E. Riva Sanseverino and Dr. P. Castellacci, from the Institute of Physiology at the University of Bologna in Italy, sought to evaluate the impact of ozone therapy on physical activity. They tested the endurance of a group of eight healthy adults between forty-two and sixty years of age on an elevated treadmill for 30 to 45 minutes, with subjects both walking and running.

Heartbeat and oxygen consumption were measured. The eight individuals were then given ozone through major autohemotherapy once or sometimes twice a week over a four-month period. In order to establish a control, some were given infusions with added oxygen only. After each treatment, the subjects were tested on the treadmill and results were evaluated.

Overall, the researchers found that physical performance twelve to twenty-four hours after one to nine sessions of autohemotherapy improved by 8 to 12 percent. Of special note was that heart rate progressively decreased as the number of autohemotherapy sessions increased.[1]

In Cuba, ozone therapy has become a routine treatment for patients suffering from angina and heart attacks. During my first visit in January 1994, I met the eighty-year-old mother of Dr. Manuel Gomez, the cofounder of the Department of Ozone. Three years before, Doña Matilde had had such severe angina that she could barely get from one room to the other without pain and shortness of breath. After much resistance (she is a very stubborn woman), her son finally persuaded her to undergo three weeks of daily major autohemotherapy, during which the angina completely disappeared. Although she hadn't changed her lifestyle one bit ("I don't like taking long walks"), she was still energetic and strong at ninety-two.

Cuban physicians have treated patients with heart disease with ozone therapy for decades. In one study investigators from the National Center for Scientific Research determined that patients who had suffered a heart attack (cardiac infarction) showed a decrease in glutathione peroxidase and superoxide dismutase activities in their blood, which are part of the body's primary antioxidant system and help protect against lipid peroxide and superoxide radicals, respectively. In this study, reported in *Free Radical Biology & Medicine,* twenty-two patients who had had a heart attack between three months and one year before the study were treated with ozone by autohemotherapy for a total of fifteen sessions.

Researchers observed a statistically significant decrease in plasma total cholesterol and low-density lipoprotein. In addition, "significant" increases of erythrocyte glutathione peroxidase and glucose-6-phosphate dehydrogenase activities were found after five sessions. There was no change in plasma lipid peroxidation levels. The researchers concluded: "Endovenous ozone therapy in patients with myocardial infarction has a beneficial effect on blood lipid metabolism, provoking the activation of antioxidant protection system."[2]

Post-Infarction Treatment

A unique Russian study at the F. E. Dzerzhinsky Central Clinical Sanatorium in Sochi was designed to estimate the influence of ozone therapy on oxygen metabolism kinetics and the circulation system during spa and resort treatment of 145 patients who survived myocardial infarction. All were given routine spa-and-resort therapy, a popular Russian tradition that usually involves therapeutic bathing and drinking mineral water, a healthy diet, exercise, recreation, and rest.

Of these 145 patients, 56 also received traditional heart medications, while the remaining 89 were given medication plus ozone therapy in the form of intravenous ozonated saline. Clinical examinations included a variety of diagnostic tools: electrocardiography, veloergometry (a type of cardiac stress test), and echocardiography (a kind of ultrasound test). Kinetics of oxygen metabolism was evaluated by transcutaneous polarography (a type of test using electrodes), laser Doppler flowmetry (LDF, a noninvasive method to estimate the blood perfusion in the microcirculation), and computer capillaroscopy.

The results of the study indicated that ozone therapy in combination with traditional medical treatment reduces the period of post-infarction rehabilitation, decreases tissue hypoxia, improves microcirculation characteristics, and improves the overall health status of the patients.[3]

Oxidative therapies work by activating red blood cell metabolism, which manifests as a rise of adenosine triphosphate (ATP) and a greater supply of oxygen to body tissues. At the same time, hydrogen peroxide and ozone can reactivate the capacity of cells that had previously been deficient to metabolize oxygen more effectively.

In Cuba today emergency rooms at many major hospitals have an ozone generator to treat victims of heart attack and stroke. In February 1996, the Reuters wire service reported that Nicaraguan president and Sandinista leader Daniel Ortega Saavedra had been treated in Cuba for a heart condition the previous year and had returned to Havana for a medical check-up. According to the dispatch, the Cuban news agency Prensa Latina said Ortega was receiving a treatment called ozone therapy to purify the blood. It seems that Ortega, a friend of former President Fidel Castro, had received ozone therapy for several months beginning in November 1994 after suffering a "silent" heart attack about three months previously.[4]

Ozone and hydrogen peroxide alter the structure of blood and the way it flows through the veins and arteries. The "pile of coins" erythrocyte (mature red blood cell or corpuscle) formation, which is typical of arterial occlusion disease, is reversed through changes in the electrical charge of the erythrocytic membrane. At the same time, the flexibility and elasticity of the erythrocytes is increased, improving the blood's ability to flow through the blood vessels.[5] This increases the supply of life-giving oxygen to the heart and other vital body tissues.

Some of the most important early research in this field was carried out at the New England College of Medicine. Investigators found that small amounts of hydrogen peroxide alter the way that blood platelets aggregate or come together. Platelets play an important role in the coagulation of blood and the formation of blood clots. In a paper published in the journal *Blood,* researchers concluded: "The generation of peroxide at a site of thrombus [blood clot] formation may alter the development of the thrombus. This alteration could occur via the changes in either aggregation or disaggregation of platelets."[6] Other studies at the Upstate Medical Center in Syracuse, New York, and the University of Massachusetts Medical School in Worcester later confirmed the role of hydrogen peroxide as a modulator of platelet reactions.[7]

There is also evidence that hydrogen peroxide oxidizes fatty substances, such as the plaque that adheres to arterial walls. In an article appearing in *Townsend Letter for Doctors* (now *Townsend Letter for Doctors and Patients*), Dr. Farr wrote:

> The oxidative benefit may include the oxidation of lipid material in the vessel wall. The benefit of oxygen saturation of tissue fluid from the oxygen produced by H_2O_2 may be of secondary importance. Cholesterol and triglycerides become elevated after the intra-

arterial injection of H_2O_2. Repeated intra-arterial infusion has been found to remove atheromatous [fatty] plaques and increase elasticity of the blood vessel wall.[8]

In her article "The Biochemical Processes Underlying Ozone Therapy," Dr. Renate Viebahn-Haensler addressed the efficacy of medical ozone in improving blood circulation in technical terms:

The so-called circulatory enhancing effects of ozone, as expressed in the form of its being administered intravascularly and intramuscularly, are the result of a direct influence exerted on the oxygen metabolism by the ozone-oxygen mixture applied:

(a) The formation of peroxides from non-saturated fatty acids, and an influence on the rheological properties of the blood
(b) Activation of the cellular enzymal protection system against peroxides, oxygen and ozone
(c) Activation of the erythrocytic metabolism and an increase of 2,3-DPG
(d) As a fourth factor, a direct influence of the ozone on the redox function of the mitochondrial respiratory chain is considered: this can be demonstrated, for example, by a significant reduction in NADH [a co-enzyme]

As a total effect, the above properties of ozone bring about a reactivation of the disturbed oxygen metabolism: this is expressed by an increase in the arterial partial oxygen pressure and an enlargement of the arteriovenous pO_2 [oxygen partial pressure] difference, as well as by an increase in deoxygenating substances producing a greater supply of oxygen to the tissues or by improving the actual processing of oxygen by the system.[9]

It was mentioned earlier that oxidative therapies also can activate important enzymes (such as glutathione peroxidase, catalase, and superoxide dismutase) that are involved in free radical scavenging. An excess of free radicals can contribute to heart disease and other circulatory disturbances.

As we'll see in this chapter, the clinical evidence regarding the effectiveness of oxidative therapies in treating different forms of cardiovascular disease is well established. Given the fact that cardiovascular disease and related circulatory problems are the primary cause of death and disability among adults in this country, it is time to explore the role that oxidative therapies can play in the prevention and treatment of heart disease and related disorders.

ATHEROSCLEROSIS

Involving the Coronary and Cerebral Vessels

Russian scientists at the Medical Academy in Nizhny Novgorod treated thirty-nine patients suffering from severe atherosclerosis. All patients exhibited symptoms of angina, nine had suffered heart attacks, one had undergone a bypass operation, and two had suffered strokes. Nearly two-thirds of the subjects had cerebral blood supply insufficiency (i.e., a deficient amount of blood to the brain), and one-quarter had a condition called "discirculatory encephalopathy," causing impaired circulation in the brain.

Over twenty days of treatment, ozonated sodium chloride was given intravenously five times a day. By the end of the study, angina attacks decreased from an average of 6.1 a day to 2.5. Doses of nitroglycerin were reduced. Tolerance to physical load increased in 82.1 percent of the patients. Of those suffering from repolarization impairments (defined by *Taber's Cyclopedic Medical Dictionary* as "re-establishment of a polarized state in a muscle or nerve fiber following contraction or conduction of a nerve impulse"), 51.1 percent recovered completely. In addition, among the group, cholesterol levels dropped 48 percent and triglyceride levels fell 53 percent. These favorable results led the researchers to conclude that ozone therapy should be considered an effective method for treatment of atherosclerosis in the medical clinic.[10]

At the end of the course of treatment, researchers observed a statistically significant decrease in plasma total cholesterol and low-density lipoprotein ("bad" cholesterol). In addition, biologically significant increases on erythrocyte glutathione peroxidase and glucose-6-phosphate dehydrogenase activities were found. There was no change in plasma lipid peroxidation level. The researchers concluded that "endovenous ozone therapy in patients with myocardial infarction has a beneficial effect on blood lipid metabolism, provoking the activation of antioxidant protection system."[11]

A team of researchers led by Dr. Gregorio Martínez-Sánchez of the Medinat SRL clinic in Camerano, Italy, investigated the use of ozone to treat patients with coronary artery disease (CAD). CAD is the most common cause of sudden death and death of people over twenty years of age.

Because ozone therapy has been found to activate the antioxidant system and improve blood circulation and oxygen delivery to tissues, the aim of this study was to investigate the therapeutic efficacy of ozone in patients with CAD who were also being treated with antithrombotic therapy, specifically aspirin and policosanol.

A randomized controlled clinical trial was performed with fifty-three patients divided into two groups: those in one group (twenty-seven patients) were treated with antithrombotic therapy, and those in the other group (twenty-six patients) were treated with antithrombotic therapy plus oxygen-ozone administered as rectal insufflation. A third group (numbering fifty individuals) of similar age and gender was used as reference for the experimental variables. The efficacy of the treatments was evaluated by comparing hemostatic indexes and biochemical markers of oxidative stress in both groups after twenty days of treatment.

The researchers found that ozone treatment significantly improved prothrombin time when compared to the patients receiving antithrombotic therapy alone, without modifying bleeding time. Combination antithrombotic therapy and oxygen-ozone improved the antioxidant status of patients, reducing biomarkers of protein and lipid oxidation.

These reactions, in turn, enhanced patients' total antioxidant status and modulated the level of superoxide dismutase and catalase, with a 57 percent and 32 percent reduction in superoxide dismutase and catalase activities, respectively. This was connected to a redox environment changing to a status of low production of oxygen with an increase in hydrogen peroxide detoxification. No side effects were observed.

Writing in the *European Journal of Pharmacology*, the authors concluded: "These results show that medical ozone treatment could be a complementary therapy in the treatment of CAD and its complications."[12]

Involving the Extremities

In the early 1990s, researchers at the Department of Gerontology, Geriatry, and Metabolic Diseases at the Second University of Naples in Italy compared the effectiveness of hyperbaric oxygen and oxygen-ozone therapy in treating patients suffering from peripheral occlusive arterial disease (POAD). In this study, researchers investigated the influence of these treatments on medical parameters that play an important role in the origin and the clinical course of arteriosclerosis. Two groups of fifteen patients suffering from POAD were assigned at random to a cycle of either hyperbaric oxygen therapy or oxygen-ozone therapy. Blood tests were done to evaluate blood viscosity, erythrocyte filterability, hematocrit value, fibrinogen concentration, and thrombin time, all of which are used to determine the nature and extent of the disease.

The researchers found that the oxygen-ozone therapy brought about a significant increase of erythrocyte filterability and a significant decrease of blood viscosity, showing that it helps relieve symptoms of POAD. By contrast, hyperbaric oxygen therapy did not produce any significant change in the blood. The researchers concluded, "The increase of lipid perioxidation, proved by raised malonyldialdehyde plasma levels, seems a likely mechanism involved in the hemorrheologic effects of O_2-O_3 therapy."[13]

A major study on the effects of medical ozone on patients suffering from symptoms of atherosclerosis in the extremities was undertaken by surgeon Ottokar Rokitansky at a major Vienna, Austria, hospital. During the early 1980s, he evaluated 372 patients whose symptoms fit the last three of four categories of the disease, as classified by French heart specialist R. Fontaine:

Stage I: rapid tiring, exhaustion, sensation of coldness
Stage II: latent pain(s), intermittent lameness or limping
Stage III: pains when lying down at night or at rest
Stage IV: gangrene

In the third and fourth stages, amputation of fingers, toes, and/or limbs is often necessary.

The participants in the study were divided into two groups of roughly similar ages and symptoms. In Group 1 (consisting of 232 participants), an oxygen-ozone mixture was added to the patients' blood and administered through intra-arterial injection. In addition, ozone gas was applied within a plastic bag that surrounded the affected limb (ozone bagging, as described in chapter 5). Group 2 consisted of a control group of 140 who received traditional vasodilation therapy—medication designed to open up blood vessels.

Dr. Rokitansky reported marked clinical improvement in up to 80 percent of the experimental group patients suffering from stage II of the disease, as compared to 44 percent of the patients receiving traditional therapy. At-rest pains disappeared for 70 percent of the people in stage III who received ozone, as compared to 39 percent of the control group. The stage IV patients in Group 1, who were all hospitalized, had a 50 percent cure rate of the ulcers and soft-tissue gangrene, which reduced their time in the hospital. By contrast, similar results were achieved by only 28.6 percent of the controls. The rate of upper thigh amputations declined from 15 percent to 10 percent for the stage III patients and from 50 percent to 27 percent for patients with gangrene (stage IV) who received ozone (see table 10.1).[14]

Table 10.1. Therapy Cases Compared

Stage	Number of Subjects		Marked Improvement %		Some Improvement %		Deterioration or No Improvement %	
Group	1	2	1	2	1	2	1	2
II	105	73	80.0	43.8	11.4	19.2	8.5	37.0
III	72	46	70.8	39.1	19.4	17.4	9.7	43.5
IV	55	21	50.9	28.6	21.8	19.0	27.3	54.0

Source: Ottokar Rokitansky, "The Clinical Effects and Biochemistry of Ozone Therapy in Peripheral Arterial Coronary Disturbances," in *Medical Applications of Ozone*, edited by Julius LaRaus (Norwalk, CT: International Ozone Association, Pan American Committee, 1983), 53.

In 1988 a study was done at the National Institute of Angiology and Vascular Surgery in Havana, Cuba, on sixty patients suffering from severe atherosclerosis. Primary symptoms included blocked blood circulation to their extremities, primarily the feet. The patients were divided up into two groups so that their age range and symptoms were similar. Of the treatment group, half received either ten daily sessions of autohemotherapy with oxygen and ozone or intra-arterial injections of oxygen and ozone. The control group was given traditional medical treatment.

By the end of the ten days, 73.4 percent of the patients treated with ozone with less severe atherosclerosis exhibited marked improvement, while the condition of 20 percent deteriorated. In contrast, 40 percent of the control group improved, while 53 percent got worse. The fifteen patients who suffered from more serious symptoms (which included severe pain, gangrene, and ischemic ulcers) and were treated with ozone showed good results as well. Sixty percent experienced clinical improvement, while only 26 percent of the control group improved. Six patients (40 percent) of the patients receiving ozone got worse as compared to eleven (73 percent) of the control group.[15]

In 1989, a study was undertaken in Poland by Dr. J. Sroczynski and colleagues at the Katedry i Kliniki Chorob Wewnetrznych i Zawodowych Sl. AM, a research hospital specializing in internal and occupational diseases. Ozone was administered intra-arterially to fifty subjects suffering from arteriosclerotic ischemia of the lower extremities and to forty-one subjects with diabetes mellitus. Serum lipids concentration was examined before and after the course of treatment. Researchers reported that the group with arteriosclerotic ischemia experienced a "significant" decrease in blood cholesterol level. At the same time, the patients suffering from diabetes showed a significant reduction of LDL (or "bad") cholesterol. In both groups, total serum lipid levels decreased. According to an abstract of this article poorly translated into English, the researchers concluded that "ozone therapy set back the arteriosclerosis progress, normalized some parameters of lipid metabolism and improved HDL to LDL cholesterol fractions relationship."[16]

Two other Polish studies carried out in the early 1990s revealed the positive effects of ozone therapy on circulatory problems of the lower limbs. In the first study, investigators at the Katedry i Zakladu Biofizyki Sl. examined fifty-three patients with occlusive arteriosclerosis of the lower limbs. Blood and plasma viscosity, total lipids, triglycerides, total cholesterol, free fatty acids, fibrinogen, lipid profile, and hematocrit levels were determined both prior to and after a course of ozone therapy. At the same time, intermittent claudication distance was measured, which evaluated lameness or difficulty in walking. The results were very positive: after ozone therapy, all patients showed a significant prolongation of the distance walked painlessly. In addition, there was a marked reduction in blood and plasma viscosity as well as a decrease in total cholesterol after therapy with ozone.[17]

The second study, which was coordinated by Dr. Sroczynski as a follow-up to his earlier research, investigated the value of intra-arterial ozone injections in the treatment of atherosclerotic ischemia. Ten injections of ozone and oxygen were administered into the femoral arteries of fifty patients suffering from atherosclerotic ischemia of the lower extremities over a period of several weeks. The same treatment was given to forty-nine diabetic patients suffering from similar symptoms. All patients were assessed clinically with standard medical tests, including the "ankle-brachial index" and measurement of intermittent claudication distance prior to and after the treatment. The results showed a significant improvement in both groups as measured by an increase in the ankle-arm index, as well as a twofold prolongation of the intermittent claudication distance. The researchers concluded that treating atherosclerotic ischemia of the lower extremities with ozone is both "valuable and safe."[18]

Researchers at the Department of Ozone Therapy at the Regional Medical Diagnostic Center in Nizhny Novgorod, Russia, also studied the effect of ozone therapy on atherosclerotic vessel disorders of the lower extremities and announced their findings at the Twelfth World Congress of the International Ozone Association in 1995. Working in cooperation with the Nizhegorodski Regional Hospital of War Veterans, 132 war invalids between sixty-two and eighty-four years of age suffering from grade 3 to grade 4 peripheral circulation disorders of the lower extremities were observed.

Although all had been receiving traditional medical care over the years, none of the patients was able to walk for a distance of more than 150 to 200 meters. All experienced chronic pain in the calf muscles and had cold lower legs and feet. Eleven war veterans suffered from crus and femur wounds of forty-seven to fifty years standing, while eight patients had been afflicted with frostbite during World War II. Thirty-one of the patients had circulation problems accompanied by chronic trophic ulcers.

Different types of ozone therapy were administered to patients, who were divided into three groups depending on symptoms. The first group was given eight to ten intravenous injections of ozone-saturated rheopolyglucin solutions (Rheomacrodex). The second group received intravenous ozone injections combined with subcutaneous injections of ozone and oxygen. The third group was given a course of three or four autohemotherapy treatments in addition to the therapies above. Patients with trophic ulcers were given external ozonation through the plastic bagging method described in chapter 5.

By the end of the courses of treatment, virtually all patients exhibited a "significant improvement in their well-being," with warming of the extremities and complete relief of muscle cramps. There was also an average ten- to fifteenfold increase in walking distance. The trophic ulcers all shrank from 2 to 4 cm^2 daily during and after treatment, eliminating the need for surgery. The researchers concluded that ozone therapy (especially the combination of the three types of ozone therapies) was "highly effective" in the treatment of peripheral circulatory disorders of the lower extremities, especially in people advanced in age.[19]

A later Russian study at the Regional Medical Diagnostic Center in Nizhny Novgorod involved eighty-one patients suffering from atherosclerosis. After treatment with ozone therapy, patients improved significantly. The researchers reported, "It was found that use of ozone-oxygen mixtures leads to hypocoagulatory changes (diminution of platelet aggregation, lowering of fibrinogen concentration, prolongation of activated partial thrombplastin time, enhanced fibrinolytic activity) which contribute to clinical response."[20]

We mentioned earlier that in Russia ozone therapy is considered part of the medical mainstream. Physicians at the prestigious Medical Academy at Nizhny Novgorod (connected to the Ministry of Health Service of the Russian Federation) not only have been pioneers in discovering of how ozone works in the body but have developed a variety of protocols for treating patients with different cardiovascular problems.

In treating patients diagnosed with atherosclerosis, they found that ozone can produce a hypolipodemic effect on blood, thus reducing total cholesterol, low-density lipoproteins ("bad" cholesterol), and trigycerides (fat in the blood) while increasing levels of high-density ("good") lipoproteins.

In addition to reducing harmful fats in the blood, ozone can also help regulate free radical processes. A small amount of ozone in the blood activates the body's antioxidant defense system, thus eliminating lipoprotein toxicity. This is why Russian physicians consider ozone therapy as an anti-sclerotic treatment.

The methods used to treat patients with atherosclerosis include intravenous infusions of 200 ml of ozonated saline solution, major autohemotherapy, and rectal insufflations. Between six and ten treatments are recommended depending on the patient. The first two procedures of intravenous infusions or rectal insufflations are done every day, while the rest are administered every second day. The six to eight procedures of major autohemotherapy are done twice a week.[21]

A Cuban study involved seventy-two elderly nondiabetic patients with obliterant atherosclerosis, compounded by intermittent claudication, or severe pain in the calf muscles while walking. The patients were randomly divided into four groups. Three of the groups were treated with ozone: one group with major autohemotherapy, another via intramuscular injection, and the last with rectal insufflation. Members of the fourth group of patients (the control group) were given conventional medical treatment. Members of the first three groups who were treated with ozone showed little difference among them; however, the three groups showed considerable improvement when compared to members of the control group. The claudication distance on the treadmill increased to 2.5 km/hour. Ankle-arm pressure rates showed a significant difference as well, which corresponds to the Polish findings mentioned earlier. Patients reported that of all methods of ozone application, rectal insufflation was the least uncomfortable.[22]

A more recent study at the Second University of Naples involved twenty-seven patients suffering from POAD, clinical stages 2 to 3. All received autohemotherapy. Thirty minutes after treatment, significant improvements in blood were recorded, while the blood of the control group (which received an autohemotransfusion without ozone) showed none. The researchers reported, "Ozonized autohemotransfusion may be useful to improve both the poor rheological properties of the blood and the oxygen delivery to tissues in patients suffering from POAD."[23]

A group of Spanish researchers from the Radiation Oncology Department at the Dr. Negrin University Hospital in the Canary Islands studied the effects of ozone therapy on muscle oxygenation. Twenty-three patients and three healthy volunteers were evaluated after three autohemotherapy treatments over one week. Tissue oxygenation (mm/Hg) was directly measured after the first and third session. The researchers concluded:

Ozone therapy can modify oxygenation in resting muscles, particularly of those that are the most hypoxic. Our results suggest that ozone therapy could be used effectively as a complementary treatment of hypoxic and ischemic syndromes and that the therapy warrants further investigation for possible application in other clinical conditions.[24]

Additional information about blood circulation can be found in chapter 16, which discusses the effects of oxidative therapies on diabetes, beginning on page 233.

HEART DEFECTS
(WITH INFECTIOUS ENDOCARDITIS)

An unusual study was carried out at the Interregional Cardiosurgical Center at Nizhny Novgorod in Russia on patients undergoing heart surgery whose cases were complicated by the presence of *endocarditis,* an inflammation of the lining of the heart and its valves. When endocarditis was present, over one-quarter of the heart patients died either during or after surgery.

During the operations undertaken as part of the study, each patient's heart was bathed in ozonated cardioplegic solutions, which are designed to stop the heart. A heart-lung machine circulated the blood (to which a mixture of oxygen and ozone was added) during the operation. The results showed that the death rate from complications of infectious endocarditis fell from an average of 26.6 percent to only 4.2 percent.[25]

HYPERCHOLESTEROLEMIA
(EXCESSIVE CHOLESTEROL)

Some of the most important research in the field of oxidative therapies took place at Baylor University Medical Center in Texas in the early 1960s, particularly in the areas of heart disease and cancer. In one study, Dr. J. W. Finney and his colleagues studied the ability of hydrogen peroxide to remove cholesterol and other fats from the arteries. They based this early research on postmortem studies of the arteries of cancer patients who had received intra-arterial hydrogen peroxide (as an adjunct to irradiation therapy) for a period of four to sixteen weeks in the late stages of their disease. The blood vessels of a similar control group of cancer patients who did not receive hydrogen peroxide were studied for comparison.

When the blood vessel samples were analyzed, it was found that the patients receiving hydrogen peroxide had approximately a 50 percent reduction in total lipids (fats) in the area that had been infused with hydrogen peroxide.[26]

A study at the Center for Medical-Surgical Research in Cuba a quarter century later involved twenty-two male patients between the ages of forty-six and seventy-two who had had previous heart attacks. All patients had elevated levels of total cholesterol as well as low-density lipoproteins, the most dangerous form of cholesterol. The only treatment given during the study consisted of fifteen sessions of autohemotherapy with ozone.

After five treatments the patients were evaluated. Cholesterol levels began falling by an average of 5.5 percent, and by the end of the treatment period of fifteen sessions, the levels of cholesterol in the blood had fallen by an average of 9.7 percent. Levels of low-density lipoproteins had decreased 15.4 percent after five sessions of autohemotherapy and fell 19.8 percent by the fifteenth session.

The researchers concluded: "Endovenous ozone therapy has beneficial effects on [the] lipid pattern of patients that have suffered myocardial infarction [heart attack], and accompanied by an effective stimulation of [the] antioxidant enzyme system."[27]

HYPOXIA

Another of the Baylor studies found that hydrogen peroxide can provide oxygen for the anoxic or ischemic heart, as well as help normalize cardiac arrhythmias and reverse cardiac arrest. Dr. Harold C. Urschel Jr., who was involved in much of the Baylor research, expounded on these findings in the journal *Diseases of the Chest:*

> Hydrogen peroxide releases dissolved oxygen equivalent to that found in solutions under oxygen at 3–8 atmosphere pressure [i.e., hyperbaric oxygen]. H_2O_2 administration does not require lung transport. It can be given continuously over long periods of time, it can be administered by a single physician without expensive equipment and large teams, and it avoids compression-decompression hazards, as well as central nervous system and pulmonary toxicity.[28]

At about the same time, another of the Baylor studies focused on the ability of hydrogen peroxide to protect the heart during ischemic episodes of heart attacks. Using pigs, Dr. J. W. Finney and his colleagues found that diluted solutions of hydrogen peroxide were able to keep the heart functioning in spite of an ischemic episode. They added DMSO (dimethyl sulfoxide) to the hydrogen peroxide mixture, and the scientists discovered that the new mixture "will afford more protection [to the heart] than either reagent alone."[29] It is interesting to note that the Baylor studies, which were supported at first by a large pharmaceutical company, have experienced little or no clinical follow-up.

Similar results were achieved with ozone. Dr. S. P. Peretyagin of the Medical Academy in Nizhny Novgorod performed a clinical study of how ozone can increase the flow of oxygen through the blood vessels.[30] This is why many of the larger Cuban hospitals routinely use ozone therapy in emergency rooms and intensive care units for patients who come to the hospital suffering from heart attacks or strokes. The ozone provides the heart and brain with the vital oxygen they need by enabling the blood to flow more freely through the circulatory system.

ISCHEMIC
CEREBROVASCULAR DISEASE

Ischemic cerebrovascular disease involves a blocking of the blood supply to the brain. Patients often become incapacitated both mentally and physically, which leads them to become a burden to other family members. This disease is also a leading cause of death among the elderly in many of the industrialized nations of the world.

A Cuban study regarding the ability of ozone to improve the health status of older adults suffering from ischemic cerebrovascular disease was carried out at the Geriatric Complex of the Salvador Allende Hospital in Havana. A group of 120 was chosen for the study.

Extensive physical, psychomotor, multidimensional psychological, and neurological tests (including CT scans and EEGs) were given before and after treatment. Special attention was devoted to the patients' mental condition, their ability to participate in daily activities, their ability to administer their own medications, and their social interaction with friends and family. Patients were then classified into three standardized groups according to their symptoms. Forty-eight (40 percent) were in an "acute" phase of the disease (meaning they entered the study with less than thirty days since the onset of symptoms), forty-two (35 percent) in an "ancient" phase (between one and six months of symptoms), and thirty (25 percent) in the "chronic" phase of the disease (between six months and one year of symptoms). Treatment consisted of fifteen sessions of ozone therapy given through rectal insufflation over a period of three weeks.

The results were impressive. The mental condition of all acute-phase patients participating in the study improved by the end of therapy, along with 91 percent of those in the ancient phase and 67 percent in the chronic phase. By the same token, the medical condition of all acute-phase patients improved, while improvement took place in 67 percent of those in the ancient phase and 47 percent in the chronic phase of the disease. Post-therapy tests revealed that the subjects' ability to participate in daily life situations improved among all of the acute-phase patients, 95 percent of the ancient phase, and 80 percent of the chronic phase.

The researchers concluded the following:

1. Ozone therapy, in the way and doses applied, produced significant improvement in the group of patients with cerebrovascular disease of the ischemic type, being more effective the faster the therapy begins.
2. The initial clinical state improved in 88 percent of the patients treated, obtaining better results in those in the acute phase.
3. In the multidimensional evaluation, all parameters measured as improved, especially daily life activities.
4. No adverse reactions were reported during the treatment.[31]

These results have led the physicians at the Salvador Allende Hospital to use ozone therapy on all patients who enter the facility for the treatment of ischemic cerebrovascular disease.

A more recent study on how ozone therapy can improve cerebral blood flow was undertaken in the Canary Islands by researchers at various departments at the Dr. Negrin Hospital, as well as by doctors from La Paterna Medical Center and the Canary Islands Institute for Cancer Research. Using five patients and two healthy volunteers, blood flow in twenty-eight arteries was measured before and after major autohemotherapy was administered three times over a three-week period. Scheduled medication was not modified. Blood flow was estimated using transcranial Doppler.

The researchers, impressed at the results, reported, "This preliminary Doppler study supports the clinical experience of achieving improvement by using ozone therapy in peripheral ischemic syndromes. Its potential use as a complementary treatment in cerebral blood flow perfusion syndromes merits further clinical evaluation."[32]

A later Spanish study found that ozone therapy can improve blood flow and metabolism in ischemia-related syndromes such as radiation-induced brain injury (RBI) or stroke. Clinical improvement was long-lasting and sustained.[33]

HYPERTENSION

In Russia, ozone therapy is considered a valuable method for treatment of hypertension or high blood pressure. Researchers at the Medical Academy at Nizhny Novgorod believe that "it corrects the decreased energy of cells, the main component of pathogenesis. No other available hypotensive preparations are known to have such properties."

Russian physicians suggest that ozone therapy can be used alone or in combination with other medications. As a monotherapy, they believe that ozone is efficient in patients at the initial stages of the disease (mild labile hypertension). In their clinical studies, positive results were obtained in 70 percent of treated patients.

Patients with more serious and chronic hypertension should receive ozone therapy along with hypotensive preparations. The researchers state: "According to our findings, conventional hypotensive preparations can be administered in lower doses when combined with ozone therapy. In combined treatment clinical manifestations of hypertensive disease, such as headaches, dizziness, heart pains—either disappeared within a shorter time period or abated."

As with treating patients with atherosclerosis, the three major treatment methods with ozone include intravenous infusions with 200 ml of ozonated saline, with an ozone concentration of 20 µg/kg of patient's weight (ozone concentration at the output from the generator); rectal insufflations with an ozone/oxygen mixture, with the ozone dose being 75µg/kg of patient's weight; and major autohemotherapy, with the ozone dose being 1 to 3 mg. Treatment with intravenous infusions or rectal insufflations involves eight to ten procedures: doctors begin with two or three daily procedures, while the remaining three or four procedures are done every second day. As blood pressure decreases, the number of procedures is diminished to two procedures a week and then one procedure a week. Major autohemotherapy is generally performed twice a week over three to four weeks.[34]

STROKE

Physicians have found that early intervention with ozone applications can help reduce the severity of symptoms for people who suffer a stroke. This is believed to be partly due to ozone's ability to increase the level of ATP to tissues, improve blood circulation, and aid in the release of oxygen to the body's cells. Ozone generators can be found in many hospital emergency rooms in Cuba, where they are primarily used to treat patients suffering from heart attack and stroke.

One of the few clinical studies of stroke patients and ozone therapy was carried out by Gerd Wasser, M.D., of the Wasser Clinic in Germany. He studied forty-five patients who had recently suffered from acute brain stroke. Although patients had already received primary treatment at the hospital, none had received the full course of traditional medical care.

Three different types of post-stroke syndrome were identified as follows:

Type 1: All functions (including fine motoric movement) are reestablished. Sensory failures are possible but not obvious at first glance.

Type 2: Patients did not restore fine motoric movement but were able to regain a basic level of motoric nerve transmission.

Type 3: Patients were confined to bed due to paralysis.

After a course of treatment with ozone therapy, the results were very encouraging. Forty of the forty-five patients moved into type 1, and five patients were classified in type 2. None of the patients remained paralyzed, and none of them died. This is far better than the average outcome for stroke patients, which normally includes a 30 percent death rate. Of the survivors, approximately 55 percent remained handicapped and 15 percent needed total care twenty-four hours a day.

In his presentation in 1995 at the Twelfth Ozone World Congress in Lille, France, Dr. Wasser recommended that ozone therapy be applied as soon as possible after the stroke occurs: "The total dosage should reach 3,000 micrograms of O_3. In the following days the same dosage will be given once a day. Edema-related paralysis disappeared in all cases within 10 minutes. Relapses are very rare and can receive the same treatment described above."[35]

Despite the tremendous promise that oxidative therapies offer to patients suffering from heart and circulatory disease, little research is being done to study ozone and hydrogen peroxide in North America. Even without the proven benefits of exercise and a plant-based diet, the therapeutic use of ozone and hydrogen peroxide appears to have a positive and lasting effect on a person's cardiovascular health.

Unfortunately, no studies have been sponsored by the American Heart Association, the National Institutes of Health, the Centers for Disease Control and Prevention, or any other major organization to scientifically evaluate oxidative therapies among large groups of people.

By the same token, no studies have been done to evaluate the preventive effects of regular ozone or hydrogen peroxide treatment among people who may be genetically predisposed to heart attack, or for individuals who are otherwise at risk for heart disease or stroke.

11
Cancer

One of the most controversial areas in oxidative therapy is the treatment of cancer. Many patients turn to therapeutic ozone and hydrogen peroxide as a last resort when conventional medical therapies have failed. In such cases, their cancer is often far too advanced for these therapies to work, which leads people to believe that the therapies are ineffective in treating cancer in general.

In addition, a small number of unscrupulous practitioners with minimal training (including some who are not licensed to practice medicine) offer ozone therapy as a "miracle" cancer cure to desperate patients for fees running into the tens or even the hundreds of thousands of dollars. These patients, who often travel to countries where oxygen therapies are totally unregulated, invariably return home sicker (and a lot poorer) than before. News reports documenting such patient abuse probably cause more harm to legitimate oxidative physicians—and the advancement of medical research in ozone and hydrogen peroxide—than any other factor.

CONTRIBUTORS TO CANCER

Cancer is generally believed to be caused by a variety of factors. In addition to genetics, these factors include behaviors such as tobacco use, diets high in meat and refined sugar, and low physical activity;

certain types of infections; chronic inflammation; age; hormones; immune suppression; and environmental exposures to radiation and different types of chemicals. The National Cancer Institute lists no fewer than twenty-five of the most common environmental carcinogens on their website.

Many cancerous tumors have been found to be hypoxic, meaning that they contain low levels of oxygen. Common sense would dictate, then, that if a tumor is deprived of oxygen, it would shrink. However, numerous studies—including one published in *Cancer Research*—have shown that tumor hypoxia, in which portions of the tumor have significantly low oxygen concentrations, is in fact linked with more aggressive tumor behavior and poorer prognosis. Rather than the tumor succumbing to the hypoxic condition, the lack of oxygen commonly created as a tumor outgrows its blood supply signals a tumor to grow and metastasize in search of new oxygen sources. This can cause a hypoxic tumor—such as in the bladder—to metastasize to the lungs.[1]

Another study by Dr. Yin Xu and his colleagues at the University of Georgia found that low oxygen levels in cells may be a primary cause of uncontrollable tumor growth in some cancers, including those of the breast, kidney, liver, lung, ovaries, pancreas, and stomach. The authors' findings run counter to widely accepted beliefs that genetic mutations are responsible for cancer growth and point to new and innovative ways to both prevent and treat certain types of cancers.[2]

Can oxygen therapies cure cancer? As we'll see in this chapter, clinical and laboratory studies show that therapeutic ozone and hydrogen peroxide can indeed play an important role in cancer therapy.

It was mentioned earlier that oxidative therapies have the ability to increase the activation of immunocompetent cells, stimulate the release of cytokines, upregulate the body's antioxidant system, and induce a mild activation of the immune system. Activating the patient's neuroendocrine system causes the patient to experience less pain and a greater sense of well-being. As a result, the patient's overall quality of life is enhanced. Although most practitioners will not make any promises that oxidative therapies will cure cancer, the more conservative leaders in the field recommend ozone or hydrogen peroxide as a complementary medical procedure[3] that can enhance the effectiveness of traditional cancer therapies and perhaps reduce the adverse side effects of surgery, radiation, and chemotherapy.

A LONG-HELD PROMISE

Physicians have treated cancer with hydrogen peroxide and ozone therapy for decades. The rationale behind the use of oxidative therapies to treat cancer is based on several important discoveries. The first discovery was made by Nobel Prize winner Dr. Otto Warburg, director of the Max Planck Institute for Cell Physiology in Berlin. He confirmed at a meeting of fellow Nobel laureates by the shores of Lake Constance, Germany, in 1966 that the key precondition for the development of cancer is a lack of oxygen at the cellular level.[4]

The second important factor was addressed in 1965 by another Nobel Prize winner, Dr. James D. Watson, the codiscoverer of the DNA double helix. He found that "among the most useful carcinogenic agents known at present are several viruses."[5] In other words, the development of cancer has a viral component that was not recognized before.

The third discovery, which was first reported by Dr. Joachim Varro of Germany in 1974, revealed a peroxide intolerance in tumor cells, suggesting that ozone and hydrogen peroxide may induce metabolic inhibition in certain types of cancerous growths.[6] This was not confirmed in an English-language publication until 1980, when an article by Dr. Frederick Sweet and his colleagues in the journal *Science* introduced laboratory evidence proving that ozone selectively inhibits the growth of cancer cells.[7]

It's important to note that Dr. Sweet's work examined the effect of ozone in tumor cell culture only. While ozone is a good cytotoxic (an element that is harmful to cancer cells) in these conditions, it has been much more difficult to translate these results in vivo. Although it has been done, physicians rarely administer a direct injection of ozone into a cancerous tumor.

One of the early mainstream physicians to offer tentative support for the use of oxidative therapies in treating cancer was Boguslaw Lipinski, M.D., of the Boston Cardiovascular Health Center and the Tufts University School of Medicine:

> Preliminary clinical studies indicate that oxidative therapy might produce desirable results in cancer treatment. . . . Exposure of patients' blood in vitro to ozone and subsequent injection is a medical procedure used for a successful treatment of cancer in one Swiss clinic [the famous Roka Clinic] since 1960. . . . Although these preliminary findings do not constitute proof in themselves, they may certainly encourage clinical researchers and practitioners to try this unorthodox but apparently promising modality.[8]

In the following pages, we will examine some of the laboratory and clinical evidence that lends support to the concept that ozone and hydrogen peroxide can assist in the treatment of cancer, either alone or as an adjunct to traditional or alternative cancer therapies.

HYDROGEN PEROXIDE STUDIES

Early cancer research at the Baylor University Medical Center in Texas began in the early 1960s with Dr. J. W. Finney and his associates. One of the first articles discussing their findings, published in the *Southern Medical Journal* in March 1962, spoke of the value of hydrogen peroxide as an adjunct to radiation therapy for treating cancer. "The Use of Hydrogen Peroxide as a Source of Oxygen in a Regional Intraarterial Infusion System" revealed that cancer cells become more sensitive to irradiation in the presence of increased oxygen tension produced by hydrogen peroxide. Phases 1 and 2 of the study involved laboratory animals. In phase 3 of the study, doses of hydrogen peroxide diluted in water were administered intra-arterially to patients suffering from a variety of carcinomas. The researchers noted increased regional oxygenation, which led them to believe that there is an "increased therapeutic ratio" in malignant tumors receiving radiation when oxygen levels of the affected area are increased with hydrogen peroxide.[9]

A related Baylor University cancer study (this time with large, inoperable abdominal tumors) was undertaken using intra-arterial hydrogen peroxide and irradiation. The researchers wanted to see if hydrogen peroxide could shrink the tumors and make them amenable to surgery. Two of the three patients in the study experienced a shrinkage of their tumors and underwent successful operations to remove them. One of the patients experienced no changes after four weeks and was sent home to die. However, to everyone's surprise, he began to improve over the next several months and the tumor began shrinking considerably. The doctors later removed the shrunken tumor with no complications. In their article in the journal *Cancer,* the researchers concluded:

> The resection of this tumor apparently was made possible by presurgical medium dose irradiation associated with regional oxygenation by the intra-arterial infusion of a solution of hydrogen peroxide into the abdominal aorta. The findings in 2 other patients with intra-abdominal tumors have been summarized in regard to the usefulness of intra-arterial hydrogen peroxide procedures. The findings justify further investigation in these areas.[10]

Another early study concerning the value of hydrogen peroxide as a complementary therapy for cancer was done at the Tottori University School of Medicine in Japan in 1966. Fifteen patients suffering from maxillary cancer (cancer of the nasal cavity and/or jaw) were given intra-arterial infusions of hydrogen peroxide daily for ten days followed by daily injection of mitomycin C (Mutamycin), an antibiotic showing anti-tumor activity. A control group of twenty-nine received the anticancer agent alone.

Operations were then done to remove and analyze the tumors. Of the fifteen cases treated with hydrogen peroxide and Mutamycin, eight showed almost a complete disappearance of the tumor, while six experienced a partial reduction. One had little change. The changes involved either an actual shrinking of the tumor or a softening of a hard tumor, so that it had, as described by the researchers (in a way that might be unique to Japanese doctors), the texture of tofu, or bean curd. By contrast, of the patients who received the anti-cancer drug alone, six experienced complete disappearance, twenty-one patients had partial reduction, and two showed no response.

In their summary, the researchers wrote: "Enhancement of the anti-cancer agent was observed. We have also proven clinically that the method [does not] cause danger in each individual patient."[11]

The anti-tumor effects of hydrogen peroxide were also studied by Dr. Carl F. Nathan and Dr. Zanvil A. Cohn at Rockefeller University in New York City. In their paper, published in the *Journal of Experimental Medicine* in 1979, they wrote, "Hydrogen peroxide contributes to the lysis [destruction] of tumor cells by macrophages [immune cells that devour pathogens and other intruders] and granulocytes [white blood cells that act as scavengers to combat infection] in vitro." (In a later in vivo experiment, they found that 8 mg of hydrogen peroxide was able to kill more than 90 percent of P338 lymphoma cells.)[12]

At the same time, Nathan and Cohn's research led them to conclude that hydrogen peroxide could exert a "direct anti-tumor effect in vivo and thereby prolong the survival of the host [the patient]." Like the Japanese, they added that "hydrogen peroxide can synergize in vivo with certain anti-tumor drugs already in use."[13]

The results of another study undertaken at the University of California at Irvine on the ability of hydrogen peroxide to kill cancer cells associated with Hodgkin's disease were published in the June 1989 issue of *Cancer*. Dr. Michael K. Samoszuk and his colleagues from the Department of Pathology took cell suspensions taken from twenty-three lymph nodes of living patients and subjected them to a low concentration of hydrogen peroxide. They found that a substantial killing of the infected cells took place after only 15 minutes of incubation. The researchers observed that "peroxidase in Hodgkin's disease sensitizes the tumor cells to killing by low levels of hydrogen peroxide" and concluded, "The significance of our observation is that it provides a rationale for investigating new therapeutic modalities designed specifically to deliver cytotoxic quantities of hydrogen peroxide to Hodgkin's disease."[14]

A study undertaken at the Carolinas Medical Center in Charlotte, North Carolina, investigated the efficiency of using hydrogen peroxide as an adjuvant therapy after extended local curettage (involving scraping away dangerous lesions) for benign cell tumors of bone. Cell cultures taken from the tumor tissue of six patients were cultured and treated with ordinary saline (as a control) or hydrogen peroxide for 2 minutes. The findings revealed that hydrogen peroxide is very effective in killing giant cell tumors of bone, leading the researchers to conclude, "The results support the theory of using a minimum concentration of hydrogen peroxide as a chemical adjuvant in the surgical treatment of giant cell tumors of bone."[15] Although this research was done on noncancerous tumors, similar results could perhaps be found with malignant tumors as well.

In 2001, a group of researchers from the Department of Life Sciences at Nottingham Trent University in England injected hydrogen peroxide solutions into solid tumors in mice and found that the solutions had the potential to cause tumor cell death without generating dangerous by-products. They were very impressed with the findings and concluded that hydrogen peroxide was a potent cytotoxic agent: "H_2O_2 can act as an anticancer drug with two distinct advantages over conventional therapeutic agents: [it] produce[s] minimal short- and long-term side effects and is relatively cheap and cost-effective."[16]

An unusual report on a study of breast cancer cells was published in the journal *Biomedical Sciences Instrumentation* in 2003. In this study, researchers at Jackson State University in Mississippi explored the combined effect of oxidative stress (with hydrogen peroxide) and *Nigella sativa* ("love-in-a-mist"), a medicinal herb from the Middle East, on breast cancer cells. Measurements of cell survival were conducted using standard cell culture techniques, which revealed that a combination of hydrogen peroxide, ethanol, and *Nigella sativa* could effectively inactivate the cancer cells. "In conclusion, *N. sativa* alone or in combination with oxidative stress were found to be effective in vitro in inactivating MCF-7 breast cancer cells, unveiling opportunities for promising results in the field of prevention and treatment of cancer."[17]

RESEARCH WITH OZONE

As in the hydrogen peroxide studies, the first cancer research in the United States concerning ozone therapy involved laboratory animals. One of the first preliminary American studies on the effects of ozone on mammary carcinomas was reported in the early 1980s by Dr. Migdalia Arnan and Lee E. DeVries at the Northern Dutchess Hospital in Rhinebeck, New York. Mice with mammary carcinomas were injected with a mixture of ozone and oxygen, while the mice in the control group were untreated. The tumors regressed in the mice receiving ozone. However, the dead tumor tissues were not removed, which was believed to present a burden on the tissue macrophages, suppressing the immune system of the ozonated mice. Nevertheless, the group of mice receiving ozone survived thirty to forty-eight days longer than the control mice.[18]

As mentioned earlier, the first report of the possible effectiveness of ozone as a cancer treatment for humans in a major scientific journal was given in the magazine *Science* in 1980 by Dr. Frederick Sweet and his associates at the Washington University School of Medicine in St. Louis, Missouri. Using in vitro studies, they found that the growth of human cancer cells from lung, breast, and uterine tumors was selectively inhibited by ozone given in a dose of 0.3 to 0.8 part per million in air over a period of eight days. Exposure to ozone at 0.8 part per million inhibited cancer cell growth by more than 90 percent and controlled cell growth to less than 50 percent. They also noted that there was no growth inhibition of normal cells, which they felt was due to the fact that "cancer cells are less able to compensate for the oxidative burden of ozone than normal cells."[19]

One of the first reports on the successful use of ozone therapy with actual patients was reported by German surgeon Joachim Varro at the Sixth World Congress on Ozone in 1983. Dr. Varro is considered one of the pioneers in the use of medical ozone to treat cancer, and his work has been admired around the world. Dr. Varro believed that cancer is not the result of an outside infection but has its source in the body itself:

> The malignant tumor is not an exogenous foreign body like a virus or bacteria, but rather a substance of the body proper, consisting of organic cells and behaving autonomously as a foreign body only because of misinformation in its growth impulses. It has removed itself from the orderly principles of the organism as a whole. Thus, the tumor is not actually the cause of metabolic chaos but should be seen as the end product of a misguided prior pathophysiological development.[20]

In his article, Dr. Varro did not provide statistical data. Since many of his patients came to his office as a last resort, many of them had undergone surgery, chemotherapy, and radiation. For those reasons, he believed that statistical evaluation would be difficult to document. However, he noted that ozone therapy had a marked effect among his patients. Patients experienced increased appetite, greater strength, higher rates of physical activity, and a reduction in pain. He offered his clinical evaluation of the patients who had undergone ozone-oxygen therapy:

1. Side effects and after effects of surgery and radiation can frequently be diminished and even completely eliminated; the same

applies to cytostatic consequences of chemotherapy [which prevents the growth and proliferation of cells].

2. The patients are free of metastasis and tumor relapses for remarkably long periods of time.

3. The survival time could be prolonged, far exceeding the usual dubious prognoses, even in cases of inoperability, radiation resistance, or chemotherapy non-tolerance, and with improved quality of life.

4. Most patients who had undergone the combination therapy *shortly* after surgery and radiation could return full time to their occupations.[21]

CURRENT THERAPIES

At the Hospital Santa Monica in Mexico, founded by Kurt W. Donsbach and believed to be the largest hospital providing holistic health care in the world, intravenous hydrogen peroxide is used extensively to treat cancer. Thousands of patients have come to the hospital as a last resort when traditional medical therapy has failed them, and many have been able to experience complete recovery. In his book *Wholistic Cancer Therapy*, Dr. Donsbach has the following to say about the therapeutic use of food-grade hydrogen peroxide:

1. Cancer cells are less virulent and may even be destroyed by the presence of a high oxygen environment.

2. Hydrogen peroxide given by transfusion and orally has the ability to increase the oxygen content of the blood stream which will increase the oxygen environment of the cancer cell.

3. Clinical evidence has overwhelmingly convinced me that the use of hydrogen peroxide is a valuable adjunct in the treatment of cancer.[22]

In addition to hydrogen peroxide, Dr. Donsbach utilizes vitamin therapy, mineral therapy, hyperthermia, and other natural modalities during the patient's course of treatment. When administering daily doses of intravenous hydrogen peroxide, he includes dimethyl sulfoxide (DMSO), a solvent used by physicians primarily to facilitate absorption of medicines through the skin. Dr. Donsbach found that DMSO helps mitigate the irritation that some patients experience with hydrogen peroxide. In addition, he believes DMSO to be a cancer treatment in its own right and also credits it with being able to retard the growth of bacteria, viruses, and fungi and reduce inflammation and swelling. He gives daily infusions of hydrogen peroxide and DMSO to every patient throughout his or her course of treatment at the hospital.

Dr. Donsbach and his associates also use medical ozone at the Hospital Santa Monica, though to a lesser extent than hydrogen peroxide. In his book *Oxygen-Peroxide-Ozone,* he wrote:

> Advances in ozone manufacture and technology have created a great interest on my part in using humidified ozone by rectal insufflation. The methodology allows repeated treatment during the day without invasive procedures such as required to give an intravenous infusion. The rectal tip is introduced and a thirty-second burst of humidified ozone is injected into the rectum, yielding about one-half liter. It is very painless and the reports I have seen indicate a higher concentration of oxygen can be achieved in the bloodstream by this method than injecting the ozone directly into the bloodstream. Our patients love it because there is almost always a feeling of well-being immediately after the treatment. We use this up to three times per day in critical patients. This treatment method is unique in that it avoids the intestinal cramps that injecting dry ozone into the rectum causes.[23]

I once asked Dr. Donsbach for statistics regarding the number of people cured of cancer at Hospital Santa Monica. He replied that statistics are an illusive factor, but added:

Approximately 70 percent of our patients are alive three years after their first visit to our facility. Some are cured, some are in remission and some are slowly dying. However, very few of these patients had more than months to live according to their doctors when they arrived. But what kind of statistics are these? We see a significant percentage of our patients become totally and completely cured as documented by medical diagnostic standards.[24]

Dr. Horst Kief has been using autohomologous immunotherapy (AHIT) extensively to treat a variety of cancers. During a surprise visit to his clinic in December 1993, I observed a woman receiving treatment for breast cancer, which had come back after traditional medical treatment had failed. Through the use of oral AHIT and AHIT injections applied around the infected part of the breast, the woman experienced a rapid remission. In an interview, Jon Greenberg, M.D., a former associate of Dr. Kief, reported that the long-term remission rate for cancer patients receiving AHIT at the Kief Clinic is 60 percent, with another 20 percent of patients experiencing improvement.[25]

In 1988 Dr. Kief studied thirty-one patients suffering from a variety of malignancies, including carcinomas, lymphomas, a sarcoma, and a kidney tumor. Most had received chemotherapy and radiation, without long-term success. AHIT therapy was given daily over a four-month period. The results showed that after four weeks of AHIT therapy, levels of gamma interferon increased by between 700 and 900 percent. Gamma interferon is a protein found when cells are exposed to viruses. Noninfected cells exposed to interferon are protected against viral infection. Overall, Kief observed dramatic subjective improvement in patients, including a decrease of pain in 70 percent and increases in vitality in 90 percent of the patients using AHIT.[26]

During my interview with Dr. Kief, one of the participants in this study, a sixty-two-year-old man, happened by the clinic for a routine examination. In 1988 he had been diagnosed with immunocytoma stage IVb, a particularly lethal cancer that involves the lymph nodes.

The oncologists who had treated him held out no hope for his recovery. After eleven months of AHIT, the patient experienced a complete remission that continued until the time I met him four years later.[27]

Since that time, Dr. Kief has refined his work with AHIT to include activated macrophages (AHIT-aM). Macrophages are white blood cells that help destroy bacteria, protozoa, and tumor cells; they also release substances that stimulate other cells of the immune system. Considered controversial in Germany, AHIT-aM has not been evaluated in double-blind studies and is viewed, even by Kief, as experimental.

As is the case with many oxidative physicians, many of Dr. Kief's patients come to him as a last resort after traditional medical therapy has failed them. Nevertheless, Kief's clinical findings merit serious study. From 2000 through 2002, Dr. Kief kept records on 108 patients who received a course of treatment in AHIT-aM. Of the total, 55 percent experienced either full remission (thirty-four patients) or partial remission (twenty-five patients). The best results took place with bronchial cancer (68 percent), prostate cancer (55 percent), ovarian cancer (57 percent), colon cancer (50 percent), and "other" cancers (85 percent), while the least favorable results were among women with breast cancer (27 percent).[28]

Dr. Bocci and other critics are often frustrated that randomized, double-blind studies have not been performed with AHIT therapy, preventing objective clinical evaluations. However, oncologists are often reluctant to objectively evaluate ozone (and AHIT) therapy and other nontraditional approaches to treating cancer. Double-blind studies are very time-consuming and expensive to carry out, and funding sources are nonexistent. Plus, as mentioned in the introduction, they often are not reliable.

OZONE AND HYDROGEN PEROXIDE: ADJUNCTS TO TRADITIONAL CANCER TREATMENT

Cuban, American, and European researchers have explored the use of ozone and hydrogen peroxide therapy as adjuncts to traditional cancer therapy since the mid-1990s. Physicians at a number of Cuban hospitals, working with scientists from the National Center for Scientific Research in Havana, undertook a study with seventy patients diagnosed with prostate cancer in 1997. All were treated with cobalt-60 therapy, but half of the patients also received rectal ozone insufflations six days per week, at a dose of 8 mg (40 mg/L and 200 ml) during the six weeks of radiotherapy.

Side effects (including radiodermatitis, cystitis, and proctitis) occurred in 84 percent of the patients treated with cobalt therapy alone, while such side effects occurred in only 52 percent of the ozone group—a significant difference. Prostatic specific antigen figures decreased to less than 10 mg/ml in 92 percent of patients treated with ozone and in 52 percent of the control group one month after completing treatment; clinical and humoral control of the disease was achieved in 88 percent of the ozone group and 80 percent of the controls after six months of treatment.[29]

Physicians at the Department of Obstetrics and Gynecology and at the Central Research Laboratory at the Medical Academy of Nizhny Novgorod in Russia observed fifty-five women who received adjuvant chemotherapy for ovarian cancer. Thirty-five underwent rectal insufflation with ozone therapy. The results showed that ozone therapy, administered on days when chemotherapy was not given, brought about marked improvement in the patients' overall well-being, including better sleep, increased appetite, and decrease in nausea and vomiting. It also produced an immunomodulating effect, mainly on humoral immunity, which refers to the production of antibodies. Ozone also helped decrease lipid peroxidation, thus improving the activity of the body's antioxidant defense system.[30]

Another Russian study focused on the blood of sixty-eight patients with colorectal cancer both before and after surgery. Researchers found that after surgery, activity of adenosine triphosphatase (ATPase) was reduced, leading to postoperative erosive-ulcerous lesions of the gastric tunica. They found that if ozone therapy is administered before surgery, ATPase activity remains normal after surgery.[31]

A recent Spanish report utilized ozone therapy for progressive radiation-induced hematuria (presence of blood in the urine). Ozonated water was inserted into the bladder of the patient with a catheter; sessions took place three times a week over several weeks for 30 minutes per treatment. The hematuria was successfully controlled, leading the researchers to recommend ozone therapy to counter this radiation-induced side effect.[32]

Radiation-Induced Proctitis

Dr. Bernardino Clavo and eleven associates from a variety of hospitals and research institutes in Spain and Italy undertook a multiyear study to see if ozone could help relieve persistent radiation-induced proctitis (inflammation of the rectum and anus) and rectal bleeding among cancer patients. Their results were published in *Evidence-Based Complementary and Alternative Medicine* in 2015.

Twelve adult males between the ages of sixty-four and seventy-seven were chosen for this study. All had received radiation for prostate cancer and experienced persistent or severe rectal bleeding after treatment. Their iatrogenic symptoms did not respond to conventional medical therapy. Ten patients (83 percent) were found to have grade 3 or grade 4 toxicity as measured by the CTCAE (Common Terminology Criteria for Adverse Events) scale.

Patients received ozone therapy via rectal insufflations and/or topical application of ozonated oil, with an average treatment of thirty-eight sessions over thirteen months. The median follow-up time after ozone therapy was 104 months.

Following ozone therapy, the median grade of toxicity improved from 3 to 1 and the number of endoscopy treatments fell from thirty-seven to four after ozone treatment. After the follow-up period, all patients achieved grade 0 or grade 1 toxicity status.

In addition to the laboratory findings, researchers also explored quality-of-life changes among the patients. At the end of treatment, the perception recorded by the patients in the study group was

100 percent improvement in seven patients (58 percent of the total), up to 75 percent improvement in three patients (25 percent of the total), and an improvement of around 50 percent for the other two patients. The researchers found that ozone therapy was well tolerated and no adverse effects were noted, except for soft and temporary flatulence for several hours after each ozone session.

The researchers concluded:

> Our results show a significant, and clinically relevant, effect of ozone therapy in the management of radiation-induced rectal bleeding. Following ozone therapy, the requirements for blood transfusions were significantly decreased as was the need for endoscopic procedures. The grades of toxicity (according to the CTCAE scale) were also reduced. These effects were maintained over the course of protracted follow-up, and no adverse impact on survival was noted. We believe the local application of ozone therapy can be useful as adjuvant treatment in managing radiation proctitis and, as such, merits further evaluation in randomized clinical trials.[33]

Actinic Keratosis

Actinic keratoses (AKs) are a precancerous condition of the skin. Also known as *solar keratoses,* AKs are scaly, crusty lesions caused by damage from the sun's ultraviolet (UV) rays. They typically appear on sun-exposed areas of the body such as the face, bald scalp, lips, and back of the hands. They are often pink or red in color, elevated, and rough in texture and resemble warts. If left untreated, about 10 percent can develop into squamous cell skin cancer (SCC).

A group of researchers from the Center for Molecular Biology and Biotechnology at Florida Atlantic University undertook a study to evaluate increased reactive oxygen species (ROS) in the mechanism of cancer killing by sulindac in the presence of an oxidizing agent. ROS are chemically reactive molecules containing oxygen, and they have the ability to kill cancer cells. Sulindac is a prescription NSAID that also appears to have the ability to reduce the growth of polyps and precancerous lesions in the colon as well as other anti-cancer properties. The researchers chose a combination of gels containing sulindac and hydrogen peroxide in the treatment of patients with AKs.

Nine patients with actinic keratosis were recruited for the three-week-long clinical study, and five completed it. The researchers performed cell culture studies using a skin SCC cell line and normal human epidermal keratinocytes. A *keratinocyte* is the predominant cell type in the epidermis, the outermost layer of the skin, constituting 90 percent of the cells found there. After treatment with sulindac and hydrogen peroxide gel, they measured cell viability and intracellular ROS levels.

They found that in SCC cells, a combination of sulindac and hydrogen peroxide gel led to between 400 percent and 500 percent increases in intracellular ROS, which resulted in significant cell death. In sharp contrast, normal keratinocytes did not show increases in ROS levels and were not killed. A total of ten AKs that were treated, and six had a measurable reduction in size or were no longer visible. Skin biopsies at the end of treatment showed that there was no residual AK involvement on five of the six histopathology specimens.

The researchers concluded that increased levels of ROS appear to be important in the selective killing of cancer cells in the presence of sulindac and hydrogen peroxide. They added, "Further studies are necessary to define the role of the combination of sulindac and oxidizing agent therapy in patients with AKs and skin cancer."[34]

Like the two studies cited in the beginning of this chapter, research by Velio Bocci and colleagues at the University of Siena in Italy suggests that in contrast to normal tissues, cancerous tumors tend to thrive in hypoxic—or oxygen-starved—environments. Based on evaluating numerous studies of patients with severe circulation disorders, they found that ozone therapy increases oxygen delivery to hypoxic tissues. While Dr. Bocci and his colleagues didn't find that ozone therapy permanently restores normoxia to the tumors of cancer patients, they believed that it could help control tumor progression: "We postulate that a prolonged cycle of ozonated autohemotherapy may correct tumor hypoxia, lead to less aggressive tumor behavior, and represent a valid adjuvant during or after chemo or radiotherapy. Moreover, it may re-equilibrate the chronic oxidative stress and reduce fatigue."[35]

While many of the clinicians cited above have reported good results with cancer patients, others have not. After reviewing this chapter, Dr. Bocci offered his candid evaluation on the ability of ozone to treat cancer patients who were seriously ill:

> However, after performing intensive ozonated autohemotherapy plus hydrogen IV infusions plus minor AHT [autohemotherapy] in advanced cancer patients with extensive metastasis in spite of 2–3 years of chemotherapy, although there was a transient improvement of the quality of life, partly due to ozone and some to a placebo effect, the tumors progressed and patients did not recover. Thus, my clinical experience does suggest that seriously ill patients do not respond to ozone therapy. This is the plain and hard truth but, in contrast to physicians mentioned above, I do not want to raise unjustified hopes and attract desperate patients in a charity clinic where my work was done without a fee.

Yet he added:

> I do not want to dismiss entirely the possible value of ozone and bio-oxidative therapies but, whenever possible, we should combine our therapies with chemo or radiotherapy from the beginning, possibly even before the surgical removal of the bulk of the tumor. In this case, the results may turn out to be different, but oncologists have never allowed me to do this study.[36]

The *Madrid Declaration on Ozone Therapy* (2015) takes a conservative view of the potential of ozone therapy to cure cancer, stating that "ozone therapy has so far not been able to show a therapeutic effect on cancer," although it suggests that ozone treatment can be effective as an adjuvant to conventional cancer treatment, especially in cases of cancer metastasis or to reduce side effects of chemotherapy or radiation. It also recommends that ozone therapy may be useful in treating cancer-related fatigue.[37]

TOWARD THE FUTURE

Ongoing research points to the suitability of medical ozone and hydrogen peroxide for cancer treatment. An article published in the British magazine *New Scientist* discussed findings presented at an April 1994 meeting of the American Association of Cancer Researchers in San Francisco that oxygen can be an important part of tumor treatment. It appears that tumors have regions that are starved of oxygen, which results when blood vessels grow haphazardly inside a developing cancer. The article reported that Dr. Beverly Teicher, of the prestigious Dana-Farber Cancer Institute in Boston, told the meeting that this lack of oxygen was hampering treatment by protecting the tumor against conventional therapies such as radiation and chemotherapy. By increasing the oxygen levels in the tumor, conventional therapy can be made more successful. Although the methods highlighted in the meetings included a synthetic blood substitute, ozone and hydrogen peroxide have similar applications.

The article added that clinical trials on patients with superficial tumors—such as melanomas—are promising, and it mentioned that other cancer therapies have been designed at Stanford University to exploit the hypoxia using anti-cancer drugs designed to work in almost anaerobic conditions. These findings appear to confirm both Dr. Warburg's conclusions and the early Baylor University studies that link cancerous tumors to low oxygen levels, as well as the ability of oxidative therapies to destroy tumors by increasing oxygen tension in malignant cells.[38]

In chapter 5 we introduced the work of Dr. Siegfried Schulz and his colleagues at the Philipps-Universität of Marburg, Germany, who used peritoneal ozone to treat cancer in rabbits. Schulz and colleagues' pilot study was reported at the Fourth International Symposia on Ozone Applications in Havana, Cuba, in 2004. The researchers infected the rabbits with a virus-induced squamous cell carcinoma, a highly malignant form of cancer. While 100 percent of infected rabbits normally die within one hundred days of infection, half of those treated with ozone were tumor-free for more than five hundred days. The researchers wrote, "Exogenously applied ozone (O_3 /O_2 pneumoperitoneum) exhibits a strong anticarcinogenic and antimetastasising effect on primary tumor cell inoculations (VX2 tumor cells), VX2 tumor and on the lymphogenic metastatic spread in rabbits."[39]

It has been reported that Dr. Schulz has developed a special medical device that delivers ozone through the peritoneum. In addition, Dr. Schulz and his colleagues are presently exploring cancer protocols for treatment of malignant tumors in human subjects, mostly in Germany and Brazil. Many feel that Schulz's method has tremendous potential for cancer treatment in the future.

It is hoped that additional clinical studies can be made with cancer patients treated by ozone and hydrogen peroxide, but that will probably not happen. Given the life-threatening nature of cancer itself, few people will agree to undergo a double-blind study in which they may have to discontinue another therapy that may be keeping them alive. In addition, the value of oxidative therapies is rarely witnessed in patients who have never received other cancer treatments, since most patients seek out therapy with ozone or hydrogen peroxide after chemotherapy, radiation, and surgery have failed them.

Despite these considerations, there is growing clinical and laboratory evidence that these therapies are of value, especially when used as an adjunct to traditional cancer therapies. Tens of thousands of European patients are becoming cancer-free thanks to ozone therapy, while hundreds of Americans are beginning to appreciate the value of hydrogen peroxide and ozone, either alone or combined with other therapies.

Many of the well-known European health spas use ozone as a routine spa treatment for guests (which may be compared to the regular tune-ups we give our cars), and a number of European physicians who treat patients with ozone also use it on themselves, even if they are not sick. These examples highlight the potential value of ozone and hydrogen peroxide as preventive therapies for cancer and many other diseases. An interesting project would be to study two groups of healthy people who may be genetically predisposed to cancer. One group could undergo oxidative therapy for several years, and any cancer cases would be documented. The results could be enlightening and could form the basis for preventive cancer protocols for years to come.

Unfortunately, the main problem in undertaking such research is a lack of money. Almost all the medical research that is taking place in industrialized nations is financed either directly or indirectly by pharmaceutical companies. In a country like the United States, representatives of the drug companies sit on Food and Drug Administration committees that decide what is to be studied. Since there is no financial incentive to study the effectiveness of ozone or hydrogen peroxide—which are both extremely cheap and cannot be patented—studies on their effectiveness as preventive therapies will probably never be done.

12
HIV/AIDS

Despite the global threats of SARS (severe acute respiratory syndrome), bird flu, and Ebola virus, AIDS (acquired immunodeficiency syndrome) is perhaps the most feared disease on the planet. Often fatal, especially in developing countries, it slowly destroys the immune system until the individual is vulnerable to a wide variety of diseases that rarely affect noninfected persons. These diseases, such as *Pneumocystis jiroveci* pneumonia and Kaposi sarcoma, may affect the brain, lungs, eyes, or other organs. Persons with AIDS also can experience debilitating weight loss, diarrhea, weakness, and depression.

AIDS has been the most controversial disease of our time. Because it first affected primarily homosexuals, bisexuals, and intravenous drug users in the United States, critics charge that society's negative feelings toward these groups led the government to be slow to respond to the growing epidemic. Today infection is greatest among intravenous drug users in North America, followed by those who became infected through heterosexual transmission and homosexual transmission. There is also a great deal of controversy surrounding the methods used to treat persons who are infected with the virus believed to cause AIDS—HIV (human immunodeficiency virus)—and those who reveal one or more symptoms of the disease.

AIDS has given birth to an entire "industry" involving physicians, nurses, hospitals, pharmaceutical companies, medical equipment manufacturers, government agencies, insurance companies, alternative therapists, testing laboratories, AIDS counselors, support groups, information networks, writers, publishers, researchers, educators, and magazines. Billions of dollars are involved in AIDS research, treatment, care, prevention, and education.

Physicians, scientists, and laypeople advocating the use of ozone and hydrogen peroxide can be included in this group. Some are motivated by altruism and the desire to serve humanity; others are primarily interested in money. For many providers of goods and services to AIDS patients, this epidemic has become an economic windfall of gigantic proportions.

By 2006 more than one hundred approved or experimental drugs for HIV-related problems were used in the United States. These included protease inhibitors (PIs), which prevent T cells that have been infected with HIV from producing new copies of the virus, as well as nucleoside/ nucleotide reverse transcriptase inhibitors (NRTIs), non-nucleoside reverse transcriptase inhibitors (NNRTIs), and entry inhibitors, all of which prevent healthy T cells in the body from becoming infected with HIV. In addition, a wide range of medications have been developed to help control opportunistic diseases associated with HIV, including bacterial infections, malignancies (cancer), viral infections, fungal infections, protozoal infections, neurological conditions, sores, low platelet counts, and wasting syndrome.

Many of these new medications have brought about suppression of symptoms, longer life, improved quality of life, and hope to millions of people who have been infected with HIV in countries where they are able to afford them. However, like all medications, those for treating HIV have side effects. Depending on the drug, they can include nausea, vomiting, rash, diarrhea, stomach pain, loss of appetite, pain in the arms and legs, anemia, muscle wasting, and tingling, pain, or numbness in the hands and feet (peripheral neuropathy). In rare cases liver and pancreatic damage can result from taking such medications. Another problem is that some of these drugs lose their effectiveness over time, so other medications are constantly being developed.

The total cost of these medications easily runs into the tens of billions of dollars each year. For example, a recommended "cocktail" of two protease inhibitors (six 400 mg tablets of Crixivan and two 100 mg tablets of Norvir) costs approximately $33 a day (more than $12,000 a year) per patient, even if no other medications are used. Some individual drugs, like Fuzeon (marketed by Hoffman-La Roche), carry an annual price tag of $20,000 a year or more. In addition to the pharmaceutical companies themselves, many physicians, hospitals, and insurance companies involved with AIDS have discovered that this disease is a big source of income and profit. For this reason, the quest to find inexpensive therapies and modalities to treat the disease has never been a high priority.

Since the late 1990s, several developing countries—such as India and Brazil—have begun developing their own medicines to combat HIV, often using the patented formulas of the pharmaceutical companies. As a result, they have been able to make the drugs available to patients at less than one-tenth the cost of patented drugs sold in developed countries like the United States. Yet even with these lower costs, the Joint United National Programme on HIV/AIDS estimated that $12.3 billion would be needed for treatment and care alone for patients living in low- and middle-income countries between 2006 and 2008.[1]

This has led people infected with the virus to explore other avenues of treatment, often using a combination of traditional and nontraditional approaches, including nontoxic therapies like acupuncture, acupressure, Chinese and/or Western herbs, ayurvedic medicine (an ancient Indian healing tradition that stresses diet and herbal medicines), homeopathy, chiropractic, ultraviolet blood irradiation (UBI) therapy, and nutritional therapy.

Oxidative therapies—especially when combined with either traditional therapies or other natural methods—make up one of these approaches. The potential of ozone and hydrogen peroxide for helping people with HIV and AIDS is enormous, because laboratory evidence has shown that ozone and hydrogen peroxide can inhibit (if not kill) the virus believed to cause AIDS. This result is deceiving because ozone can inactivate HIV only in a saline solution in vitro. How does this happen?

Figure 12.1 depicts a chemical model of a virus that is about to infect a cell. It also shows how ozone can affect the process of infection. The virus is encapsulated in an envelope made of lipids (fats or fat-like substances). Tiny bulbs on the virus spikes are known as *receptors*. It is through these receptors that a virus can connect with, and eventually infect, other cells.

Figure 12.1. Chemical model of a virus and its encounter with ozone. (From Siegfried Rilling and Renate Viebahn, *The Use of Ozone in Medicine* [Heidelberg: Haug Publishers, 1987], 43. Reprinted courtesy of Dr. Siegfried Rilling and Haug Publishers.)

With the application of ozone or hydrogen peroxide, several events rapidly take place. The virus spikes are inactivated because the addition of ozone to the blood changes the structure of the receptor. Although still alive, the virus cannot join with the cell. At the same time, the ozone oxidizes the virus's outer envelope.[2] Without this envelope, it cannot survive.

In addition to the effects of hydrogen peroxide introduced from outside the body, the threatened cell naturally defends itself by producing its own hydrogen peroxide. In some cases, especially when the cell is unhealthy to begin with, the hydrogen peroxide produced by the cell causes it to "burst" before reproduction of the virus can take place. In other cases the peroxides introduced by added ozone or hydrogen peroxide act synergistically with the hydrogen peroxide inside the cell, destroying any virus that has penetrated it.[3] Stated more simply, if the cell is unhealthy to begin with, it is destroyed by a hydrogen peroxide burst. If it is strong, it kills off the virus and becomes even stronger than before due to the increased oxygenation brought about by added ozone or hydrogen peroxide. As a result, the virus is either inhibited or destroyed.

Another possible benefit of ozone therapy for people with HIV is its ability to stimulate the production of superoxide dismutase, a vital enzyme that catalyzes the conversion of two molecules of superoxide into one molecule of oxygen and one molecule of hydrogen peroxide. According to a report in *American Medical News,* researchers at the Webb-Waring Institute in Denver, Colorado, discovered that HIV inhibits the body's natural production of superoxide dismutase. Indeed, HIV, like many other viruses, induces a chronic oxidative stress that aggravates the disease. The news release added that researchers are testing human cell cultures to determine whether a drug can inhibit HIV's ability to suppress the enzyme. They believe that if they are able to safeguard the enzyme's levels in cells, the time during which HIV stays inactive could be prolonged. This finding points to the value of ozone therapy in helping prevent HIV-related symptoms from manifesting.[4]

As immunomodulators, ozone and hydrogen peroxide can also

strengthen a compromised immune system. They can help guard against opportunistic infections and enable persons suffering from the disease to lead longer, more active, and more productive lives. While oxidative therapies should not be considered a cure for AIDS, they may open the door to long-term remission, especially when used in synergistic combination with other immune-strengthening therapies. Investigations are now taking place to delineate such combinations, including ozone and/or hydrogen peroxide and oral alpha interferon, staph vaccine, lentinan (shiitake mushroom extract), and Chinese herbs. Readers interested in updates regarding these combinations may contact an organization called Keep Hope Alive (see the list of organizations in appendix 2).

ONE CAUSE?

Although few people disagree that AIDS destroys the body's immune system, many researchers, physicians, and patients have taken issue with the "one cause" theory for AIDS and the established approaches for treatment. One approach states that the person is *already* immunosuppressed and that the HIV virus, if it is a factor at all, is only taking advantage of a previously compromised immune system rather than being the cause of it.

Michael Ellner, from the former New York alternative AIDS organization HEAL (Health Education AIDS Liaison), regarded "AIDS as a condition of toxicity rather than a viral disease; it is a disturbance of immune function caused by a lifetime of toxins."[5] His view was also proposed to me during a 1994 interview with Dr. Juliane Sacher of Frankfurt, Germany, who had one of the largest medical practices treating AIDS patients with ozone in Germany. She placed special emphasis on the combined effects of air pollution (especially in the large cities), the growing number of pesticides in our food supply, the widespread use of antibiotics and other immune-suppressing drugs, recreational drug use such as "poppers" (isobutyl nitrite, butyl nitrite, and amyl nitrite), eating heavily processed and devitalized foods, and a variety of vitamin and mineral deficiencies that occur as a result. For this reason, she believed that a greater emphasis should be placed on building up the person's immune system while assisting the patient to become (and remain) as free of toxins as possible.[6] However, some researchers, like Dr. Bocci, believe that to dismiss the relevance of the virus is untenable, although other immunosuppressive factors can accelerate the progression of the disease.[7]

Although I cite laboratory evidence that ozone can inactivate the human immunodeficiency virus (and that some people who once tested HIV-positive revert to HIV-negative), I reiterate that neither ozone, hyperbaric oxygen, nor hydrogen peroxide is a cure for AIDS. However, if correctly applied, they can play an important role in a holistic approach to treatment. This perspective was succinctly expressed in a communication from Frank Shallenberger, M.D., H.M.D., of Nevada, who was among the first practitioners to treat HIV patients with ozone and other natural therapies:

1. Ozone therapy does *not* cure AIDS. [It] never has and probably never will.
2. AIDS has a multifaceted causation and is *not* an infectious disease. Therapy for AIDS will *never* work if it is only aimed at anti-infectious protocol.
3. Ozone therapy works in AIDS by acting as an immune system modulator. In this capacity, it is very effective, safe, inexpensive, and readily available.
4. Proper therapy for AIDS will be directed at:
   - Early intervention (i.e., CD4 count >300)
   - Ozone plus other synergistic immune-augmented therapy
   - Intestinal cleansing, which is paramount due to the immunosuppressive aspect of parasites[8]

In the following pages, we will explore the laboratory and clinical findings related to HIV, plus the ways in which ozone and hydrogen peroxide are being used by patients today.

IN VITRO STUDIES

In vitro studies to evaluate the ability of ozone to kill HIV in the test tube have been undertaken by eminent scientists in the United States, Russia, and Canada. The first researchers in the world to prove that ozone can inactivate HIV were the late Michael T. F. Carpendale, M.D. (chief of medicine and research services at the Veterans Administration Hospital in San Francisco and professor at the University of California School of Medicine, San Francisco), and his associate, Dr. Joel K. Freeberg of the Veterans Administration Hospital. They first presented their findings at the Fourth International Conference of AIDS in Stockholm, Sweden, and later published their report in the peer-reviewed journal *Antiviral Research*. Carpendale and Freeberg showed that HIV could be 99 percent inactivated with only 0.5 µg ozone/ml of human serum, and completely inactivated by ozone concentrations of 4 µg/ml of human serum. Those concentrations of ozone did not harm healthy cells.[9]

Another in vitro study, supported in part by the U.S. Public Health Service and Medizone International, a manufacturer of a patented medical ozone delivery system, was reported in the October 1, 1991, issue of the medical journal *Blood*. Using ozone generated from medical-grade oxygen and delivered into a cultured cell medium of HIV-1, a team of four scientists from the State University of New York Health Science Center in Syracuse, the Brooklyn Hospital, and Merck Pharmaceutical found that ozone deactivated the virus completely, yet without causing significant biological damage to noninfected cells. In evaluating their findings with HIV, the researchers concluded, "The data indicate that the antiviral effects of ozone include viral particle disruption, reverse transcriptase inactivation, and/or a perturbation of the ability of the virus to bind its receptor to target cells."[10]

In Russia, scientists at the Institute of Virology in Moscow also used a concentration of 4 µg ozone/ml on an infected culture containing HIV. Within minutes, the cells of the virus decomposed and died. The researchers noted that "complete deactivation of [the] extra cell virus is achieved by putting gaseous ozone through [the] virus-containing [liquid]."[11] This will not happen in vivo.

In chapter 4, brief reference was made to a major study in Canada coordinated by the surgeon general of the Canadian Armed Forces to determine the ability of ozone to kill HIV, hepatitis, and herpes viruses in blood used for transfusion. After a three-minute ozonation of serum spiked with one million HIV-1 particles per milliliter, a 100 percent deactivation of the virus (in vitro) was achieved.[12] Referring to this study during his interview in the video documentary *Ozone and the Politics of Medicine*, Captain Michael E. Shannon, a scientist and medical doctor with the Canadian Department of National Defence, said: "We are dealing not with concentrations that are toxic to the human, but are in fact concentrations of ozone that have been used in clinics in Germany for the last thirty years with thousands of patients without any evidence of any harm."[13]

Despite the importance of the results (which would indicate that simple ozonation of the blood supply would render it free of HIV, as well as herpes, hepatitis, and other viruses), these Canadian findings received little notice in the North American press.

CLINICAL EXPERIENCE

Germany

Dr. Horst Kief, who is perhaps best known for his work with patients suffering from cancer and neurodermatitis, as well as the development of autohomologous immunotherapy (AHIT), is believed to have been the first physician in the world to treat AIDS patients with hyperbaric ozone "blood washings" in the early 1980s. His standard AIDS protocol was a session of autohemotherapy once a week for three months, to be repeated if necessary.

In a monograph published in the German medical journal *Erfahrungsheilkunde* in July 1988, Dr. Kief recalled that the patients experienced a near-complete alleviation of various AIDS-related symptoms, including thrush and oral hairy leukoplakia. In addition, their

T4-cell count increased dramatically, as did the T4:T8 ratio over a time period of sixty-five days.[14] In an interview shown in *Ozone and the Politics of Medicine,* Dr. Kief said that a seven-year follow-up of his first patients found them alive, working, and "doing very, very well."[15]

However, the first documented cases of using ozone to treat AIDS were reported by German physician Alexander Pruess in 1986. In his work with four patients, Dr. Pruess used ozone in combination with Suramin (a reverse transcriptase inhibitor), immunomodulation therapy, vitamin and mineral supplementation, and the hygienation (cleansing) of intestinal flora (bacteria present in the intestines). He wrote the following about his decision to use ozone: "As it is well-known that the actual disease(s) occurring through AIDS consists of a combination of viral, fungal and bacteriological infections, I searched for a substance which is virucidal, fungicidal and bactericidal at the same time. Ozone was here the obvious choice."[16]

Dr. Pruess noted immediate improvement in all four patients, including the elimination of HIV-related problems like skin diseases, fungal infections, gastrointestinal problems, and low energy. More than a year after treatment, all subjects were considered clinically healthy.

In a monograph published in 1993, Dr. Kief wrote about a study comparing thirty patients from the Kief Clinic who were given ozone in the form of AHIT and twenty patients from the University of Frankfurt School of Medicine who received conventional treatment, including AZT (azidothymidine). Dr. Kief's patients were observed for 251 days while the Frankfurt patients were observed for 363. T4:T8 ratios rose from 0.324 to 0.352 among Kief's patients, while they fell from 0.293 to 0.223 among the Frankfurt patients.

In a related study of twenty-seven AIDS patients receiving AHIT, the percentage surviving after eighteen months was 80 percent, and the percentage surviving after 45 months was 70 percent. This represented a much higher percentage than patients receiving conventional medical therapy anywhere.[17]

While these figures were encouraging, I learned that Dr. Kief is no longer using AHIT to treat people with AIDS. In 1992 German health authorities ordered him to create and maintain a separate (and highly secure) laboratory to make AHIT for his HIV and AIDS patients. Since the cost to build and secure a new facility was considered prohibitively expensive, Dr. Kief decided to stop using AHIT, and his HIV/AIDS practice became confined to treating patients with major autohemotherapy.

United States

In the United States, pilot studies were developed by Dr. Carpendale and Dr. John Griffiss of the Department of Laboratory Medicine at the University of California School of Medicine in San Francisco to find out if there is a role for medical ozone in the treatment of HIV and associated infections.

The study focused on two asymptomatic persons infected with HIV, one (known as "Patient G") who began with a T-cell count of 309, and one ("Patient I") who began with a T-cell count of 907. The treatment protocol consisted of doses of ozone and oxygen given via rectal insufflation daily for twenty-one days, once every three days for sixteen weeks, and once weekly for fifteen weeks, for a total of seventy-three treatments over a period of thirty-four to thirty-six weeks. For the next two years, the subjects treated themselves with a three-week "booster dose," which was repeated from time to time, as seen in figure 12.2 on page 171.

The researchers reported that T-cell levels remained acceptable (i.e., over 430) over the next six years, and both individuals "remained in the best of health, with increased feeling of well-being and energy, while on ozone therapy and with no infections and no adverse symptoms of malaise for the first five years." By that time, Patient I, who began the study with a higher T-cell level, not only attained a T-cell count of 1,185 but later tested HIV-negative. However, three months into the sixth year, Patient G died suddenly from lobar pneumonia (not the AIDS-related *Pneumocystis jiroveci* pneumonia) after getting soaked in a storm while recuperating from the flu. When he died, Patient G was still HIV-positive, yet he had maintained a T-cell count between 500 and 700.

Figure 12.2. Absolute CD4 ("T") cell count in HIV+ patients treated with ozone plotted against time. (From Michael T. Carpendale, M.D., and John Griffiss, M.D., "Is There a Role for Medical Ozone in the Treatment of HIV and Associated Infections?" in *Ozone in Medicine: Proceedings of the Eleventh Ozone World Congress*, Stamford, Conn., International Ozone Association, Pan American Committee, 1993, M–1–39, 40.)

In their report, which was published in *Ozone in Medicine: Proceedings of the Eleventh Ozone World Congress,* the researchers concluded:

> These normalizing results support the hypothesis that ozone may be effective in suppressing and possibly eliminating HIV, especially in the stages of the disease when the patient is asymptomatic and has a CD4 cell count in the normal range. It also indicates the potential for self treatment [via rectal insufflation] for long term prophylaxis, treatment or care.[18]

In a related study, which was published in the *Journal of Clinical Gastroenterology,* Dr. Carpendale and his associates gave five AIDS patients suffering from intractable diarrhea daily rectal insufflations of ozone (at doses from 2.7 to 30 mg) for twenty-one to twenty-eight days. By the end of the study, three of the four patients were completely relieved of their symptoms, while one patient, whose diarrhea was the result of the parasite *Cryptosporidium,* experienced no change. Relief from secondary infections including herpes simplex, folliculitis, and sycosis barbae was also reported. Patients experienced less toxicity, less discomfort, and more energy than they had before being treated with ozone. No adverse side effects were reported.[19]

Dr. Carpendale was so encouraged by the results of these studies that he attempted to secure government funding for additional ozone studies involving many more people. He met with no success.

The results of another pilot study with ozone were presented at the Fourth International Bio-Oxidative Medicine Conference in April 1993 by Dr. Frank Shallenberger. He administered intravenous ozone over a period of fourteen days to five randomly selected men diagnosed with AIDS. The total daily dose was calculated to be 0.15 μg ozone/kg of body weight. On the first day, one-quarter the daily dose was given; on the second, one-half; and on the third, three-quarters. From the fourth to the fourteenth day, the full dose was administered. Patients were carefully monitored and evaluated before and after each treatment. During the period after therapy, no other therapies were given, except for one patient who began taking ddI (didanosine) after the fourth month.

Before the ozone treatments began, each patient participated in a holistic protocol including a whole-food nutritional program, meditation and deep breathing, lymphatic drainage massage, nutritional supplements, safer sex practices, and regular exercise.

Although Dr. Shallenberger considered the sample too small to be statistically significant, the results included at least a six-month period of overall survival, an immediate increase in the number of T cells, relief of symptoms from opportunistic infections among most patients, and higher energy levels overall. Dr. Shallenberger's clinical observations follow:

1. S.W. (34 years old): Diffuse cutaneous Kaposi sarcoma of two-year duration went into clinical remission for six months before the lesions returned. Otherwise continues to be in good health.

2. S.S. (27 years old): Chronic diarrhea (cryptosporidium), chronic fatigue, and weight loss >20%. All symptoms disappeared within two months, and the patient remains healthy one year later. CD4 count remains at 7.

3. R.J. (34 years old): Oral thrush, fatigue, and mild lymphadenopathy [swollen lymph nodes]. Thrush disappeared for six months. Fatigue is gone. Lymphadenopathy has not progressed, and the patient remains in good health one year later.

4. T.B. (32 years old): Hairy leukoplakia and mild lymphadenopathy. Neither of these symptoms changed. He remains in otherwise good health one year later.

5. M.P. (41 years old): Neuro-leukodystrophy. Needs assistance to walk, has urinary incontinence and impotence. Within one week of treatment his incontinence and gait improved considerably. One month later, he was walking easily without assistance and had no incontinence. MRI remains stable, showing no progression of lesions, as does the patient at a ten-month interval.[20]

Dr. Shallenberger's findings support the hypothesis that ozone therapy can have long-term positive effects on AIDS patients. While not a cure, ozone therapy can play a role in improving the quality of life of persons living with AIDS. Soon after the results of the Shallenberger study were released, the Nevada medical authorities attempted to close down his practice.

Positive results from oxidative therapies were also reported by John C. Pittman, M.D., from North Carolina, who worked extensively with HIV and AIDS patients over several years. Pittman's holistic treatments, including ozone and hydrogen peroxide, reportedly helped a number of patients to become HIV-negative. He also began to collect data relating to HIV-infected patients who received oxidative therapy throughout the country.

One of these patients was a thirty-four-year-old man referred to as "D.M." He was diagnosed HIV-positive in March 1991 and had a CD4+ T-cell count of 600, considered to be in the low range of normal. In April 1991 he began receiving autohemotherapy once a day for ten days, along with intravenous hydrogen peroxide and intravenous vitamins, including especially large amounts of vitamin C. In July, he repeated a thirty-day treatment protocol with ozone, hydrogen peroxide, vitamins, and antiviral compounds, as well as nutritional therapies designed to aid in intestinal cleansing and metabolic detoxification. During the first two weeks of therapy, D.M. experienced fever and a drop in his T-cell count to 400, which Dr. Pittman attributed to a die-off of virus particles and infected lymphocytes. Following the thirty-day protocol, D.M. reported that his enlarged neck and inguinal lymph nodes became much smaller. Laboratory tests showed that his CD4+ T-cell count rose to 900.

D.M. continued receiving occasional treatments with ozone and vitamin C, and by November 1992, his helper T-cell count reached 1,400 and his enlarged lymph nodes had returned to normal. Although D.M. still tested positive for the HIV antibody, there was no sign of viral activity by P24 antigen testing.[21] (An antigen is a substance that induces the formation of antibodies.)

Like Dr. Shallenberger, Dr. Pittman's treatment protocol encompassed a holistic approach. Dr. Pittman recommended using intravenous ozone, intravenous hydrogen peroxide, intravenous vitamin C, EDTA (ethylenediamine tetra-acetic acid) chelation, external oxygenation (baths with ozone and hydrogen peroxide), hyperbaric oxygen, metabolic and intestinal detoxification, a raw and living food diet, nutritional supplements, and exercise.[22]

It was mentioned earlier that hyperbaric oxygen (HBO) therapy has also been found useful in the treatment of AIDS. In 1990 Michelle R. Reillo, R.N., began a six-year research program on three hundred patients with late-stage AIDS who underwent HBO treatment for diverse AIDS-related complications, primarily in the Baltimore, Maryland, area. Reillo investigated how HBO works in the manifestation of peripheral vascular insufficiency, pulmonary complications, neurological manifestations, dermatological manifestations, metabolic disorders, and liver problems. Although their life expectancy was just two years at the time the study was begun, more than half of the patients were still alive and enjoying a good quality of life six years later, although they did not take antiviral drugs.

In her book *AIDS under Pressure,* Reillo offered many case studies. The following case history of a thirty-five-year-old male who received HBO treatments three times a week for eight months is typical. The initial tests recorded plasma viral load at 28,550 copies/ml. After three months, another test indicated a viral load of 15,000 copies/ml. Three months later, the results were negative (less than 4,000 copies/ml), even though the patient was not taking antiviral drugs or other medications. Reillo reported, "Clinically, the patient gained ten pounds, felt an increase in energy and stamina, and had relief of fatigue. He reported no adverse effects from HBO [therapy]."[23] She not only found the treatment cost-effective and without adverse side effects, but also concluded:

Managing AIDS with hyperbaric medicine restores immune function, enhances the body's ability to fight infections, directly destroys microorganisms that the immunosuppressed body cannot eliminate, and ameliorates complications related to the presence of HIV. . . . As a primary and adjunctive therapy, hyperbaric oxygen therapy is a technology that prolongs and enhances the quality of life of people with AIDS.[24]

Reillo also found that HBO therapy enhanced the effectiveness of antiviral drugs, as well as other drugs used to manage opportunistic infections or drug-related side effects such as anemia, yeast infections, nausea, liver toxicity, anorexia, and leukopenia.[25]

Yet in spite of the research, mainstream physicians have not embraced the use of HBO therapy to treat AIDS. As is the case for other oxygen therapies, the scope of HBO therapy is often misunderstood, and many physicians do not fully appreciate its possibilities. In the United States and Canada, most hyperbaric chambers are hospital-based (where conservative treatment is the norm), and the use of HBO therapy must be recommended by a licensed physician, who may know very little about hyperbaric oxygen in the treatment of AIDS. In her book *AIDS under Pressure,* Reillo wrote: "Regardless of the beliefs of the health care practitioner, the responsible position is to share all options with the patient. Often, however, it is the patient who educates and encourages the health practitioner to explore all options."[26]

Canada

Heartened by the in vitro blood studies done by the Canadian Armed Forces, the Canadian government decided to sponsor a study with actual AIDS patients. Coordinated by Captain Michael E. Shannon, M.D., in collaboration with Dr. Michael O'Shaughnessy, a virologist with the Laboratory Centre for Disease Control in Ottawa, the study employed twenty-four volunteers suffering from AIDS in two trials using minor autohemotherapy. The Phase I study, which involved ten patients, showed an increase in T cells among those who had 300 or more to begin with, while those who had 90 T cells or fewer experienced a decrease.[27] A Phase II random study was then begun with fourteen patients, with half to receive ozone treatments and the other half a placebo. The findings were inconclusive, however, because the ozone generator used in the study failed to produce ozone. Since the study was double-blind, no one knew about the defect until it was too late.

However, in a private communication I received in January 1994, Captain Shannon wrote: "Of interest, however, the three patients (out of ten volunteers) who responded to minor autohemotherapy in the *first trial,* are still alive after four years post-treatment, with CD4 counts in excess of two hundred. These patients theoretically should have succumbed to AIDS within a year post-treatment."[28] Captain Shannon added that although these initial results must still be explained, there was little interest within the Health Protection Branch of Health and Welfare Canada to pursue the matter further.

In a letter dated January 13, 1995, and addressed to Ed McCabe, Dr. Shannon (who by that time was both promoted to the rank of commander and appointed deputy surgeon general of Canada) offered his candid evaluation of the future of ozone in treating patients with HIV and contradicted the views of one of the other researchers who participated in the second study. At Dr. Shannon's request, the letter is reproduced here in its entirety.

Notwithstanding the negative findings of Dr. Garber's 1991 clinical trial, I firmly believe that ozone therapy has potential to play a valuable role in the medical management of AIDS. From a regulatory point of view, it is clear that not all forms of ozone therapy will be considered sufficiently safe and/or efficacious in this regard; however, there is no doubt in my mind that a protocol will eventually emerge with proven benefit.

Looking back at my past experience with minor autohemotherapy in the treatment of AIDS, there still remains a discrepancy between the Phase 1a and 1b trial results, which may, in part, relate to the lack of sophisticated technology to control for O_3 concentrations in both trials. Given the lack of any significant therapeutic breakthroughs in the treatment of AIDS since that ill-fated trial and the growing testimonial support for its efficacy, the need for further clinical research with ozone is certainly indicated. It is indeed unfortunate that the North American medical community and its funding agencies could not take a more neutral stance on this subject; tragically, professional opinion has been somewhat polarized on this issue. I believe that it is time to take the emotion out of the arguments, both pro and con, and commence a systematic examination of the evidence currently available on the merits of this therapy. Where information gaps exist (particularly in peer-reviewed scientific studies) which might preclude any regulatory decision on the validity of certain claims, properly designed research initiatives should be encouraged with the same kind of public support normally afforded any other scientific endeavour of this import.[29]

At the time of this writing, no large-scale research is being done on the ability of ozone to treat either HIV infection or AIDS.

Cuba

AIDS has not been a major health problem in Cuba. When the AIDS epidemic first came to light, everyone on the island was tested for HIV infection, and the several hundred who tested positive (many of whom were believed to have contracted the virus in Angola, where Cuba was involved in military operations) were quarantined by the government. They were placed in campus-like settings and given free housing, medical care, and healthy food but were not allowed to leave the area. By 1998 this policy became liberalized for those who were not likely to spread the virus to the general population, which had received a crash course in HIV prevention by the Cuban health authorities.

During my interviews with scientists from the National Center for Scientific Research in Havana, I learned that ozone had been given to several of the detainees with some success, although undertaking a study of ozone to treat AIDS was not a high priority due to the low number of infected people.

Dr. Silvia Menendez, a chemist who cofounded the Ozone Research Center with Dr. Manuel Gomez in 1985, told me that ozone works best when administered as soon as possible after infection, before the virus has penetrated the lymphatic system and bone marrow. She believed that, if caught early, ozone could deactivate the virus in the blood and prevent it from infecting other cells. She added that ozone therapy could help prevent and treat some of the opportunistic infections that are common among AIDS patients.[30]

Her comment regarding the early use of ozone for those infected with HIV is very important. If a person could be treated with ozone *as soon as possible after infection,* perhaps the normal progression of the disease could be interrupted. The economic and social ramifications of this possibility cannot be underestimated.

Africa

Concerned with improving and maintaining health through homeopathy and complementary and alternative therapies, Abha Light Foundation (affiliated with Ananda Marga Universal Relief in India) has been treating a limited number of African patients with HIV and AIDS with a combination of intravenous hydrogen peroxide and ultraviolet blood irradiation (UBI)—also known as photo-oxidation—for years.

Patients are treated in a doctor's office. A normal treatment usually takes two hours and is done in two parts. First, hydrogen peroxide is added to a glucose or normal saline IV solution and is slowly infused into the patient. In the second part of the procedure, about 50 ml of the patient's blood is taken out and passed over an ultraviolet light source. It is then transfused back into the patient in a sterile "closed circuit" system.

The clinic reports that treatments are usually given once or twice a week in the case of chronic illness, with one to twenty treatments administered depending on the condition of the patient and the illness being treated. The patient is evaluated periodically for progress, and the physician determines if additional treatments are necessary. It's important to point out that no one has been cured of AIDS at Abha Light, although hydrogen peroxide therapy appears to be a useful adjunct in helping prolong life and increase the quality of life among AIDS patients.

UBI therapy has also been used in other countries either alone or as an adjunct to oxidative therapies in treating patients with HIV/AIDS. UBI treatment produces a number of therapeutic benefits often related to ozone and hydrogen peroxide: inactivation of toxins, destruction and inhibition of growth of bacteria, increase in the oxygen-combining power of the blood and oxygen transportation to organs, activation of steroid hormones, vasodilation (the dilatation of blood vessels, which decreases blood pressure), activation of white blood cells, stimulation of cellular and humoral immunity, removal of blood clots, decreased viscosity of blood, improved circulation, stimulation of corticosteroid production, and decreased platelet aggregation. Some physicians have found that UBI is effective in the treatment of pneumonia and other respiratory diseases.

Although few people have heard of UBI, scientific research has documented its powerful effects for many years. Early articles attesting to the antibacterial and antiviral properties of ultraviolet light appeared in reputable medical journals like the *Archives of Physical Medicine* (1946), *Review of Gastroenterology* (1948), *Experimental Medicine and Surgery* (1950), and the *American Journal of Surgery* (1955).[31] More recent articles about how ultraviolet light can inactivate viruses (including HIV and cytomegalovirus) and bacteria can be found in professional journals related to blood and blood transfusion, including *Blood Cells* (1992), *Vox Sanguinis: International Journal of Transfusion Medicine* (2004), and *Transfusion* (2004, 2005).[32] One of the best reviews of this modality was written by Robert J. Rowan, M.D., and published in the *International Journal of Biosocial Medical Research* in 1996. In reviewing the promise of UBI and other nonspecific healing modalities like ozone and hydrogen peroxide, he wrote:

> Modern medicine has focused on drugs to suppress symptoms or inhibit certain physiology (NSAID drugs as prostaglandin inhibitors, hypertensive drugs as enzymatic blockers) to treat disease. As a result, we have seen the frightening rise of resistant organisms and

the side effects of chemical pharmacology. Perhaps medicine should consider the concept of nonspecific modalities that encourage the body's healing response and immune system.[33]

Anecdotal Findings

Over the years, hundreds of anecdotal reports have surfaced regarding the positive results of oxidative therapies for the treatment of HIV infection and AIDS. A number of these reports come from patients themselves and their physicians, many of whom must remain anonymous. The use of medical ozone generators remains illegal in most states and Canadian provinces, and physicians—if discovered—can lose their medical licenses or be put in jail.

J.P. of Milwaukee was first diagnosed HIV-positive in 1988 and had a T4-cell count of 237 in June 1992. He decided to use Viroterm (a type of oral alpha interferon) and ozone through the sauna bag method over a period of several months. After three weeks of using ozone daily, J.P. found that his lymph nodes, which had been swollen for three years, subsided to normal. In addition, his T-cell counts increased from 237 in June to 292 in October. In June, he had tested positive for P24, a protein found in the core of the human immunodeficiency virus, and by October, his doctor told him that he had tested negative for P24.[34]

Brad J. is a registered nurse who was stuck with a needle while taking blood from an AIDS patient in June 1991. By November he had tested positive for HIV, as well as hepatitis B and C. His T-cell count dropped substantially and by February he had lost thirty pounds, was extremely fatigued, and suffered from severe diarrhea, making it almost impossible to work. Despite his physician's advice, he refused to take AZT and began intravenous infusions of vitamin C five times a week, which caused the diarrhea to abate from twenty movements a day to six. In December 1992, he met Ed McCabe, who told him about ozone, and the following February Brad traveled to Germany to become a certified practitioner in ozone therapy. However, it was not until April 1993 that Brad began taking ozone via autohemotherapy that he administered to himself every seventy-two hours. By the second treatment the diarrhea was eliminated and he felt his old energy return. His hepatitis symptoms disappeared and his viral load index became undetectable after six months of treatment.

Brad has continued using ozone sporadically since that time, augmenting it with Chinese herbs, vitamin C, and other nutritionals. Since he finds the needle stick for autohemotherapy uncomfortable, Brad currently administers ozone in each ear once or twice a week and takes ozone saunas and occasional rectal insufflations. His health situation is stable: after twelve years, he has been free of HIV-related symptoms and his T-cell counts are normal. His energy level is astounding. In addition to his full-time job as a nurse and rebuilding an old house in the country by himself, he has been assisting physicians in setting up ozone clinics. Although Brad credits his good health partly to a spiritual awakening and the use of vitamins and herbs, he says bluntly, "Ozone saved my life."

Another man, whom I will call Bill, tested HIV-positive in 1982 and by 1993 had a T-cell count of 36. In August of that year, he began using the sauna bag method, and he reported that the breathing difficulties he had disappeared after three treatments. Bill also experienced relief of a chronic herpes problem. He began rectal insufflation with humidified ozone in November twice a day and reported relief of abdominal pain and an improved ability to sleep.

Although the exact dose of ozone to be given via rectal insufflation for each individual should be determined by a physician, Dr. Carpendale disclosed the protocol he used in his San Francisco clinical investigations with AIDS patients at the Eleventh Ozone World Congress in 1993:

Ozone was produced from a portable medical ozone generator (Hansler, Iffezheim, Germany), and was insufflated through a Teflon catheter into the colon. This is a simple, safe, inexpensive and well-documented method for treatment with ozone. Dosage concentration was 22–30 mg O_3/ml O_2; average volume was 1100 ml for a total dose of 26.2–33 mg O_3 per treatment. The treatment program was daily for twenty-one days, once every three days for sixteen weeks, and once weekly for fifteen weeks, for a total of thirty-four to thirty-six weeks and seventy-three treatments containing 2065–2137 mg ozone.[35]

Further information regarding the rectal insufflation method to treat HIV/AIDS can be found in the literature published by Keep Hope Alive.

John from Illinois had a T-cell count in the 200 range and began taking five drops of 35 percent food-grade hydrogen peroxide in water three times a day about three hours after meals. He gradually increased the dose to twenty drops, which he maintained for another two months. He then reduced it to five drops and got tested again. His T-cell count had risen to 800. In his comments on the case, Mark Konlee, the author of *AIDS Control Diet* and *Immune Restoration Handbook,* did not recommend using oral hydrogen peroxide. However, he added that these same results could also result by adding a pint of food-grade hydrogen peroxide to warm bathwater and soaking in it for 20 minutes a day.[36]

Like Dr. Silvia Menendez of the National Center for Scientific Research in Cuba, Dr. Bocci suggested that if ozone therapy is applied as soon as possible after exposure to HIV, the patient stands a good chance of avoiding illness.

Writing in the journal *Mediators of Inflammation*, Dr. Bocci stated:

> Our working hypothesis is that ozone acts mainly by inducing blood mononuclear cells to produce immunoregulatory cytokines, particularly those produced by lymphocytes with TH1 phenotype. After incubation of ozonized blood we have shown the release of small amounts of practically all cytokines so far tested, particularly GM-CSF, IL-2, IL-8, IFN, TNF and IFN. After reinfusion of ozone-treated blood, mononuclear cells are supposed to home in various lymphoid (spleen, lymph nodes, thymus, Peyer's patches) and non-lymphoid (lungs, liver) organs thus priming and activating other immune cells. The prolonged repetition of autohemotherapy favors a progressively amplified activation of the immune system via numerous pathways such as activation of either major histo-compatibility complex restricted cytolysis,

or nonspecific killing via activation of natural-killer cells, macrophages and neutrophils, that ultimately represents the most efficient system of destruction of viral infected cells.

He concluded, "Optimized autohemotherapy after a brief exposure of blood to ozone may today afford the trick of reprogramming the immune system to keep HIV at bay. The autohaemotherapeutic procedure is simple, safe, inexpensive and most likely is more effective than conventional approaches."[37]

HIV AUTOVACCINE

In 2010 Dr. Bocci, along with Drs. Iacopo Zanardy and Valter Travagli of the Department of Pharmaceutical Sciences at the University of Siena, offered a novel proposal for a universal HIV autovaccine for both the prevention and treatment of HIV infection. They proposed collecting HIV-infected plasma samples from HIV-infected individuals from five continents around the world. They outlined the procedure in the medical journal *Virulence*:

a) Collection of human HIV plasma samples

b) Centrifugation of the pooled plasma samples and filtration through an antibacterial filter

c) Five cycles of freezing (−196°C) and thawing (+4°C) within a week

d) Inactivation of HIV with ozonation (800 μg ozone per ml of plasma)

e) Addition of both human albumin (200 mg/ml) and ozonated ethyloleate, corresponding to 20 μg of ozone

f) Laboratory tests. Preclinical evaluation in animals. Evaluation in volunteers of a mock vaccine and of the actual ozonated vaccine

g) Vaccination schedule

They added, "A potential advantage of this procedure is that a vaccine made of virions obtained from a great variety of patients will contain all possible HIV genetic diversity at the present and possibly in future times. If the immune system is able to efficiently respond to the ozonated antigens, the vaccine could be used as preventive and possibly curative vaccine."[38]

HIV, AIDS, AND THE POLITICS
OF OXIDATIVE THERAPIES

The use of oxidative therapies for patients with HIV/AIDS is still fraught with controversy. Pharmaceutical companies—which have been earning billions of dollars in profits from anti-AIDS medications—are completely opposed to the use of cheap, safe, and potentially effective oxygen healing therapies in treating this disease, even as an adjunct to traditional medical therapy. In addition, many physicians are either ignorant of or hostile toward using therapies that can be self-administered, like the sauna bag method, steam cabinet method, ear insufflation, or rectal insufflation methods mentioned earlier.

Many reputable and caring physicians who have treated AIDS patients with ozone and hydrogen peroxide have been threatened by state licensing authorities and have had their practices closed down. The U.S. Food and Drug Administration and the National Institutes of Health have refused to sponsor human trials for ozone and hydrogen peroxide and have made it extremely difficult for small, independent companies like Medizone International to undertake such research. Despite the fact that over ten million patients (including thousands of AIDS patients) have received ozone therapy in Europe and that reliable data on the use of ozone and hydrogen peroxide is supported by hundreds of scientific articles and clinical studies, the Food and Drug Administration still maintains that oxidative therapies like ozone have not been proven either safe or effective. Dr. Randolph F. Wykoff, the director of the Office of AIDS Coordination and the acting associate commissioner for science for the U.S. Food and Drug Administration, testified before the Subcommittee on Crime and Criminal Justice of the Committee on the Judiciary at the House of Representatives in Washington on May 27, 1993, saying:

Ozone therapy has also been used to treat AIDS patients without any scientific data to support the agent's safety or effectiveness. Ozone therapy and ozone generators have been promoted in magazines and newspaper advertisements and in books, videos, and audiocassettes. The introduction of ozone into immunosuppressed AIDS patients without careful study of probable toxicities places the patients at unreasonable and significant risks.[39]

The political and economic situation in the United States and Canada has led many patients to seek treatment elsewhere, primarily in Mexico. While there are several reputable clinics in Mexico, some unethical promoters have held out promises for a cure at a price approaching $20,000. One scheme even offered patients six-figure salaries if they could promote their success to other prospective patients later on, especially to those who owned homes that could be mortgaged to pay for treatment.[40]

Until health care consumers speak out to their elected representatives, we will continue to be denied the right to choose the forms of health care we want. Large-scale clinical studies regarding the effectiveness of ozone and hydrogen peroxide to treat AIDS will never be done, and the task of securing research funding will continue to fall on individual researchers themselves. Doctors will be forced to continue to administer these therapies illegally and surreptitiously, and many people without access to these physicians will continue to self-administer ozone or hydrogen peroxide.

While amazingly few adverse side effects have been reported, no one should ever be forced to self-medicate without the benefit of supervision by a qualified health professional. Entrepreneurs eager to fill their pockets will offer magical cures costing tens of thousands of dollars, while many individuals who are infected with HIV or who are dying of AIDS will decide to "go for broke" and try untested treatments from clinics of dubious reputation. Those with the strength and the financial resources will choose to leave their family and friends and seek reliable care in Germany or Cuba.

13
Infectious Diseases

Medical science has long recognized that ozone and hydrogen peroxide destroy viruses, bacteria, and fungi. Unlike many individual drugs developed to fight specific diseases caused by viruses, bacteria, and fungi, oxidative therapies target a broader spectrum: they simply kill all of them. According to a recent article in a European medical journal:

> Ozone exerts a positive effect on oxygen and nutrient supply of cells, it enhances immunological processes, inhibits inflammatory processes, has a bacterio-, fungi- and virusostatic action when there is impaired resistance to microorganisms, improves rheological properties of the blood and exhibits no side effects in patients. Consequently ozonotherapy may be regarded as an effective method of treatment.[1]

On the following pages, we'll take a look at the effectiveness of oxidative therapies in treating some common infectious diseases.

BACTERIAL DISEASES

Lyme Disease
Lyme disease has become a major health problem in many rural and suburban areas of the United States. Caused by the bacterium *Borrelia*

burgdorferi, which is passed on to humans through the bite of a deer tick, Lyme disease is a multisystemic persistent disease that produces a wide range of symptoms, including chronic fatigue, joint pain, dizziness, sore throat, sleep disturbances, memory loss, headache, and abdominal pain.

In a talk presented at the Eighth International Conference on Bio-Oxidative Medicine in 1997, Kenneth Bock, M.D., a physician from rural Dutchess County, New York, and author of *The Road to Immunity,* spoke of his experience in successfully treating over a thousand patients suffering from Lyme disease, many referred to him by other physicians.

Although Dr. Bock found that an aggressive course of antibiotics works best at the onset of Lyme disease, a combination of alternative modalities, including hydrogen peroxide, hyperbaric oxygen therapy, immune-boosting herbs, and nutritional supplements, is more useful in treating chronic and "late" Lyme disease. In his presentation, Dr. Bock stressed the importance of a careful medical diagnosis to determine the nature and extent of the malady and the need to continue oxidative and other treatments for five weeks or more, even if symptoms disappear. He concluded that "oxidative modalities offer much promise for treatment of these patients with recurrent and/or chronic Lyme disease."[2]

Peritonitis

Peritonitis is a life-threatening infection affecting the peritoneum, which is the internal lining of the abdomen. At the Scientific Research Institute of Emergency Aid in Moscow, doctors used a mixture of oxygen and ozone on a variety of patients suffering from diffuse peritonitis. In their report, presented at the First All-Russian Scientific and Practical Conference on Ozone in Biology and Medicine in 1992, they commented: "Ozone therapy . . . caused [an] increase of phagocyte activity [the cell that kills bacteria and viruses] and digestive ability of the leukocytes ["scavenger" white blood cells that fight infection]; hemogram [blood count] indexes improved, the process of healing was accelerated, [and] the period of treatment was reduced."[3]

Another Russian study, undertaken by a team of surgeons, involved a test group of 94 patients aged thirteen to eighty-nine and suffering from acute peritonitis, along with a control group consisting of 174 patients with the disease. The test group received washings of the abdominal cavity with an ozonated solution under pressure, while the controls received conventional therapy.

After one or two procedures of intestinal ozone dialysis, the number of microbes in the lumen of the small intestine had decreased by 50 to 66 percent. The researchers reported that "rapid dynamics of elimination of the endogenous intoxication syndrome was detected" and that the death rate among the patients receiving ozone was 37.23 percent, while mortality among the controls was 62.07 percent.[4]

VIRAL DISEASES

Hepatitis

Among the first physicians to treat hepatitis with medical ozone therapy was Dr. Heinz Konrad of São Paulo, Brazil. During the 1970s, he began a study of fifteen adults suffering from acute type A hepatitis and seven adults with chronic type B hepatitis. Major autohemotherapy was administered twice a week.

The most significant improvement took place among those with hepatitis A: 80 percent (twelve patients) recovered after an average of five ozone applications, while three patients required an average of eleven treatments. The latter three were also given steroids after the course of ozone therapy was completed.

Hepatitis B proved more problematic. Treatment was successful in four cases (57.1 percent) and unsuccessful in three cases (42.9 percent). The patients who recovered received an average of 8.1 ozone treatments. Nevertheless, Dr. Konrad felt that medical ozone therapy "has more success and less side-effects than any other method available today [in 1982]."[5]

A more recent study was undertaken by Cuban physicians at the Octavio de la Concepcion y de la Pedraja Hospital in Camaguey in cooperation with researchers from two other Cuban health agencies.

Eighty patients between the ages of seventeen and forty-five diagnosed with hepatitis A, B, and C were chosen for the study, even though each hepatitis type has a different origination and development. Conventional treatment (which consisted primarily of bed rest and a special diet) and fifteen sessions of ozone therapy via rectal insufflation were given to forty patients. The other group received conventional therapy only.

The doctors reported that patients receiving ozone saw their symptoms go into remission during the first week and were diagnosed as cured at the end of the three-week trial. The control group began to experience a remission of symptoms after ten days and were diagnosed as cured approximately six months later. Presenting their findings at the Second International Symposium on Ozone Applications, which was held in Havana in March 1997, the researchers concluded: "Comparing these results we can say that ozone therapy is a suitable treatment against hepatitis, improving the patients' health and the healing time of the disease."[6]

There is also clinical evidence that hydrogen peroxide infusions can treat patients suffering from hepatitis C. A paper presented at the International Bio-Oxidative Medicine Association Conference in 1995 by Ronald M. Davis, M.D., described using hydrogen peroxide to treat a thirty-eight-year-old man who had been experiencing symptoms of hepatitis three months before actually being diagnosed with hepatitis C. The hydrogen peroxide IVs consisted of 0.03 percent solution mixed by giving 2.5 cc of 3 percent hydrogen peroxide in 250 cc D5W (saline solution), with 1.5 cc $NaHCO_3$ (sodium bicarbonate) added. The infusions were administered over a two-hour period.

Dr. Davis reported that the first infusion was given on September 8, 1995, and three days later the patient noted a slight worsening of nausea and fatigue. However, after the second infusion, symptoms began to improve. Symptoms of fatigue, anorexia, and weight loss resolved and the patient (an air-conditioning repairman) returned to work after the fourth treatment. Dr. Davis reported that "laboratory findings went from originally grossly abnormal to entirely normal after a dozen IV hydrogen peroxide treatments over a ten month time-span. This patient was last seen in the office [in] March 1996. He is in good health, feels well and has no complaints. One year after initiating treatment the patient is free of symptoms, feels well, and is at work full time."[7]

In 2005 Dr. Velio Bocci reported the promising findings of an Egyptian clinical trial performed by Prof. M. Nabil Mawsouf of the Cancer Institute at Cairo University and his colleagues. The study included sixty women and men (ages thirty-four to sixty-five) with chronic hepatitis C infection. They were treated with oxygen-ozone via autohemotherapy and rectal insufflation three times a week during the first two months, and twice weekly during the next four months. Tests performed after eight weeks and after twenty-four weeks showed a "highly significant" decline of the viral load (up to 95 percent) and a marked improvement in trans-aminases plasma levels. No side effects were reported. Though encour-aged by these results, Dr. Bocci called for a longer-term, double-blind placebo study to truly prove ozone's effectiveness.[8]

Prof. Mawsouf reported the findings of a related study at the First International Congress of Ozone in Medicine held in Cairo in 2006. This study included fifty genotype 4 hepatitis C patients (forty-four males and six females) between twenty-three and fifty-eight years of age. They were given a complete blood count, liver function tests, AFP (alpha-fetoprotein) tests, serological tests for bilharziasis, quantitative PCR (polymerase chain reaction) tests for hepatitis C, prothrombin time and concentration tests, and abdominal ultrasonography before treatment, after eight weeks, and after twenty-four weeks of treatment with ozone. Patients received combined treatment of major autohemo-therapy in a dose ranging from 2.8 mg to 8.4 mg, and rectal insufflation in a dose range from 6 mg to 12 mg per visit. Treatments were given three times per week for the first twelve weeks and two times a week for the following twelve weeks. Prof. Mawsouf reported that the general condition of 94 percent of cases improved, both in clinical terms and by evaluation of quality of life and overall well-being.

There was a decrease in the quantitative PCR (viral load) in 71.8 percent of cases, and of this number, 24 percent reached negative PCR after eight weeks of treatment. The number of negative PCR cases for hepatitis C virus (HCV) increased to 36 percent after twenty-four weeks of treatment. Dr. Mawsouf and his colleagues reported that there was a statistically significant improvement regarding the parameters of SGOT (serum glutamic oxaloacetic transaminase), SGPT (serum glutamic pyruvic transaminase), albumin, bilirubin, and prothrombin eight weeks after the beginning of the study. He concluded, "Ozone therapy was found to be an effective, safe and less expensive method in hepatitis C patients."[9]

Russian physicians have been using ozone therapy to treat patients with chronic hepatitis for over ten years. The mechanism is believed to involve ozone's antiviral properties, whereas virus cell receptors are destroyed and cannot penetrate the host cell. The failure in the virus multiplication process is also caused by a breakdown in the virus's RNA. At the same time, ozone activates both cellular and humoral immunity (the humoral part of the immune system includes antibodies and immunoglobulins in blood serum).

A 2008 clinical study found that a two-month course of ozone therapy destroyed all viral signs in 66 percent of patients with chronic hepatitis B and in 60 percent of cases suffering from chronic hepatitis C.

The four primary methods of treatment include rectal insufflation, minor autohemotherapy, intravenous infusions with ozonated saline, and major autohemotherapy.[10]

A group of researchers from the Department of Tropical Medicine and Gastroenterology at Assiut University in Egypt undertook a study to evaluate the role of ozone therapy in decreasing the HCV ribonucleic acid (HCV RNA) load and its effect on the liver enzymes among patients suffering from chronic hepatitis C.

This study included fifty-two patients with chronic hepatitis C (positive PCR for HCV RNA and raised serum alanine transaminase [ALT] for more than six months). All patients were subjected to a meticulous medical history and clinical examination before the clinical trial. The examination included a complete blood count, liver function tests, and abdominal ultrasonography for all patients. The ozone group included forty patients who received major autohemotherapy, minor autohemotherapy, and rectal ozone insufflation. The other twelve patients (conventional group) received silymarin (a standardized extract of milk thistle seeds) and/or multivitamin therapy. Silymarin is often used in conventional medicine for the prevention and treatment of liver diseases, including hepatitis and liver cancer.

Writing in the *Journal of Alternative and Complementary Medicine*, the researchers reported "significant improvements" of most of the symptoms of the patients in the ozone group in comparison to those in the conventional group. ALT levels normalized in 57.5 percent of the ozone group and 16.7 percent of the controls. Aspartate transaminase (AST) levels normalized in 60 percent of the ozone group and 8 percent in the conventional group. The researchers also reported that the PCR for HCV RNA was negative among 25 percent and 44.4 percent of the ozone group after thirty and sixty sessions of ozone therapy, respectively, in comparison to 8 percent among the conventional group.

The researchers concluded: "Ozone therapy significantly improves the clinical symptoms associated with chronic hepatitis C and is associated with normalized ALT and AST levels among a significant number of patients. Ozone therapy is associated with disappearance of HCV RNA from the serum (-ve PCR for HCV RNA) in 25%–45% of patients with chronic hepatitis C." They added: "Ozone, because of its special biologic properties, has theoretical and practical attributes to make it a potent hepatitis C virus (HCV) inactivator, which suggests an important role in the therapy for hepatitis C."[11]

A team of Chinese researchers from the Department of Liver Diseases at the Wuxi Hospital for Infectious Diseases in Jiangsu studied the effects of ozone therapy on patients suffering from severe hepatitis. In the introduction to their article, which appeared in the *Chinese Medical Journal,* they noted that one of the causes of death of patients suffering from severe hepatitis is the complication of renal damage or hepatorenal syndrome. The goal of their study was to observe the effects of medical ozone therapy on plasma renin activity (PRA), angiotensin II (AII), aldosterone (ALD), renal blood flow, and renal function of patients with chronic severe hepatitis and to explore the mechanisms of what made ozone therapy work in the treatment of severe hepatitis.

Eighty-five patients diagnosed with chronic severe hepatitis were chosen for this study. They were randomly divided into two groups: the ozone therapy group (forty-three patients) and the control group (forty-two patients). Patients in the control group received conventional treatment alone, while patients in the ozone therapy group were given conventional medical treatments plus ozone therapy delivered as major autohemotherapy. One hundred milliliters of venous blood was drawn from each patient and was mixed with 100 ml (35 µg/ml) of medical ozone. The treated blood was then reinfused into the patient intravenously, once every other day for twenty days. PRA, AII, ALD, renal blood flow, and damage to renal function tests were given to members of both groups before treatment and twenty days after treatment. Test results and survival rates of the two groups were compared.

Tests showed that in the ozone therapy group, PRA, AII, and ALD levels all decreased significantly after twenty days of treatment when compared with levels before treatment. These figures were also lower than those of the control group twenty days after treatment began. In addition, renal blood flow was found to have increased in the ozone group after twenty days of treatment; these figures were also statistically higher than those of the control group after twenty days of treatment. Renal damage occurred in two cases (5 percent) in the ozone therapy group, which was significantly less than in the control group (nine cases, 21 percent). Thirty-three patients (77 percent) in the ozone therapy group versus sixteen patients (38 percent) in the control group survived.

The researchers concluded: "Basic treatment plus medical ozone therapy for patients with chronic severe hepatitis could decrease PRA, AII and ALD levels, significantly increase renal blood flow, prevent renal damage to [a] certain extent and improve survival rate of the patients."[12]

Influenza

Many of us have experienced influenza at least once in our lifetime. Symptoms of fever, coughing, chills, body aches, sore throat, headache, and nausea are familiar to many flu sufferers. However, some people—especially the very young, the very old, and others who are immunosuppressed—can die from it. New strains of the virus appear every year, requiring the development of new vaccines. Health authorities fear that some influenza strains will prove extremely difficult to control, especially avian influenza, commonly known as "bird flu."

We mentioned earlier that the first known treatment using intravenous hydrogen peroxide for influenza was reported by Dr. T. H. Oliver in the British medical journal *Lancet* in 1920. Since that time, hydrogen peroxide has been a valuable yet little known treatment for this common, debilitating, and sometimes fatal disease.

A landmark study to examine the effectiveness of intravenous hydrogen peroxide to treat patients with type A/Shanghai influenza was undertaken by Dr. Charles H. Farr in January 1989. Symptoms of this strain of flu are very pronounced and typically last for forty-eight to seventy-two hours. Full recovery takes an average of twelve to fifteen days.

Dr. Farr took forty flu sufferers between the ages of sixteen and seventy-eight. They were divided into two groups of twenty, so that age groups and gender were similar. The control group received the conventional medical protocol for influenza, which included antibiotics, decongestants, and pain relievers. Some patients supplemented these medications with over-the-counter cold and cough preparations of their choice. The treatment group was given 250 ml of 0.0375 percent intravenous hydrogen peroxide over a period of one to three days, according to the patient's needs. Painkillers were also given if desired. Of this group 35 percent required a second infusion while two patients (10 percent) needed a third.

The results were impressive. Half of the control group got better after 4.1 days, and 75 percent improved in 7.8 days, with 90 percent reporting improvement after 11 days. Among the group treated with hydrogen peroxide, half got better in 1.9 days, 75 percent in 3.2 days, and 90 percent experienced a complete recovery after only 5.5 days. Overall, the group receiving hydrogen peroxide lost a cumulative 5 days of work, while the controls were absent for a cumulative 41.5 days.[13] Figure 13.1 displays the results in more detail.

Colds and Flu

Dr. Joseph Mercola, an osteopathic physician based in Utah, has reported what he calls "remarkable" anecdotal results (in the 80 percent range) in treating cold and flu symptoms with 3 percent hydrogen peroxide, the kind easily available in pharmacies and convenience stores.

Noting that treatment should begin as soon as symptoms appear, Dr. Mercola suggests administering a few drops of 3 percent hydrogen peroxide into each ear (this can easily be done with an eye dropper while the patient lies down on his or her side).[14] As the liquid penetrates the inner ear, it begins killing the virus that caused the flu or cold;

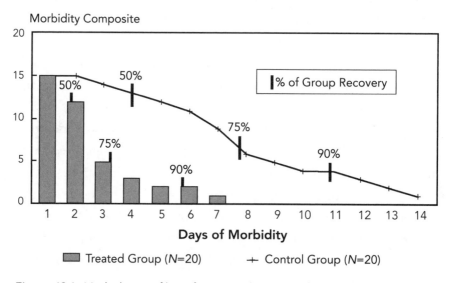

Figure 13.1. Morbidity profiles of type A/Shanghai influenza. Treated group: H_2O_2/analgesic. Control: Antibiotic/decongestant/analgesic. Treated group given 250 ml 0.0375% H_2O_2 first day. Seven required repeat treatments second day. Two required a third. (Reprinted courtesy of Charles H. Farr.)

the patient is asked to wait to drain the ear until any bubbling (and occasional stinging) has subsided, which usually takes from five to ten minutes. While this simple home treatment is also recommended for children, the loud bubbling and possible stinging sensation may be distressing. In such cases, a trusted adult should administer the hydrogen peroxide and make sure it doesn't get into the child's eyes: if this happens, flush the eyes immediately with water.

Given that millions of North Americans come down with different varieties of influenza every flu season, the time, suffering, and money lost to absenteeism that can be saved through hydrogen peroxide therapy can be significant indeed.

Because ozone can kill all influenza virus strains, research should begin immediately to find possible preventive and therapeutic applications of ozone therapy on the avian influenza strain (bird flu). Both Dr. Silvia Menendez of the National Center for Scientific Research in Cuba and Dr. Bocci have expressed in personal communications that ozone has global potential in controlling this disease among birds and humans alike.

FUNGAL INFECTIONS

Candidiasis

Dr. Charles H. Farr successfully treated hundreds of patients suffering from candidiasis with intravenous hydrogen peroxide at the Genesis Medical Center in Oklahoma City, Oklahoma, for more than fifteen years. In his monograph *The Therapeutic Use of Intravenous Hydrogen Peroxide,* Dr. Farr offered a case history of one of his patients:

> Ms. P.M., a 34 y/o w/f, has been treated repeatedly over the past 5 years for Chronic Systemic Candidiasis. Her history and symptoms are classic. Her current problems had an onset after several episodes of upper respiratory infections, about 5 years ago, which were treated with large doses of various antibiotics. Following this she had repeated episodes of yeast vaginitis and intermittent problems

with diarrhea. These episodes were then followed with the development of chronic fatigue, acne, lethargy, migratory arthralgia [joint pain], frequent headaches, menstrual irregularities, mental confusion, difficulty concentrating and a poor tolerance to environmental and exercise stress.

She was treated with various elimination and rotation diets, nystatin, nizoral, monostat, allergic desensitization, and various natural anti-yeast preparations. Each time the therapeutic modality was changed, she would have a temporary subjective improvement for a few days or weeks [and] then relapse to her pretreatment morbid level. She had been unable to work for over two years and had become totally dependent on her mother for financial and physical support. She often did not feel able to dress or feed herself.

She was started on weekly injections of 250 mL of 0.15% H_2O_2 and after two treatments reported a significant improvement in alertness, ability to concentrate and had an improved feeling of well-being. After the third treatment, she pointed out how her complexion was improving and her acne was considerably better. A menstrual period, the previous week, had been normal and previous signs of vaginitis had disappeared. Her bowel function was becoming more regular and normal and she was talking about wanting to return to work.

Her 4th, 5th and 6th treatments were scored with continued subjective improvements from her previous complaints. After 8 treatments she was free of symptoms for the first time in 5 years. Objectively she appeared much healthier and had more vitality, smiling and happy for the first time since we saw her as a new patient. When tested for candida sensitization subcutaneously, she now tested a 1 dilution compared to her usual 4 to 6 dilutions during her more morbid times. Two months after her last infusion, she was seeking employment, had redeveloped her self-confidence and had shown no signs of relapse. Follow-up evaluations are continuing.[15]

Mucormycosis

Mucormycosis is a devastating and often lethal fungal disease that mainly affects diabetics and immunosuppressed patients. Physicians at Virginia Commonwealth University/Medical College of Virginia in Richmond reported two interesting cases that did not respond to treatment with intravenous amphotericin B, the medication most often used to control this disease. Both patients underwent soaks with topical (3%) hydrogen peroxide, diluted to half-strength, which destroyed *Mucor* fungi and the surrounding host tissue, thus apparently eradicating the disease. The researchers proposed adding half-strength topical hydrogen peroxide soaks to the list of possible adjunctive treatments of mucormycosis.[16]

Onychomycosis (Nail Fungus)

Onychomycosis is a fungal infection that affects the nails of the hands and feet. Affecting more than three million patients a year in the United States alone, onychomycosis is the most common disease of the nails and constitutes about half of all nail abnormalities. It is often highly resistant to traditional medical therapy. A group of researchers from the National Center for Scientific Research and the Carlos J. Finlay Hospital in Cuba studied two hundred adult outpatients suffering from onycho-mycosis. They were divided into two equal randomized groups: one group received one drop of ozonated sunflower oil (Oleozon) on each infected nail twice a day, while the other group was treated twice a day with tolnaftate solution. The course of treatment lasted three months. Other medications were added for the control patients suffering from yeast infections and filamentous mycosis.

A patient was considered "cured" when the affected nail completely regained normal color, growth, and thickness and no fungi were detected; a patient "improved" when a decrease of symptoms was present and there was a positive finding of fungi; "same" symptoms were based on no changes in the nails and a positive finding of fungi; and "worse" when nail lesions increased and fungi was found. The results can be seen in the table on page 200.

Results of Patients Treated with Oleozon

Group	Worse	Same	Improved	Cured
Experimental	0	0	31	69
Control	0	68	25	7

Researchers concluded that this study demonstrated the fungicidal power of ozonated oil and recommended it as superior to conventional medical treatments.[17] I would like to add that my ninety-year-old aunt had suffered from onychomycosis on one nail that was resistant to conventional therapy for over ten years. After she applied Oleozon for a week, her symptoms completely disappeared.

Sixteen years later, an article in the medical journal *Mycoses* showed the results of a randomized control phase II trial in Cuba involving the use of Oleozon in the treatment of onychomycosis.

Under the direction of Dr. Silvia Menéndez, a total of four hundred outpatients diagnosed with onychomycosis were randomly divided into two groups: the "experimental" group was treated with topical Oleozon, two times per day for three months, while the controls were treated two times per day for three months with ketoconazole 2 percent cream, a popular over-the-counter antifungal medication. A patient was considered cured when the infected nails regained the normal color, growth and thickness, along with a negative mycological study.

In the group receiving Oleozon, a regression of symptoms was achieved during the first month of treatment, while in the control group, it was obtained after the third month of treatment. At the end of the study, all patients treated with Oleozon were either cured (90.5 percent) or showed improvement (9.5 percent). However, in the control group, only 13.5 percent of patients were cured, 27.5 percent improved, and 59 percent remained the same. After a one-year follow-up, the researchers found that 2.8 percent of patients in the experimental group and 44.4 percent of patients in the control group had experienced relapses. They concluded: "Topical Oleozon demonstrated effectiveness in the treatment of onychomycosis, superior to that of ketoconazole. No side effects were observed."[18]

PARASITIC DISEASES

Giardiasis

Giardia lamblia is a parasite that can infest the small intestine. For those unfortunate enough to contract the parasitic disease giardiasis, symptoms include diarrhea, weight loss, nausea, cramps, and vomiting. *Giardia lamblia* is often highly resistant to medical therapy. While giardiasis is usually managed with drugs, there is no known cure.

At the General Calixto Garcia Hospital in Havana, Cuba, fifty adults suffering from giardiasis who did not respond to traditional medical treatment were given two cycles of therapy with ozonated water over a twenty-seven-day period. Each patient drank four glasses of ozonated water per day for ten days, which was followed by a seven-day period without treatment. The second cycle consisted of another ten days of drinking four glasses of ozonated water daily.

Researchers reported that twenty-three patients (46 percent) experienced a remission of symptoms during the first cycle of treatment, while twenty-four others (48 percent) became asymptomatic by the end of the second cycle. Unlike many receiving drug therapy, subjects reported no adverse side effects from ozone. The researchers concluded, "Ozone's easy availability and low cost, as well as its great effectiveness in the treatment of *Giardia lamblia,* permits its recommendation to be used on a greater scale and to substitute it for conventional treatments used to treat giardia."[19]

After the success of the previous investigation, another team from the National Center for Scientific Research developed a study with physicians from the Department of Parasitology at the Central Havana Pediatric Hospital to see whether ingestion of ozonated sunflower oil could help cure giardiasis in children. A group of 222 children from seven months to fourteen years of age who had been diagnosed with infantile giardiasis were selected for the study. Of the patients, 76 percent (169) had been previously treated with antigiardastic medications without success. Children were given drops or capsules of ozonated sunflower oil (marketed as Oleozon-A in Cuba) at age-dependent doses at bedtime over a ten-day period. After a break of ten days, another ten-day course of therapy took place.

After the second course of treatment, a duodenal gavage (a procedure using a stomach tube) was performed and feces were examined. The absence of cysts or trophozoites of *Giardia lamblia* in feces and the duodenal gavage would indicate a cure. The results were very encouraging: 79 percent of the patients treated with Oleozon-A were cured. Of the remaining 21 percent, nine out of ten children reported a disappearance of all symptoms, of which abdominal pain and diarrhea were most common. A third cycle of treatment for the noncured patients brought further improvement. No adverse reactions to the therapy were observed.[20]

Malaria

Studies at the Middlesex Hospital Medical School in England revealed that blood-stage murine malaria parasites were killed in vitro by hydrogen peroxide at even tiny concentrations. In vivo studies (on mice) in 1983 showed that hydrogen peroxide was able to kill the lethal varieties of *Plasmodium yoelii* and *Plasmodium berghei*, although the latter proved more difficult to kill. The researchers concluded, "We propose that hydrogen peroxide is in fact a possible contributor to the destruction of at least some species of malaria parasite."[21]

The first in vitro study with ozone and the malaria parasite *Plasmodium falciparum* was done seventeen years later at the University of Tublingen's Institute of Tropical Medicine in Germany. A laboratory strain of the parasite was ozonated with 80 µg/ml ozone, and parasitic growth was evaluated for four days. They discovered that ozone had a strong inhibitory effect on *Plasmodium falciparum*, even when parasites were added after ozonation of the culture medium took place.[22]

Like many other laboratory findings regarding the ability of hydrogen peroxide and ozone to kill strains of malaria-related parasites, studies on human beings suffering from malaria have not yet been done. Given the prevalence of malaria in tropical countries (many strains of which have become resistant to traditional antimalarial drugs), oxidative therapies—whether alone or as adjuncts to traditional medications—may offer promise to help heal thousands of infected people yearly.

OZONE AND HUMAN PANDEMICS

Ebola

Ebola virus disease (EVD) is a severe, often fatal illness in humans. The Ebola epidemic of 2014–2015 is believed to have been transmitted to people from wild animals in Africa and spread through human-to-human transmission. Mortality rates during the height of the epidemic were estimated to vary between 83 percent and 90 percent.

According to the World Health Organization (WHO), there are no proven treatments available for EVD. However, a range of potential treatments including blood products, immune therapies, and drug therapies are currently being evaluated. At the time of this writing (2016), no licensed vaccines are available, although two potential vaccines are undergoing human safety testing. Some are currently being used on an experimental basis, with mixed results.

The three primary mechanisms of action of therapeutic ozone include:

- The inactivation of bacteria, fungi, yeasts, viruses, and protozoa by disrupting the integrity of the cell envelope through oxidation of the cell phospholipids and lipoproteins. Ozone also has been found to upset their reproductive cycle.
- Stimulation of oxygen metabolism, causing an increase in the red blood cell glycosis rate. It also stimulates the production of enzymes that act as free radical scavengers and cell-wall protectors.
- Activation of the immune system through the production of

interferon, tumor necrosis factor, and interleukin-2, which launches a cascade of beneficial immunological reactions throughout the body.

During the height of the Ebola epidemic, Dr. Adriana Schwartz of the International Medical Ozone Federation (IMEOF) appealed to WHO to consider utilizing ozone therapy as a safe, low-cost, and effective treatment for Ebola virus disease.

In a well-documented scientific report released to the health care community in October 2014, Dr. Schwartz wrote: "It is an absolutely safe treatment that stimulates the immune system. It may be available in large quantities at low cost, even in the poorest areas of the world. The antiviral and antibacterial properties of ozone are well recognized. The Ebola virus has little chance to survive [when] directly exposed to its gas."

When used according to established protocols, Dr. Schwartz believes that medical ozone can:

1. Kill the Ebola virus
2. Reduce the patient's level of oxidative stress brought on by the disease
3. Reduce patient pain and discomfort due to its analgesic properties
4. Boost the patient's overall immune system
5. Help maintain a sterile environment in the hospital or clinic[23]

Her appeals were largely ignored by WHO and other sectors of the mainstream medical community. Why was this? We mentioned earlier that a major reason for a lack of interest is that ozone is a *non-patentable* substance that is inexpensive to manufacture and use. The net cost of the materials for a treatment of rectal insufflation can be less than $10, especially in a clinic designed to treat large numbers of people in a developing country.

In a health care industry that is largely driven by profit, ozone poses a threat to the continued dominance of the medical establishment: the pharmaceutical industry, medical centers, and physicians who are accustomed to providing expensive drugs, complex medical procedures, and long hospital stays.

Zika

The Zika virus is spread to people through bites from the *Aedes aegypti* mosquito. The most common symptoms of Zika virus disease are fever, rash, joint pain, and conjunctivitis (red eye). The illness is usually mild, with symptoms lasting from several days to a week. Severe disease requiring hospitalization is uncommon.

In May 2015, the Pan American Health Organization (PAHO) issued an alert regarding the first confirmed Zika virus infection in Brazil. The outbreak in Brazil led to reports of Guillain-Barré syndrome and pregnant women giving birth to babies with birth defects and poor pregnancy outcomes.

The most serious birth defect connected to Zika is *microcephaly,* an abnormal smallness of the baby's head associated with incomplete brain development. For this reason the U.S. Centers for Disease Control and Prevention (CDC) recommends that women who are pregnant (and those who are planning to become pregnant) should take special precautions against being bitten by mosquitos that could spread the Zika virus, for which there is no known cure. The World Health Organization declared the Zika virus outbreak in the Americas a public health emergency in February 2016.

Advocates of ozone therapy believe that ozone can be an effective treatment for those infected by the Zika virus when administered as soon as possible after exposure. As it is with Ebola, ozone can be used to:

1. Kill the Zika virus
2. Reduce the patient's level of oxidative stress brought on by the disease

3. Reduce patient pain and discomfort due to its analgesic properties
4. Boost the patient's overall immune system

By 2016, a number of clinics in Latin America had begun treating Zika patients with ozone. They have reported positive results, including disappearance of symptoms after three days of autohemotherapy. Although this is good news, Silvia Menéndez Cepero, head of the clinic of the National Center for Scientific Research in Cuba, cautions that anecdotal evidence regarding treatment of Zika with ozone means very little. As the coordinator and chief writer of more than forty scientific studies involving ozone therapy, she wrote, "You need to do a controlled clinical trial in order to say that ozone is good in Zika treatment."[24]

Dealing with a health threat like Ebola or Zika is a major challenge for humanity. When effective treatments are not available—or are beyond the financial means of most patients—it is time to consider safe, effective, and inexpensive alternative treatments. It is especially important to have the interest and the ability to fund controlled clinical trials to evaluate their effectiveness. It is time for ozone and hydrogen peroxide therapy to be seriously considered as two such alternatives when dealing with human pandemics of bacterial, fungal, or viral origin.

14

Musculoskeletal Problems

Ozone and hydrogen peroxide have been used to treat musculoskeletal problems for more than forty years. One of the major methods used involves injections of small amounts of ozone or hydrogen peroxide, either alone or with other therapeutic substances. Medically, it is known as either regenerative injection therapy (RIT) or proliferative therapy. In some cases, this therapy is used with other oxidative modalities like autohemotherapy.

An article in *Medical Hypotheses* addressed the safety and effectiveness of RIT in treating painful ligaments and joints. The authors wrote that ozone dissolves in body fluids and immediately reacts with biomolecules that generate biochemical messengers responsible for biological and therapeutic activities. They continued, "The results are an anti-inflammatory response, which also results in a similar trophic [promoting cellular growth or survival] reaction to that of RIT. It is logical to expect that combining these two modalities [RIT plus minor or major autohemotherapy] would result in enhanced healing and therefore improved clinical outcomes."[1]

A broad-spectrum German study of the value of ozone therapy in treating orthopedic problems was undertaken by C. H. Siemsen, M.D., a specialist in orthopedics and sports medicine and a lecturer in biomedical technology at the Polytechnic College in Hamburg. Fifty-nine male and female patients were chosen for the study. Patients were suffering from acute and chronic joint diseases including active inflammatory gonarthrosis, stiffness of the shoulder and shoulder area, and chronic diseases of the shoulder joint with calcification and painful restrictions of movement. Patients also suffered from lateral and medial epicondylitis (tennis elbow), chronic adductor insertion endopathy (known as "footballer's hip" in Europe), and malformations of the hip, including acute and chronic trochanteric bursitis. Ozone treatment was carried out after all other forms of medical therapy were deemed unsuccessful.

Over a period of several weeks, fifty patients were given an average total of ten intra-articular injections of ozone and oxygen in the affected areas, preceded by a local anesthetic. Nine patients suffering from therapy-resistant systemic conditions were given a course of autohemotherapy as well. Patients were examined the day after each treatment.

The patients were assessed with scores by adding the numbers 1 to 6 to form quotients: a value of 1.9 (i.e., good) was a measure for the knee joint (activated gonarthrosis) and a value of 2.5 (i.e., good to satisfactory) was assigned to shoulder joint problems. After the course of treatment, all patients improved to a "good" quotient level. It was noted that none of the patients required corticosteroids. Dr Siemsen concluded, "The application of ozone in orthopedics and in the treatment of acute, chronic or therapy-resistant painful diseases of the joints with involvement of the articular and periarticular regions is a good alternative treatment method for obtaining rapid pain relief, subsidence of inflammation and an increase in motility."[2]

HOW DOES OZONE RELIEVE MUSCULOSKELETAL PAIN?

A study by researchers of the University of Ancona in Italy and Cairo University in Egypt focused on understanding the mechanism behind ozone's proven clinical ability to reduce pain. Fifty-two patients suffering from shoulder, cervical, and low back pain were chosen for this study, and each received subcutaneous injections of oxygen and ozone.

Although pain among patients was relieved, the focus of this study was on how pain was mediated with ozone. The researchers concluded that the analgesic mechanism of ozone involves two important steps:

1. A short-term mechanism that may correspond with the direct oxidation on biomolecules
2. A long-term mechanism that may involve the activation of anti-oxidant pathways

The authors stressed that deeper research is needed to clarify the biochemical pathways that are involved in the short- and long-term pain-reducing process.[3]

ARTHROSIS

Arthrosis is a disease that involves the progressive degeneration of cartilage in the spine, knees, and other joints. Like arthritis, arthrosis causes intense pain and limits movement. In 1990 Cuban researchers studied 234 patients complaining of pain and related problems in the spine, lumbar-sacrum, knee, and other joints. A total of twenty intramuscular injections of oxygen and ozone were given over a period of thirty days, with one injection daily for the first ten days, and an additional ten on alternate days. All patients were carefully examined, diagnosed, and evaluated before the study.

The results were impressive: 208 patients (89 percent) reported complete disappearance of pain; 24 (10 percent) reported some degree of relief; and 2 patients (1 percent) reported no changes in their health status. In their follow-up examinations, the researchers found that most of the patients remained symptom-free for three to six months, while some did not feel pain for up to eleven months after treatment. People with herniated spinal discs also felt relief with ozone therapy.[4]

Due to improved treatment methods, these results were even better than an earlier Cuban study of 122 arthrosis patients, in which 71.8 percent of the patients treated with ozone reported complete relief of pain, while 21.8 percent reported improvement.[5]

HERNIATED DISC PAIN

Herniated disc pain is a common problem among many adults. Conservative treatment usually calls for the injection of steroids and painkillers, while surgery is often recommended for more difficult cases. Ozone therapy has been considered effective in bringing about pain relief when other methods fail.

A major controlled clinical trial on oxygen-ozone therapy to treat pain from a herniated lumbar disc was done at Bellaria Hospital in Bologna, Italy, and reported in the *American Journal of Neuroradiology* in 2003. Six hundred patients suffering from herniated discs were treated with a single session of oxygen-ozone therapy. The first group of three hundred (Group A) was given only ozone. In addition to ozone, the other half (Group B) received a corticosteroid and an anesthetic.

Both groups were evaluated six months later. In Group A treatment was a success (i.e., excellent or good outcome) in 70.3 percent and considered a failure in the remaining 29.7 percent of patients. In Group B treatment was successful in 78.3 percent and a failure in 21.7 percent. The researchers concluded that the combined use of ozone and steroids provides the best results and added: "Oxygen-ozone therapy is a useful treatment for lumbar disc herniation that has failed to respond to conservative management."[6]

A double-blind study comparing the effectiveness of using steroids alone and steroidal therapy in addition to ozone to treat pain related to acute herniated lumbar discs was undertaken by physicians in the Departments of Radiology and Neurosurgery at the University of L'Aquila in Italy.

The researchers randomly divided 159 patients (eighty-six men and seventy-three women between eighteen and seventy-one years of age) into two groups. Seventy-seven patients (Group A) underwent intradiscal and intraforaminal injections of a steroid and an anesthetic, and eighty-two patients (Group B) underwent the same treatment with the addition of an oxygen and ozone mixture. Procedures were performed with computed tomographic guidance. An Oswestry Low Back Pain Disability Questionnaire was administered before treatment and at intervals during the study, with the final follow-up done six months after the first treatment. Both patients and clinicians did not know which treatment was performed.

After six months, treatment was considered "successful" in thirty-six patients (47 percent) in Group A and in sixty-one patients (74 percent) in Group B. The researchers concluded, "Intraforaminal and intradiscal injections of a steroid, an anesthetic, and O_2-O_3 are more effective at 6 months than injections of only a steroid and an anesthetic in the same sites."[7]

A study undertaken by Chinese physicians at the Department of Interventional Radiology at Nanfang Hospital (part of Southern Medical University) in Guangzhou evaluated the effects of oxygen/ozone injections to treat herniated lumbar discs.

Fifty-eight patients (forty-eight men and thirteen women between the ages of twenty-two and seventy-eight) suffering from large herniated lumbar discs were selected for the study. Patients received injections of ozone and oxygen into the facet joints (joints in the spine that make our spine flexible and enable us to bend and twist) on the first and fifth days of the study. Follow-up exams were given over the next six to eighteen months, with the results evaluated by the Macnab criteria, a primary outcome assessment of patient satisfaction. The outcome was "excellent" in thirty-seven cases (63.8 percent), "good" in sixteen cases (27.6 percent), and "fair/poor" in five cases (8.6 percent). The researchers concluded: "Percutaneous intradiscal ozone injection via the posterior-lateral route and inner margin of the facet joint is effective and safe for treatment of large lumbar disc herniation."[8]

Another Chinese study involved a group of ten physicians from three hospitals in Guangzhou (Guangzhou General, Zhujiang, and Nanfang) comparing the effectiveness of one-, two-, and three-week treatments of oxygen-ozone injections for patients suffering from herniated lumbar discs.

Between November 2003 and October 2008, 187 patients (115 male and 72 female) with diagnostically confirmed lumbar disc herniation were chosen for the study. Their average age was 45.8 years (ranging from 21 to 75). All patients complained of sciatica and low back pain lasting from one month to twelve years. Physical examinations showed that all patients showed a positive reaction to Lasègue's sign (a standard straight leg raising test to diagnose herniated lumbar disc problems). Diagnostic verification by CT and MRI exhibited disc protrusion with nerve root or thecal sac compression. The disc lesions in all patients occurred between the L4/5 and L5/S1 vertebrae of the spine.

Patients were placed into three groups for one-week, two-week, and four-week treatment sessions to compare the difference in the clinical curative effect of oxygen-ozone therapy.

- Group 1: a one-week treatment course in which the patient had only one interventional procedure and dehydration medicine venous injection treatment for three days.
- Group 2: a two-week treatment session in which the patient had one interventional procedure and dehydration medicine venous injection treatments for three days, and repeated seven days later.
- Group 3: a four-week treatment session in which the patient had two interventional procedures and dehydration medicine venous injection treatments for three days, and repeated twenty-eight days later.

They followed up with all patients for three months to forty-eight months after the procedure. The results showed that the effective rate of oxygen-ozone therapy was 85.02 percent (159/187 patients) in all groups. The effective rate was 82.52 percent (85/103) with one week of treatment, 85.24 percent (52/61) with two weeks of treatment, and 95.65 percent (22/23) with four weeks of treatment.

The researchers concluded that while oxygen-ozone therapy was indeed effective in relieving symptoms of lumbar disc herniation, the number of treatments didn't make much of a statistical difference. For this reason, they recommended that doctors should "advocate a single treatment session as the first choice, and postpone a second injection after one month's observation. This strategy will not only guarantee the curative effect, but also reduce the cost of treatment."[9]

Several years later, another group of Chinese researchers in Guangzhou studied the effectiveness of injecting ozone into the spinal cord and dural sac under CT guidance to treat patients suffering from herniated lumbar discs. Their findings were published in the Chinese *Journal of Southern Medical University*.

A total of 262 patients diagnosed with lumbar disc herniation were recruited for this study. Medical oxygen-ozone was injected under CT guidance into the lumbar intervertebral disc by the posterior paramedian approach 1 to 2 cm from the spinous process, targeting the affected lumbar discs, protruded nucleus pulposus, and ipsilateral lateral recess. The concentration of ozone was 40 to 50 μg/ml in the disc/protruded nucleus pulposus and 30 μg/ml in the lateral recess (around the nerve root).

Treatment was successfully completed in all patients. The average JOA scores (a clinical symptom score for patients with herniated lumbar disc developed by the Japanese Orthopedic Association; a higher score denotes improvement) and VAS scores (visual analog scale for measuring back pain; a lower score indicates improvement) before treatment were 8.30 and 8.73. They changed significantly to 24.16 and 2.41 after treatment, respectively. According to the modified Macnab criteria, the therapeutic effect was "excellent" in 165 cases, "good" in 64 cases, "fair" in 20 cases, and "poor" in 13 cases. The researchers claimed a success rate of 87.4 percent. No patients showed serious complications after the treatment.

The researchers concluded that when compared with routine ozone therapy by the traditional posterior-lateral approach, targeted ozone injections into the intervertebral disc by the modified posterior approach is safe and yields better therapeutic results for patients diagnosed with lumbar disc herniation.[10]

A 2014 study by researchers at the Biotechnological and Applied Clinical Sciences Department at the University of L'Aquila in Italy found that injections of oxygen and ozone can help shrink herniated lumbar discs, affording pain relief and greater mobility to patients.

One hundred fifty-four patients suffering from lumbosciatica (eighty-nine men and sixty-five women between the ages of twenty-three and sixty-two years) were chosen for this study and randomly assigned to two groups. Seventy-seven patients (control group) underwent conservative treatment with intraforaminal injections of steroid and anaesthetic. The remaining seventy-seven patients (study group) underwent the same treatment with the addition of oxygen-ozone. During the following six months, an MRI follow-up with the same sequences was performed. An intervertebral disc volumetric analysis (IDVA), DWI signal score, and post-treatment clinical outcome evaluation were performed for an assessment of hernia reduction.

The researchers found that approximately 20 percent of patients in both groups experienced pain reduction at the two-month follow-up, which increased to 40 percent for the study group and 32 percent for the control group after four months. By six months, however, the statistics changed markedly. The researchers found that fifty-eight of seventy-seven patients (approximately 75 percent) treated with oxygen and ozone discolysis had successful clinical outcomes and statistically significant herniation volume reduction, compared with thirty (38.9 percent) of the seventy-seven control group patients.[11]

Intramuscular Application

Clinical findings have shown that oxygen-ozone therapy can be used to treat herniated lumbar discs that fail to respond to traditional medical management. Most of these findings are based on intradiscal/intraforaminal oxygen-ozone injection, whereas intramuscular-paravertebral (*paravertebral* refers to the space located next to the spinal column) injection is a technique that is used more often in clinical practice in Italy and other Western countries.

A double-blind randomized study was undertaken by eight spinal specialists from three Italian medical rehabilitation centers to determine whether intramuscular-paravertebral oxygen-ozone injections were effective in treating lumbar disc herniation (LDH).

Sixty patients suffering from acute lower back pain (LBP) caused by LDH were randomized to an intramuscular oxygen-ozone group (study group) or a control group. Patients were observed to assess pain intensity, LBP-related disability, and drug intake at fifteen and thirty days after treatment started and two weeks, three months, and six months after treatment ended.

Patients in the study group received three oxygen injections weekly for five consecutive weeks. Members of the control group were given simulated injections using a false needle that pricked the skin without piercing it, applied at the lumbar paraspinal (paraspinal muscles are those that run roughly parallel to the spine) level. This was followed by hand-applied pressure on the same site, which was designed to reproduce the load sensation commonly described after O_2-O_3 injections. A bandage was applied to each patient in the study, which was removed before a new injection (or simulated injection) was given.

A significant difference between the two groups was observed at six months after treatment; 61 percent of the study group versus 33 percent of the control group reported that they were pain-free. Patients who received oxygen-ozone had a lower mean pain score than patients who received simulated therapy throughout the observation period. In addition, the researchers observed significant improvement in LBP-related disability in the study group patients when compared with the control group patients. Active oxygen-ozone therapy was followed by a significantly lower number of days on nonsteroidal anti-inflammatory drugs at fifteen days and thirty days after treatment started, and by a lower number of days at two weeks after treatment ended. No adverse events were reported among participants in the study.

The researchers concluded: "[Oxygen-ozone] intramuscular lumbar paravertebral injections, which are minimally invasive, seem to safely and effectively relieve pain, as well as reduce both disability and the intake of analgesic drugs."[12]

LUMBAR DISC PAIN AND ASSOCIATED MOTOR WEAKNESS

In this chapter we have shown that intradiscal injection of oxygen and ozone is an effective treatment for pain caused by protruding disc disease and nerve root compression due to bulging or herniated disc.

In Italy the most widely used therapeutic combination involves an intradiscal injection of an oxygen-ozone mixture followed by peri-radicular injection of oxygen-ozone close to the nerve root, plus a steroid and a local anesthetic to enhance the anti-inflammatory and analgesic effect. The treatment is designed to resolve pain and is administered to patients without motor weakness.

Thirteen patients were recruited for a study on this treatment that took place between March 2009 and August 2013. Patients all suffered from low back pain and cruralgia (nerve pain starting in the lower back and spreading along a leg; it differs from sciatica by the affected nerve root), low back pain and sciatica, and subacute partial motor weakness caused by nerve root compression. All participants in the study had not responded to conventional medical treatment.

Patients were managed by physicians at the Neurosurgery Unit of Bellaria Hospital (part of the IRCCS Institute of Neurological Sciences) and the University of Bologna in Italy. One treatment was given to all patients, and a follow-up treatment was administered between one month and three months after the first.

The researchers reported that all of the patients had experienced a complete resolution of motor weakness, and 84.6 percent had complete pain relief. Two patients opted for surgery because their pain was not reduced by the oxygen-ozone treatments.[13]

HOW DOES OZONE WORK IN TREATING HERNIATED DISC PAIN?

Writing in the journal *Pain Physician,* Vahid Eslami, M.D., and Vafa Rahimi-Movaghar, M.D., of the Tehran University of Medical Sciences in Iran outlined the four major ways that oxygen-ozone injections are successful in treating herniated intervertebral disc (HID) disorders:

1. Ozone has an effect on the inflammatory cascade by altering the breakdown of arachidonic acid to inflammatory prostaglandins. As a result, by reducing the inflammatory components, there is a subsequent decrease in pain.
2. Herniation can impinge on the venous and arterial flow and cause phlebostasis and arteriostenosis, which leads to a serious

hypoxemia of the area. By applying the ozone to the herniated site, hyperoxygenation of the area occurs, which reduces the pain by direct and indirect mechanisms.

3. This mechanism of action is the direct effect of the ozone as a rapid and strong oxidizing agent. The ozone molecule breaks down some of the glycosaminoglycan chains in the nucleus pulposus and reduces their ability to hold water, thereby diminishing the size of the herniation and subsequently contributing to pain relief.

4. The stimulation of fibroblastic activity by ozone will result in the initiation of the repair process by stimulating collagen deposition.[14]

LUMBAR SCIATIC PAIN

From September 1995 to April 1997, physicians at the Istituto Chirurgico Ortopedico Traumatologico in Latina, Italy, treated over one thousand patients suffering from lumbar sciatic pain with oxygen-ozone injections as an alternative to surgery. Of this group, fifty patients were studied who had received periodic injections of oxygen and ozone. Three- and six-month follow-up examinations were conducted. The results showed 68 percent positive results (40 percent excellent and 28 percent good) and 32 percent negative results (10 percent underwent surgery and 22 percent had to continue medical and physical treatment). Computed tomography (CT) scans (which apparently use different criteria) revealed 82 percent positive results (36 percent excellent, 46 percent good), with no major changes between pre- and post-treatment scans in the remaining 18 percent. The researchers concluded:

Ozone therapy, thanks to its ease of execution and noninvasiveness, permits the successful outpatient treatment of lumbar sciatic pain. Moreover, the lack of major complications and the good results obtained compared to other methods, such as chemonucleolysis, percutaneous automated discectomy, microsurgery and conventional surgery, suggest that ozone therapy can be considered the treatment of choice for lumbar sciatic pain and a valid alternative to surgery in many cases.[15]

A later Italian study involving 2,200 patients was carried out by physicians at the neuroradiology department at the Antonio Cardarelli Hospital in Naples. Most patients received treatment with oxygen-ozone injections and physical therapy for at least two months. No side effects were reported. After six months, researchers found an impressive 80 percent success and 20 percent failure rate among 1,750 patients; after eighteen months, the rate dropped to 75 percent success and 25 percent failure among 1,400 patients.[16]

Similar results were reported by Dr. Matteo Bonetti and colleagues at the Istituto Clinico Citta di Brescia, also in Italy. In this randomized, controlled study, a total of 306 patients suffering from low back pain and sciatica (161 with primary disc disease and 145 with nondisc vertebral disease) were treated either with oxygen-ozone injections or with steroids. Results were evaluated after six months. Clinical outcomes were poor among 15.1 percent of the eighty-one patients with disc disease receiving ozone and in 22.5 percent of eighty patients receiving steroids. Among the patients without disc disease, 8.6 percent of seventy patients receiving ozone had a poor outcome, while 21.4 percent of the seventy-five patients taking steroids had a poor outcome. The researchers concluded: "Oxygen-ozone treatment was highly effective in relieving acute and chronic lower back pain and sciatica. The gas mixture can be administered as a first treatment to replace epidural steroids."[17]

SPONDYLOLYSIS

Dr. Bonetti and his colleagues later undertook a clinical trial on patients with first-degree spondylolisthesis and spondylolysis, two very painful lower-back conditions. They chose eighteen patients with low back pain and sciatica (with radiological and CT scan diagnoses of spondylolisthesis and spondylolysis) who had had no success with physical therapy and traditional medical management. Following oxygen-ozone injections into the lysis points guided by CT scan, fifteen (83.3 percent) experienced a complete remission of pain. Follow-up visits at one, three, and six months after treatment revealed no reported recurrence of pain.[18]

Cervical spondylosis normally occurs in adults aged fifty or older. It is a disorder in which there is abnormal wear on the cartilage and bones of the neck (cervical vertebrae). It is a common cause of chronic neck pain.

A group of physicians at the 316th Hospital of the People's Liberation Army in Beijing studied the effect of a unique newly patented therapeutic ozone and laser combined puncture needle on patients.

A total of fifty-eight patients diagnosed with cervical spondylosis were chosen for this novel study. All were treated with the ozone and laser combined puncture needle between August 2008 and February 2010. Visual analog scale (VAS) scores were evaluated before treatment and at one month, three months, and six months after treatment. *The visual analog scale is a psychometric response scale used in patient questionnaires. It is an instrument for measuring a patient's feelings or attitudes regarding pain.*

The VAS score of preoperative neck and shoulder pain was (6.57±1.34), which decreased to 1.80±0.65 at one week after treatment. Pain was completely alleviated by the end of one month (with VAS scores of 0~2 after one month, three months, and six months after treatment). VAS scores did not exhibit any significant rebound within six months after treatment. After six months, 29 patients were rated "excellent," 23 were "good," and 6 were "fair," with the overall "excellent" and "good" rate at 89.6 percent.

The doctors concluded: "Ozone and laser combined therapy via puncture needle for the treatment of cervical spondylosis is safe and effective."[19]

JOINT PAIN AND PROLOZONE THERAPY

Derived from the word *ozone* and the Latin word *proli* (to regenerate or rebuild), Prolozone therapy was developed by Dr. Frank Shallenberger. It involves injecting a mixture of ozone gas, procaine, vitamin B_{12}, and selected homeopathic preparations into soft tissues, ligaments, and/or tendons where they attach to the bone. This causes a localized inflammation and anabolic (muscle-building) effect in these weak areas, which then increases the blood supply and stimulates the deposition of fibroblasts, the cells that the body uses to repair damaged connective tissue. Dr. Shallenberger writes:

> Ozone stimulates the cells called fibroblasts and chondroblasts to lay down more collagen and cartilage, and in this way actually heals damaged joints and ligaments. Many patients who were told, "you need a total knee or hip replacement," are still out running around years later after a series of ozone injections. Injecting ozone into injured or degenerated backs, hips, knees, shoulders, or necks is very rewarding.[20]

Shallenberger uses this method to treat patients suffering from a wide variety of chronic pain syndromes, including neck pain, whiplash, degenerated or herniated discs, carpal tunnel syndrome, torn tendons, TMJ (temporomandibular joint) syndrome, sciatica, heel spurs, neuromas, tennis elbow, rotator cuff tears, knee injuries, and other sports injuries. He also finds Prolozone useful in reducing scar tissue due to accidents or surgery. Shallenberger writes, "When Prolozone therapy is administered correctly, there is an 85 percent chance for the chronic pain sufferer to become completely pain free."[21]

In October 2005 I attended a seminar devoted to Prolozone therapy conducted by Dr. Shallenberger for physicians and witnessed impressive results. Many of the patients complaining of chronic joint pain found almost immediate relief, although a series of four or five treatments is recommended over a period of several months. Figure 14.1 on page 223 shows a patient receiving a Prolozone injection.

MANDIBULAR OSTEOMYELITIS

Mandibular osteomyelitis is an infectious inflammation of the lower jaw marked by local death and separation of tissue. Russian physicians studied a group of patients suffering from this disease and treated them both locally and generally with oxygen-ozone. They concluded: "Medical ozone exposure promoted more complete and rapid normalization of nonspecific resistance and T-cellular immunity, thus accelerating clinical cure and reducing the incidence of complications."[22]

OSTEOARTHRITIS

Osteoarthritis, sometimes called degenerative joint disease, is a slowly progressive disease in which joint cartilage breaks down. When osteoarthritis (OA) occurs, cartilage becomes thin and irregular, resulting in symptoms of joint pain and stiffness. It most often affects the hips, knees, hands, and spine.

At the Center of Medical-Surgical Studies in Cuba, sixty patients with osteoarthritis (mostly affecting the knee) were given one intra-articular injection of ozone per week for a total of ten weeks. Of the sixty patients, only four experienced the return of painful symptoms after two months, while the majority (93.3 percent) were symptom free. The researchers concluded that this easily applied and low-cost therapy produced "disappearance of pain after the first several ozone applications, as well as diminished clinical inflammation of the joints and restoration of normal joint movement."[23]

One of the current trends in oxygen therapy research has involved evaluating the value of medical ozone as an adjuvant to other types of medical therapy. *Adjuvant* has been defined as a substance or therapy that enhances the effectiveness of another medicine or form of treatment.

One such a study was carried out by researchers at the Beijing Geriatric Hospital to evaluate the clinical effectiveness of ozone therapy in combination with fugui gutong granule (FGG, a traditional Chinese medicine prepared with eight different herbs) in treating middle-aged and elderly patients with knee osteoarthritis (KOA) due to what the Chinese call "yang-deficiency induced cold-damp syndrome (YDICDS)."

Two hundred patients diagnosed with knee osteoarthritis were randomly assigned to four groups: the control group (Group A), the Chinese medicine treatment group (Group B), the ozone group (Group C), and the Chinese-medicine treatment plus ozone group (Group D). Patients in Group A took oral Voltaren, a nonsteroidal anti-inflammatory drug. Those in Group B took FGG. Patients in Group C received an oxygen-ozone injection (10 to 18 ml) in the knee joint cavity at 25 mg/L, once weekly for four weeks. Those in Group D received oxygen-ozone injections plus FGG. The therapeutic course for all participants in the study was one month. The efficacy of the various treatments was assessed using the visual analogue scale (VAS) and Western Ontario and MacMaster Universities Osteoarthritis Index (WOMAC).

The researchers found that the VAS score was markedly lower in Group D than in Group B and Group A at twenty-four hours and one week after the first treatment. After one month of treatment, the VAS score was markedly lower in Group D than in Groups A, B, and C. After treatment, the WOMAC score was 25.34 in Group D, which was substantially lower than that in Group A (44.72), Group B (40.58), and Group C (38.53). The pain score, the joint stiffness score, and the score for daily activities were lower in Group D than in Group A. The level of cure was 76.0 percent in Group D, which was much higher than that of Group A (25 percent), Group B (25 percent), and Group C (43.8 percent). Ozone therapy alone worked better than any other method tested but was even more effective when combined with fugui gutong.[24]

An article appearing in *ScienceDaily* highlighted a study done at two Brazilian institutions—the Federal University of São Paulo and the Paulista School of Medicine—designed to find out if ozone and oxygen injected into joints would reduce pain, increase joint function, and improve the quality of life of patients diagnosed with osteoarthritis.

The researchers followed ninety-eight people through the course of the study. Sixty-three of the participants received 10 ml injections of oxygen-ozone throughout the study, and thirty-five received 10 ml injections of air as a placebo. The researchers evaluated the participants at the beginning of the study, after their fourth and eighth injections, and eight weeks after their last injection. They paid special attention to changes in pain, joint function, and the ability to sit, stand, and walk.

Timed up and go tests (known as "TUG tests") were performed on members of both groups to determine the time it took to stand up, walk a set distance, return, and sit. The researchers found no significant differences in how the two groups performed in these tests. However, the group receiving oxygen-ozone injections had significantly better results in tests that measured pain, function, and overall health throughout the course of the study. At the end of the study, participants were given a quality-of-life survey (obtained using the Short Form-36 Health Survey). Participants in the ozone group reported improvement in all areas that pertain to quality of life after their fourth injection.

The researchers, who presented their results at the annual meeting of the American College of Rheumatology in San Francisco in November 2015, concluded, "We think the work means that ozone can give the patient a better quality of life with less pain and more independence in daily life activities. . . . Ozone is also capable of delaying the need for joint replacement surgery. It is a tool for the clinician to reduce pain or to help control it."[25]

Figure 14.1. Patient receiving a Prolozone injection for lower back pain. (Photograph by Nathaniel Altman.)

OSTEOPOROSIS

Dr. Kief has also treated patients suffering from osteoporosis, a degenerative disease involving a lack of calcium and the resultant softening of the bones. During my visit to his clinic, he spoke of a seventy-two-year-old patient suffering from both immune vascularitis (inflammation of the blood vessels) and advanced osteoporosis. The patient was first given autohemotherapy, followed by long-term autohomologous immunotherapy (AHIT), which Dr. Kief believes is more effective.[26] After one year, X-rays showed the normal calcification of bones, as seen in figure 14.2 on page 225.

RHEUMATOID ARTHRITIS

Rheumatoid arthritis is a chronic, systemic disease that causes one's joints to swell up and become painful. It is usually treated with anti-inflammatory drugs. Research carried out at Cuba's Institute of Rheumatology in 1988 compared the effectiveness of ozone and anti-inflammatory drugs on seventeen patients. In this study doctors administered a very low dose (0.7 mg) of ozone intramuscularly each day to ten patients for eight weeks, while the control group of seven patients was given traditional anti-inflammatory drugs. In all areas of criteria (including morning stiffness, painful movements, onset of fatigue, strength of handclasp, and joint swelling), the patients who received ozone scored approximately 25 percent better than those receiving drug therapy. In addition, these patients suffered no adverse side effects, while all the nonozonated patients either had to receive additional steroids or suffered symptoms of gastritis.[27]

Approximately 10 percent of all patients seeking care at the Kief Clinic in Germany suffer from rheumatoid arthritis. In a statistical study of eighty-four such patients receiving AHIT therapy, Dr. Kief reported the following results: 16 percent experienced a full remission of symptoms, 36 percent showed significant improvement (including a

Figure 14.2. X-ray photographs of a seventy-two-year-old patient with osteoporosis, before and after major autohemotherapy. (Photographs courtesy of Dr. Horst Kief.)

decrease in swelling, improved mobility, and less pain), 32 percent experienced some improvement, and 12 percent had no improvement at all. Apparently 4 percent dropped out of the study.[28]

TMD/TMJD PAIN

Temporomandibular joint dysfunction (TMD or TMJD)—also known as *temporomandibular joint dysfunction syndrome*—is a general term covering pain and dysfunction of the muscles that move the jaw and the joints that connect the jaw to the skull. A pioneer study carried out by researchers at the Cumhuriyet University School of Medicine in Turkey found that high-frequency bio-oxidative therapy proved more effective than medication in treating painful temporomandibular joint (TMJ) disorder.

Sixty-three patients were chosen for this study. Thirty were given three medications—Ketoprofen, Bi-Profenid, and thiocolchicoside—for seven days. The thirty-three others received oxygen-ozone therapy through an Omega probe to both joint sides. The researchers wrote about this novel delivery method: "Inside the glass probe, which is formed by a double glass camera, is a mixture of noble gases that conducts and emits electromagnetic energy. When the tip of the probe comes into contact with the body, it emits energy around the treated area and splits environmental, diatomic oxygen into singular atomic oxygen and ozone." These treatments were administered for ten minutes three times during the week. There were no reports of pain, although patients felt a mild increase in temperature in the areas treated.

After a week of treatments, the researchers found that 24 percent of the medicated group showed a significant reduction in TMJ pain, while the figure for patients treated with ozone was 29 percent. Four patients in the group treated with ozone did not complain of any pain after treatment, while none of the patients treated with medication had complete relief. The authors concluded, "The study showed that bio-oxidative therapy was a more effective treatment than medication therapy for relieving TMJ pain."[29]

FAILED BACK SURGERY SYNDROME

A pilot study was undertaken by researchers at the School of Medicine of the University of São Paulo to evaluate the effects of ozone administered by spinal endoscopy in patients with chronic pain related to failed back surgery. Spinal endoscopy is a procedure in which a small endoscope is passed up through the tailbone into the epidural space. It is sometimes used to allow medications to better reach the affected areas, especially the spinal nerve roots.

The investigators studied thirteen patients of both sexes between the ages of eighteen and seventy suffering from persistent chronic pain (i.e., for more than six months) in the lumbar region and in the lower limbs related to failed back surgery. Pain was classified as neuropathic (nerve-related) and non-neuropathic of the lumbar spine and legs, based on the DN4 (Douleur Neuropathique 4) questionnaire. The patients received the ozone gas in the lumbar epidural space via spinal-sacral endoscopy. Clinical evaluations were performed before, twenty-four hours after, and one month, three months, and six months after intervention using both a visual analog scale and the Oswestry Disability Index (ODI).

The researchers found that overall, at six months patients had a 43.7 percent reduction in lumbar pain and a 60.9 percent reduction in leg pain, followed by a 44.0 percent improvement in ODI scores. They also found that reduction of pain and better scores in the disability index were markedly greater in patients with non-neuropathic predominant pain; patients saw 95.2 percent, 80.6 percent, and 75.3 percent improvement in lumbar pain, leg pain, and ODI respectively. By contrast, patients with neuropathic predominant pain experienced only 12.5 percent, 42.4 percent, and 20.9 percent improvement, respectively. No infectious complications were observed during either treatment or follow-up.

The researchers concluded, "The present data suggests that epidural ozone might be a therapeutic option for persistent low back pain, especially in non-neuropathic predominant pain patients, but double-blind controlled studies are still required to prove its efficacy."[30]

FIBROMYALGIA

Fibromyalgia is a chronic disease affecting over five million Americans. Its exact cause is unknown but is believed to involve psychological, genetic, neurobiological, and environmental factors. Although generalized pain is considered to be the primary symptom, many other associated symptoms are common, especially sleep disturbance, chronic fatigue, anxiety, and depression.

A pilot study was undertaken by researchers at the Universities of Granada and Almeria in Spain along with scientists from the National Center for Scientific Research in Cuba to evaluate the effectiveness and tolerability of ozone therapy by rectal insufflation as an add-on therapy in fibromyalgia management.

A total of thirty-six patients diagnosed with fibromyalgia (thirty-three women and three men) were recruited for this study. They received twenty-four sessions of ozone therapy during a twelve-week period. At each session, the administered dose of ozone was 8 mg (200 ml of gas, at a concentration of 40 µg/ml). Ozone sessions were given five days a week during the first two weeks, twice a week from weeks three through six, and weekly from weeks seven through twelve. The Fibromyalgia Impact Questionnaire was the main measure of outcome, and it was administered when the study began and at weeks four, eight, and twelve. Secondary outcome measures, administered at the beginning and end of the study, included the Pittsburgh Sleep Quality Index, the Beck Depression Inventory, the State-Trait Anxiety Inventory, and the SF-12, the abbreviated form of the Short Form Health Survey. Adverse reactions to treatment were also recorded.

The researchers found that the total scores of the Fibromyalgia Impact Questionnaire decreased significantly during the study period, with the decrease being observed in the first four weeks of the study. Significant improvement was also seen both in depression scores and in the physical summary score of the SF-12. Most of the positive effects of ozone therapy had to do with a reduction of physical symptoms, but depression was reduced in 47 percent of the patients. Transient meteorism (distension of the abdomen due to air or gas in the intestine) after ozone therapy sessions was the most frequently reported side effect, and it impacted approximately 36 percent of the patients at some point during treatment.

The researchers concluded, "At the dose and number of sessions used in this study, ozone therapy by rectal insufflation seems to be beneficial for physical symptoms and depression of fibromyalgia."[31]

15
Neurodegenerative Disorders

PARKINSON'S DISEASE

A pioneer study to determine the effectiveness of ozone therapy in the treatment of Parkinson's disease was undertaken by researchers at the 10 de Octubre Clinical-Surgical Hospital and the National Center for Scientific Research in Cuba. Eighty elderly patients between sixty and seventy-nine years of age diagnosed with Parkinson's syndrome were given fifteen sessions of rectal ozone insufflation plus physical therapy over a three-week period. Complete neurological and psychometric exams were given before and after therapy.

According to the researchers' report at the Second International Symposium on Ozone Applications in 1997: "The results demonstrated that all symptoms and signs improved after the treatment, fundamentally the rigidity (95.7%), the gait (95.3%) and the bradiphrasia (88.8%). The Daily Life Activities improved in 95% of the treated patients. [No] side-effect or intolerance were observed during the treatment. In general, an improvement in the quality of life of these patients, increasing their autonomy for a much longer period was achieved."[1]

SENILE DEMENTIA

A double-blind study was carried out at the Department of Geriatrics of the Salvador Allende Hospital in Havana, Cuba, on sixty elderly patients suffering from senile dementia. The first group of thirty received ozone-oxygen therapy via rectal insufflation for twenty-one days, while the second group (the controls) received insufflations of oxygen alone. Before and after the study, all patients were carefully evaluated by clinical examination (including CT scans and electroencephalograms), psychometrical tests (which measured intelligence, aptitude, behavior, and emotional reactions), and other standardized diagnostic tests for senile dementia.

Among members of the first group, 85 percent of the patients showed overall improvement in their symptoms of vascular and degenerative dementia. Specifically, 73 percent experienced marked improvement in their medical status, 83 percent showed improvement in their mental condition, 83 percent were better able to self-administer their medications, and 80 percent had a greater ability to interact socially and manage their daily activities. By contrast, there was no improvement among any of the members of the control group in any of the categories. No adverse side effects were noted among the patients receiving ozone therapy.[2]

Another Cuban study evaluating the long-term benefits of ozone therapy on patients suffering from senile dementia was carried out at the Camilo Cienfuegos Provincial hospital in Sancti Spiritus. Thirty patients were chosen for the study; all were diagnosed with Alzheimer's dementia, multi-infarction dementia, and vascular epilepsy. Ozone (typically between 100 and 200 ml at a concentration of 30 to 40 mg/L) was administered for twenty sessions via rectal insufflation every three months over a two-year period. The findings substantiated the results of the other Cuban studies: although complete cures were not achieved, clinical improvement was noted in twenty-one patients (70 percent), seven patients (23 percent) remained the same, and two patients (7 percent) got worse.[3]

By 2006 over eight hundred elderly patients had been treated with ozone at the Salvador Allende Hospital for senile dementia and Alzheimer's disease. While Cuban physicians do not believe that ozone therapy is a cure for senile dementia, the marked improvement in the overall quality of life of the patients (and their families) has made ozone treatment a standard part of the therapeutic protocol at the Department of Geriatrics. Doctors note greater physical energy among the patients and an improved ability to manage their daily lives. There is also a marked relief of symptoms of depression among patients suffering from Alzheimer's disease.

After an initial two-week cycle of treatment, patients often return to the hospital once a year for an additional week of ozone therapy. No other medications are given.[4]

MULTIPLE SCLEROSIS

In Europe ozone therapy is an emerging therapeutic technique that is gaining increasing importance in treating neurological disorders. Dr. Filippo Molinari of the Politecnico di Torino and colleagues from other research institutions in Italy sought to find a validated and standard methodology to assess the effect of ozone therapy on brain metabolism and circulation. They decided to use a near-infrared spectroscopy (NIRS) system to monitor the cerebral metabolism and a transcranial Doppler (TCD) to monitor the blood flow velocity in the middle cerebral arteries before and after the administration of ozone therapy. The results of their study were published in the *International Journal of Immunopathology and Pharmacology*.

Fifty-four subjects (thirty-two neurological patients and twenty-two controls) were tested before, during, and after major autohemotherapy (MAHT). The researchers monitored the concentration changes in the level of oxygenated and deoxygenated hemoglobin (hemoglobin is a protein in red blood cells that carries oxygen throughout the body) and in the level of cytochrome c oxidase (CYT-c). Cytochrome c is an intermediate in apoptosis, a controlled form of cell death used to kill cells in the process of development or in response to infection or DNA damage. As a primary endpoint of the work, the researchers showed the changes in the brain metabolism and circulation of the group of study participants.

They found that the concentration of oxygenated hemoglobin increased after MAHT and remained higher than it had been at the beginning for another 1.5 hours. The concentration of deoxygenated hemoglobin decreased during the therapy and the CYT-c concentration markedly increased about one hour after MAHT. No significant changes were observed on the blood flow velocity.

As a secondary endpoint, researchers compared the NIRS metabolic pattern of twenty remitting-relapsing multiple sclerosis (MS) patients against twenty controls. They found that the MS subjects showed a marked increase of CYT-c activity and concentration about 40 minutes after the end of MAHT, possibly revealing a reduction of the chronic oxidative stress level that is typical of MS sufferers.

From a technical point of view, this preliminary study showed that NIRS could be useful to show the effects of MAHT at the cerebral level, which could be monitored over the long term. The researchers concluded: "The clinical result of this study is the quantitative measurement of the CYT-c level changes in MS induced by ozone autohemotherapy."[5]

16
Diabetes

Diabetes mellitus is reaching epidemic proportions in many industrialized nations, particularly the United States. While diet, exercise, and insulin are all useful in controlling this incurable degenerative disease, therapeutic ozone has been shown to be of benefit as well.

A study was carried out with forty-seven diabetics who suffered from "neuroinfected diabetic foot" at the National Institute of Angiology and Vascular Surgery in Havana, Cuba, during the 1990s. Amputation is sometimes required if the patient does not improve in these cases. The participants in this study, who had all suffered from diabetes for nine to nineteen years, were divided into three groups and treated for a total of ten days.

Group 1 (sixteen subjects) was given ozone therapy, which consisted of a combination of regular wound cleansing with ozonated water followed by daily treatments with an ozone bag for two hours. Ozonated sunflower oil was then applied to the foot. Patients in this group also received alternating daily sessions of either intra-arterial injections or autohemotherapy, totaling three to five treatments with each method. Group 2 (sixteen subjects) was treated externally with cane sugar in the form of a syrup. This folk remedy was applied to the wound daily. A bandage was applied to keep the syrup in contact with the skin for twenty-four hours. Group 3 (fifteen patients) received oral, parenteral (outside the intestines), and intravenous antibiotics as well as traditional medications applied externally to the wound.

The results were classified simply as "good" or "bad." "Good" meant that surgery was avoided, while "bad" indicated that some type of surgical intervention was needed to amputate the infected area.

Treatment	Good	Bad
Group 1 (ozone therapy)	15 (93.75%)	1 (6.25%)
Group 2 (cane sugar)	13 (81.25%)	3 (18.75%)
Group 3 (antibiotics)	10 (66.67%)	5 (33.33%)

The researchers concluded that ozone therapy was the most effective method of treatment for neuroinfected diabetic foot, while sugar cane was a good alternative when ozone therapy was not available. Conventional treatment with antibiotics was considered the least desirable therapy for this particular symptom.[1]

As it is in many Western countries, diabetes is a major health problem in Russia. A group of Russian physicians investigated the therapeutic use of medical ozone in treating patients with diabetes and reported their findings at the Second International Symposium on Ozone Applications, which took place in Havana in March 1997.

A total of thirty-eight adults who were diagnosed with diabetes in varying degrees of severity were selected; twenty suffered from diabetes mellitus type 1, and eighteen were diagnosed with diabetes mellitus type 2. Twenty-two of the patients (58 percent) suffered from related health complaints such as dry mouth, low resistance to infection, and cardiovascular problems. Patients were given intravenous injections of ozonated saline solution as well as rectal insufflations of oxygen and ozone. The course of therapy lasted for several weeks and included a total of seven to ten treatments, depending on the patient.

All subjects showed improvement over the course of therapy. Many stopped complaining of dry mouth, thirst, frequent urination, and itching, tingling, and numbness in the hands and feet. Tests showed a 50 percent average reduction of glucose levels in the blood several hours after the first treatment. After the course of therapy, glucose levels among the patients had dropped an average of 30 percent. This led the majority of the patients to reduce their doses of insulin. Positive dynamics involving lipid spectrum, coagulagram and immunogram, a rise in antioxidant activity in the blood, and lowering of lipid peroxidation products were found as well. The researchers concluded: "Ozone therapy may be used in a complex treatment of people suffering from diabetes and allows them to lower doses of the usage of sugar reduced preparations."[2]

In Russia, ozone therapy has become popular in treating vascular complications brought about by diabetes. A study to determine the efficacy of various methods of ozone treatment involved twenty-one patients with diabetes mellitus type 1 and ninety-seven patients with diabetes mellitus type 2, complicated by angiopathy of the lower limbs and diabetic retinopathy. Ninety-six patients received sugar-reducing drugs and three forms of ozone therapy. These included the ozone "boot" method as an external application, and IV infusions of ozonated saline solutions and rectal insufflations as internal applications. Some patients received both internal and external therapies. Researchers found that the combined external and internal methods brought superior results, while the internal and combined methods proved better for treating retinopathy.[3]

Russian physicians at the Medical Academy at Nizhny Novgorod have extensive clinical experience using ozone in the treatment of diabetes. They believe that ozone therapy is effective because it improves the penetration of cellular membranes for glucose. It is achieved by stimulating the pentose-phosphate pathway and aerobic glycolysis, which are inhibited when diabetes mellitus is present. They also found that ozone can help decrease hyperglycemia due to the improved transport of glucose into body tissues.

In one study, physicians observed a group of seventy patients with insulin-dependent and non-insulin-dependent diabetes. After the course of ozone therapy, they found that the average level of hyperglycemia had a 26 percent decrease. They wrote:

Ozone activates glucose metabolism that results in increasing content of 2,3 diphosphoglycerate in erythrocytes which provides better oxygen supply into the tissues. Patients with diabetes mellitus have the so called glycosylated hemoglobin forming very strong bonds with oxygen, thus, inducing hypoxia and determining the severity of the disease. That is why hypoxia control with the help of ozone therapy is of the key importance in the course of treatment.[4]

In *Ozone Therapy in Practice: Health Manual,* the authors mentioned six methods of ozone treatment:

1. Intravenous infusions with ozonated saline solutions
2. Rectal insufflations
3. Major autohemotherapy
4. Minor autohemotherapy
5. Subcutaneous microinjections with ozone/oxygen mixture
6. Stimulation of biological active points with ozone/oxygen injections[5]

Protocols

The recommended basic treatment for diabetes mellitus includes eight to ten intravenous infusions of ozonated saline or rectal insufflations every second day. If autohemotherapy is chosen, treatments are done twice a week over a period of three to four weeks.

In cases of diabetes mellitus type 2 they recommend also stimulating biologically active points with oxygen-ozone injections. In signs of secondary immune deficiency (pustular inflammatory diseases), in addition to the basic course of treatment subcutaneous microinjections with an ozone/oxygen mixture are done in the area of diseased tissue. Minor autohemotherapy is done every second day, totaling six to eight procedures for the course.

In their clinical research, doctors found that ozone therapy was successful in 92 percent of insulin-dependent cases and 89 percent of non-insulin-dependent cases. They saw a decrease of hyperglycemia and a reduction in thirst, as well as a disappearance of polyuria, pruritus, and general weakness among treated patients.

They also found that patients who underwent the course of ozone therapy could reduce doses of glucose-reducing preparations by 20 to 25 percent for a period of three to six months after treatment. They also found that ozone therapy proved to be effective in the treatment of diabetes mellitus patients with complications. For example, in patients with diabetic foot syndrome, ozone therapy—when combined with traditional topical treatments—helped heal diabetic ulcers in half the normal time. This helped reduce the number of limb amputations, crippling, and death.[6]

Perhaps the most ambitious clinical research to date was reported in the *European Journal of Pharmacology* in 2005 by a team of scientists affiliated with the University of Havana, the National Center for Scientific Research, and the Institute of Angiology and Vascular Surgery in Cuba and the University of Ancona and the University of Milan in Italy.

The randomized clinical trial involved 101 patients with type 2 diabetes and diabetic foot who were divided into two groups. One group of fifty-two subjects was treated with ozone (both locally and through rectal insufflation), while the other group of forty-nine subjects was treated with topical and systemic antibiotics. Both groups were evaluated after twenty days of treatment.

The results among the patients treated with ozone were impressive, even though they were given only fifteen insufflations over the three-week period. In the group treated with ozone, there was a greater decrease in the size of lesions, along with an increase in the number cured, with fewer amputations. The average duration of hospital stays decreased among this group, and the cost of the therapy was approximately 25 percent less than treatment with antibiotics. The researchers reported: "Ozone treatment improved glycemic control, prevented oxidative stress, normalized levels of organic peroxides, and activated superoxide dismutase,"[7] which catalyzes the dismutation of superoxide into oxygen and hydrogen peroxide and therefore is important in antioxidant defense.

The glucose concentrations of the group treated with antibiotics did not change, while hypoglycemia decreased and glucose concentrations moved to within the normal range in the group treated with ozone. The researchers concluded: "This 'antidiabetic' effect produced by ozone treatment seems to be associated with the antioxidant properties of ozone, increasing insulin sensitivity even when taking into account the resistance to hypoglycemic drugs that these patients demonstrated before the beginning of the ozone treatment."[8]

European scientists have found that type 2 diabetes mellitus is associated with multiple metabolic disturbances that result in the excessive production of reactive oxygen species and oxidative stress. These reactive oxygen species set in motion a host of redox reactions that can contribute to additional redox stress. (The term *redox* refers to a chemical reaction between two substances in which one substance is oxidized and the other reduced.)[9]

Researchers from the departments of Biotechnology, Chemistry, and Physics at the University of Siena in Italy and the Maastricht University Medical Center in the Netherlands pointed out that while orthodox Western medicine has made great strides in managing the symptoms of type 2 diabetes, it has not been able to reestablish a normal redox system in the body because diabetes medications cannot reactivate the body's cellular antioxidant system.

Writing in the journal *Annals of Translational Medicine,* they proposed that physicians integrate ozone therapy with orthodox medicine in order to interrupt this vicious circle. They cited the safety and effectiveness of the "chemical messengers" produced by medical ozone, specifically hydrogen peroxide and alkenal adducts (a type of enzyme) transferred to billions of cells of the organism to strengthen the body's antioxidant system and normalize the redox system. They added, "The activation of the Nrf2 protein [a protein that protects against oxidative damage triggered by injury and inflammation] and the upregulation of the synthesis of some 220 genes allow the enzymatic activation of the defense system in all organs."

They suggested that one treatment of ozone therapy per week performed for several years could definitely improve recovery for type 2 diabetes patients.[10]

These remarkable clinical results show that medical ozone treatment can be an effective, safe, and cost-efficient way to help manage diabetes and its related complications, either alone or as a complementary therapy. It would be useful to explore if ozone, when combined with diet and exercise, can also be an effective form of preventive therapy for the growing number of individuals who are predisposed to this debilitating and often devastating disease.

17
Gynecology and Obstetrics

GYNECOLOGICAL INFECTIONS

By 1990 over a dozen clinical studies had been carried out in Cuba regarding the effects of ozonated sunflower oil on a variety of gynecological infections, including leukorrhea, herpes, and vulvovaginitis. One such study took place at the Pasteur Polyclinic in Havana with a group of sixty women suffering from vulvovaginitis. Of these women, 97 percent had *Candida albicans, Trichomonas,* and *Gardnerella vaginalis.*

Thirty patients were treated with ozonated sunflower oil, twenty received normal medical therapy, and the remaining ten were given a placebo consisting of oil without ozone. The criteria for cure was determined by examination with a colposcope, a special instrument used to examine the vagina and cervix.

All of the patients who used ozonated oil were completely cured within five to seven days. In the control group, 20 percent were cured within ten to fifteen days. All of the subjects receiving the placebo experienced a worsening of symptoms.[1]

Other studies have been carried out in Russia. One study at the Department of Obstetrics and Gynecology at the Sechenov Medical Academy in Moscow evaluated the effectiveness of ozone on 112 women suffering from a variety of infections, including inflammation of the fallopian tubes, genital herpes, condyloma (wart-like growths on the genitals), and pelvic peritonitis. Depending on the case, patients received either 5 mg of vaginally insufflated ozone daily, topical applications of ozonated oil, or irrigation or intra-abdominal injections of ozonated solutions at a concentration of 4 to 6 mg/ml. The treatments brought substantial relief, leading the doctors to declare that ozone has strong immunomodulative, antiviral, and analgesic properties.[2]

Research in the effectiveness of ozone on acute condyloma was undertaken at the same institute with fifty-three women. They were given from eight to ten local applications of different ozonated solutions, such as oil and water. Symptoms in all patients disappeared by the end of treatment. All but two patients remained free of symptoms after eight months. One of the two was retreated and never experienced condyloma symptoms again.[3]

British researchers at the Maidstone General Hospital in Kent undertook a clinical study involving thirty women diagnosed with recurrent bacterial vaginosis. All were treated one time with a vaginal infusion of 3 percent solution of hydrogen peroxide, which was left for 3 minutes and then drained. Patients were reassessed three weeks after treatment.

A total of twenty-three women completed the study, and of this group, symptoms cleared completely in eighteen (78 percent), improved in three (13 percent), and remained unchanged in two (9 percent). Vaginal acidity was restored to normal in all but one patient, and no side effects were observed in any of the treated women. The researchers concluded: "Hydrogen peroxide (3%) used as a single vaginal wash was as effective as any other agent in current use in clearing the vaginal malodour of bacterial vaginosis at 3 weeks after treatment."[4]

THREATENED MISCARRIAGE

An unusual Russian study was undertaken by physicians at the Medical Academy in Nizhny Novgorod to determine whether ozone therapy could help pregnant women avoid miscarriage. One hundred and ten pregnant women were selected for the study. All had had previous miscarriages and were determined to be in danger of another miscarriage by their physicians. Terms of pregnancy ranged from eight to twenty-two weeks.

After a complete physical exam, it was found that many of the women had low levels of several important hormones, including estriol, progesterone, placental lactogen, and cortisol. Researchers also discovered that many had poor immune levels, indicated in part by low phagocytic activity and deficient IgM (immunoglobulin gamma M) levels in the blood. Some of the expectant mothers also suffered from hormonal imbalances, infections like chlamydia, and immune disorders.

Ozone therapy was provided by intravenous applications of 0.9 percent ozonized sodium chloride (NaCl) solutions. A total of five infusions were given over a five-day period. The results were very encouraging. The researchers found the following:

1. Fetoplacental hormones (including estriol, progesterone, placental lactogen, prolactin, and cortisol) in the blood became normalized.
2. Immune levels improved, as evidenced by normalized levels of phagocytic stimulation and immune complexes in the blood.
3. Lipid peroxidation normalized, which appeared to help preserve the membranes of the placenta's cells from free radical damage.

Pregnancy was conserved in 89 percent of the women, who gave birth to healthy babies. The researchers concluded: "We didn't note any complications. . . . This allows us to recommend ozone in appropriate dose[s] for the treatment of the sick with threatened abortion of I–III trimester of pregnancy."[5]

A more recent Russian study was carried out at the I. M. Sechenov Moscow Medical Academy. Two groups of pregnant women diagnosed with placental insufficiency were studied. The placenta is the vascular organ that unites the fetus to the mother's uterus and mediates its metabolic exchanges; villi are small, slender vascular processes that help form the placenta. The larger and healthier the villi, the stronger the placenta and its ability to function properly.

One group received traditional therapy; the other was treated with ozone. The researchers concluded: "After ozone therapy, enlargement of terminal villi with true syncytiocapillary membranes was noted. A stimulating effect of ozone therapy on the growth and differentiation of terminal villi was established."[6]

Another clinical trial on threatened miscarriage was reported by Guennadi O. Gretchkanev of the Department of Obstetrics and Gynecology at the Medical Academy of Nizhny Novgorod. He and his associates observed 130 patients with threatened miscarriage, with ninety receiving daily ozone for five days (via IV saline drip) plus traditional medications, and forty getting conventional treatment only. Seventy women in their first trimester were placed in Group I, while sixty in their second trimester were placed in Group II.

The women receiving ozone showed a "credible decrease" in lipid peroxidation and an increase of total antioxidant activity after the second day. There was also evidence that there was a much faster easing of pain among those receiving ozone, plus improved sleep and appetite. Appearance of early toxicosis decreased or disappeared in 90 percent of the women receiving ozone. As a result, their traditional medications to control these problems were reduced or eliminated.

Speaking at the Fifteenth Ozone World Congress in London in 2001, Dr. Gretchkanev observed:

> We established quite favorable influence of ozone therapy on the efficiency of treatment of threatened abortion. So, owing to the complex therapeutic procedures with ozone the pregnancy was preserved and prolonged to the physiological terms of labor in 86% of patients inside I group [Group I] and in 85% inside II group [Group II]. In the control subgroups of I and II groups it was possible to preserve the pregnancy in 65% and 60% of cases, respectively.[7]

FALLOPIAN TUBE OBSTRUCTION

It has been estimated that between 8 and 10 percent of couples are infertile, which affects an estimated 60 million to 168 million people worldwide. Fallopian tube obstruction is the single major cause of female infertility, contributing to approximately 25 to 35 percent of cases.

A team of researchers at the Second Affiliated Hospital of Shaanxi University of Chinese Medicine enlisted four hundred infertile women in a clinical study that took place between August 2006 and January 2012. The patients were chosen from a group of 2,600 admitted to the hospital for recanalization surgery. The inclusion criteria were angiography-mediated preoperative diagnosis of tubal obstruction and concurrent exclusion of other potential causes of infertility. After surgery, half of the women were given conventional interventional treatment, while the other group received ozone.

The women in the conventional intervention treatment group had 20 ml of saline solution, which contained 5 mg of dexamethasone, 4,000 units of chymotrypsin, and 80,000 units of gentamicin, injected into their fallopian tubes.

Women in the ozone group were given between 5 ml and 10 ml of medical ozone, which was slowly injected via a 3F catheter under pressure to observe whether there was gas shadow in the pelvic cavity or whether the patient had any discomfort. Fallopian tube recanalization was indicated when the operator felt no resistance during injection, and then a contrast agent was injected to confirm the non-obstruction of the oviduct. Ozone was injected every other day in the treatment group one to two times after surgery, and ozone was injected three to seven days after menstrual clean in the next menstruation for one to two times, with no concurrent anti-inflammatory treatment.

No difference was observed between postoperative *proximal tube* (the opening located within the uterus) recanalization rates in the two groups. However, the researchers found that the postoperative *distal tube* (the opening located by the ovary) recanalization rate and the recanalization rate after six months were significantly higher in the treatment group. Importantly, the adhesion rates were significantly lower and conception rates were significantly higher in the treatment group when compared to the control group after six months. The pregnancy rate after twelve months was also significantly higher among the women who were treated with ozone. These results led the researchers to conclude that ozone therapy can potentially become a viable treatment modality for distal tubal obstruction patients.

Table 17.1. Outcome Measures in the Treatment and Control Intervention Groups

	Recanalization Rate after Operation (Total)		Recanalization Rate after 6 Months	Readhesion Rate	Pregnancy Rate after 12 Months
	Proximal segment	Distal segment			
Treatment group	85% (170/200)		93%	5%	59%
	94%	56%	(186/200)	(10/200)	(108/200)
Control group	81% (162/200)		79%	21%	43%
	93%	45%	(158/200)	(42/200)	(86/200)

The researchers outlined the advantages of using ozone in the field of gynecology:

- Ozone has high oxidative potential and ozone therapy can stimulate production of immunoglobulins in the blood, thus making it a potent agent to treat microbe-mediated gynecological inflammation.
- Ozone treatment improves the rheological properties and oxygen transportation mechanism of the blood, in turn destroying contact points of virus with body cells.
- Ozone does not have adverse effects commonly associated with other antimicrobials and microbes cannot develop resistance to ozone.

- Ozone treatment does not change the pH of the female reproductive system, thus preserving the beneficial vaginal flora.

The doctors concluded: "Our results are highly encouraging and hold promise for treating distal tubal obstruction in infertile females. The large number of patients involved in the current study also makes the conclusions more robust."[8]

18
Lung and
Bronchial Diseases

Few clinical studies have been done on the impact of oxidative therapies on pulmonary diseases, primarily because most scientists believe that breathing air polluted with ozone is always bad for health. Unfortunately, this belief carries over to other applications of ozone. Yet practitioners have discovered that ozone—administered as autohemotherapy or rectal insufflation—can be very useful in treating a wide range of pulmonary diseases, including asthma, emphysema, chronic obstructive pulmonary disease (COPD), pulmonary fibrosis, and acute respiratory distress syndrome.

Dr. Bocci believes that pulmonary diseases respond to ozone for numerous reasons. First, there is improved transport of oxygen with a consequent better oxygenation of ischemic tissues; the effects of lipid oxidation products (LOPs) and the release of prostacyclin, nitric oxide (NO), and interleukin-8 (IL-8) are able to enhance pulmonary function and reduce recurrent infections. Second, there are therapeutic effects of mild, calculated oxidative stress linked to repeated bland ozonated applications of authohemotherapy, which induce an adaptation to the chronic oxidative stress present in these diseases. Such adaptation is characterized by an intracellular enhancement of several antioxidant enzymes (SOD [superoxide dismutase], GSH-peroxidase [hepatic glutathione peroxidase], catalase, etc.) and, most importantly, heme oxygenase I, resulting in mild, continuous, stimulatory effects on the immune system. Dr. Bocci has also noted patient reports of frequent improvement of cenesthesia, the general feeling of inhabiting one's body that arises from multiple stimuli from various bodily organs.[1] Of course, such therapy must be performed without the patient ever breathing a trace of ozone, which can be exceptionally harmful.

BRONCHIAL ASTHMA

Only a small number of ozone studies have been undertaken with patients suffering from bronchial asthma. However, during a research visit to Cuba in 1994, I was introduced to an eleven-year-old boy attending a special school for the hearing-impaired whose asthma had been cured with ozone. Ricardo was originally treated for hypacusis, a disease of the inner ear that causes deafness. The ozone treatments he received provided a modest degree of hearing improvement, which was consistent with the results of the other students of the school who were also given ozone for hypacusis. However, along with improved hearing, Ricardo's parents and teachers noticed that his frequent asthma attacks gradually began to diminish, to the point that they almost completely disappeared.

Dr. Gilbert Glady, a French physician, reported his clinical experience with an asthma patient at the Eleventh Ozone World Conference, held in San Francisco in 1993 (the English in his written report has been corrected where necessary):

> Mrs. Nicole B., born in 1947, had been suffering from bronchial asthma since 1981. She was treated with Lomudal and Aminophylline as well as with antibiotics every time she was suffering from ear, nose, or throat infections. The tests showed an allergy to house dusts. We met her for the first time in December 1987 at a period when she had attacks of asthma nearly every day. An ozone treatment involving alternate doses of minor autohemotherapy in

the form of subcutaneous injections at the top of the lungs and major autohemotherapy was started in February 1988. . . .

After about ten sessions, the frequency of attacks of asthma had decreased substantially, although some secondary symptoms came up like moderate fever, moderate attacks of tetany [a nervous affection that can include numbness and tingling in the extremities], reintensification of asthma, and eczema. This was followed by general improvement.

The asthma vanished and the Lomudal treatment was stopped for good in November 1988, nine months after treatment began. Since then, this patient has not suffered from a single attack of asthma.[2]

Autohomologous immunotherapy (AHIT) has been used for patients suffering from bronchial asthma in Germany since 1987. Dr. Horst Kief, the developer of AHIT, reported on a study of sixty-five patients who were treated over a period of seven months. Dr. Kief found marked improvement in many patients, as indicated by a sharp decrease in or complete elimination of the medications they required to control asthma flares. Table 18.1 shows the results of his study.

Table 18.1. Asthma Medication Use

| Medication | Patients Using Medication | | | |
| | Before AHIT | | After AHIT | |
	No.	(%)	No.	(%)
Anti-allergic drugs	13	(20.0)	2	(3.1)
Mediator antagonists	21	(32.3)	8	(12.3)
Secretolytic drugs	19	(29.2)	7	(10.8)
Theophylline derivatives	25	(38.5)	15	(23.1)
Beta-2 agonists	46	(70.8)	12	(18.5)
Systemic cortisone derivatives	35	(53.8)	4	(6.2)
Inhalant cortisone derivatives	28	(43.1)	4	(6.2)

Source: Horst Kief, "Die Behandlung des Asthma bronchiale mit der autohomologen Immuntherapie (AHIT)," *Erfahrungsheilkunde* 9 (1990).

Dr. Kief added: "It may be very encouraging that the consumption of systemic corticoids could be reduced by almost 90% (relative to the exclusive administration of this drug group) and of inhalant cortisone derivatives by more than 85%."[3]

A more recent study, reported in the peer-reviewed *Archives of Medical Research,* was undertaken at the National Center for Scientific Research in Cuba. The goal was to determine the effect of ozone therapy on serum immunoglobulin E (IgE) levels, human leukocyte antigen DR (HLA-DR) expression in peripheral blood mononuclear cells (PBMC), and the erythrocyte glutathione pathway in asthma patients. High IgE levels are common with people suffering from asthma.

The researchers worked with 113 asthma patients between the ages of fifteen and fifty. They were divided into three groups, with members of the first two groups treated using major autohemotherapy and the other group treated with rectal insufflation. Major autohemotherapy was administered at doses of 4 mg for the first group and 8 mg for the second group, with fifteen sessions per cycle; the third group received rectal insufflation at a dose of 20 mg, with twenty sessions per cycle. Blood tests were given before and at the end of each cycle, and lung function and symptoms tests were recorded at the beginning and after the third cycle of treatment.

By the end of the study, IgE and HLA-DR had decreased with all three treatments; increments in reduced glutathione, glutathione peroxidase, glutation reductase, and glutathione S-transferase were achieved with all treatments as well. Lung function and symptoms were "markedly" improved. However, the group receiving the higher concentration of ozone through autohemotherapy had the best results, followed by the group receiving lower-dose autohemotherapy and then the rectal insufflation group.

The researchers concluded: "This study demonstrates the effectiveness of ozone therapy in reducing IgE and inflammatory mediators along with the induction of antioxidant elements. The study raises the role of systemic ozone therapy in atopic asthma by means of its immunomodulatory and oxidative stress regulation properties."[4]

A later double-blind study done by scientists at the National Center for Scientific Research in Cuba evaluated thirty-three patients suffering from severe bronchial asthma; all patients had low tolerance for exercise and often required four or more treatments with bronchodilators daily. Emergency room visits were frequent.

The patients were divided into two groups. Fifteen were treated with rectal oxygen-ozone insufflations for twenty sessions (five per week for four weeks) in addition to their regular asthma medications. The eighteen members of the control group were given twenty applications of rectal oxygen insufflations in addition to their normal medications over the same four-week period.

The researchers found that members of the ozone group experienced a marked improvement in their respiratory capacity, with reduced immunoglobulin E (IgE) levels (IgE plays a major role in the body's hypersensitivity to allergens) and a reduction in their need for asthma medications. Among ozone patients, incidents of hoarseness and wheezing—two of the most common symptoms—fell by between 30 and 60 percent. The group treated with oxygen reported no change in respiratory capacity, overall symptoms, IgE levels, and the need for asthma medication.

When asked about their symptoms, all of the patients treated with ozone reported improvement, while 72.2 percent of the patients treated with oxygen reported no change in symptoms, and several reported a worsening of symptoms over the four-week period.[5]

TUBERCULOSIS

Studies in Russia have shown that ozone can be an important method of treatment for tuberculosis. One study, carried out by Dr. A. A. Priimak and his colleagues, investigated the impact of a gaseous ozone-oxygen mixture on *Mycobacterium tuberculosis* (MBT) and opportunistic microorganisms. One group of patients was given ozone therapy; the other group received traditional medical therapy.

The researchers found that after 15 and 30 minutes of exposure, the mixture of ozone and oxygen caused a "significant decrease" in the number of colonies of microorganisms as compared with the controls. They also observed that the ozone and oxygen mixture produced the highest effect of MBT suspension, which the researchers felt was probably related to a greater surface of ozone contact with a cell than with a dense medium, and higher concentration of ozone and its highly active radicals that arise from the treatment process. Specifically, after treatment with ozone, between 80 and 90 percent of the microbial cells lost their reproductive ability. They also found that the strains grown after ozone and oxygen action retained the drug sensitivity of the original strain. The researchers concluded, "The results suggest that the use of a gaseous ozone-oxygen mixture is promising in the treatment of tuberculosis to cleanse the destruction cavities and pleural empyemas [the presence of pus in a pleural cavity] including those of nonspecific etiology."[6]

Another Russian study compared various treatments of tuberculosis patients suffering from pleural empyema. Surgery is often used to correct this problem. Fifty-five patients with pleural empyema received local washings of an ozonated solution with furacilin and chlorohexidine before surgery, as opposed to another group of fifty-nine, which received the medicated solutions without ozone. The researchers discovered that purulent postoperative complications among the group pretreated with ozone was 17.7 percent versus 30.4 percent for the controls; the treatment group also had reduced mortality of 9.5 percent.[7]

RESPIRATORY FAILURE

A group of Polish physicians evaluated the effectiveness of therapeutic ozone in treating patients who experience respiratory failure after they have been on mechanical respirators for a long length of time. The doctors observed: "Ozonotherapy application[s] improve pulmonary gas exchange [and] increase production of surfactant [and] alveoli elasticity" and noted that ozone's bacteria- and virus-killing properties are useful in treating lung infections that are resistant to antibiotics. They concluded: "Ozonotherapy application in patients with severe respiratory failure gives a possibility for [the] rescue [of] human life."[8]

PULMONARY EMPHYSEMA

A team of researchers from three Cuban institutions—the National Center for Scientific Research, the Victoria de Girón Institute of Basic and Preclinical Sciences, and the Center for Medical-Surgical Research—sought to assess the effects of rectal ozone therapy in patients with pulmonary emphysema.

Sixty-four patients between forty and sixty-nine years of age diagnosed with pulmonary emphysema were chosen for this study. They were randomly assigned to three groups: one group received rectal ozone in twenty daily sessions, another group received rectal medicinal oxygen, and the third group received no treatment. Treatments were repeated three months later in the first two groups. At baseline and at the end of the study, spirometry (used to assess how well your lungs work by measuring how much air you inhale, how much you exhale, and how quickly you exhale) and other clinical assessments were performed.

Fifty patients completed the protocol. Twenty received ozone therapy, twenty were given rectal oxygen, and ten didn't receive any therapy. Before the first treatment, patients on ozone therapy had significantly lower values of forced expiratory volume in the first second (FEV1) and of forced vital capacity (how much air is exhaled). At the end of the treatment period, these parameters were similar in the three treatment groups: they only improved significantly in the group on ozone therapy. No differences were observed in other spirometric parameters. In contrast to the other groups, 40 percent of the subjects treated with ozone reported a decrease of emphysema symptoms, a finding the researchers also considered important.

The researchers concluded "Taking into account the positive results achieved in this study, we recommend the use of ozone therapy as a beneficial therapeutic alternative or as an adjuvant therapy to conventional treatment of patients with pulmonary emphysema."[9]

19
Diseases of the Skin

As with other health problems, oxidative therapies have been found to be useful in treating a wide range of skin diseases. Clinical research with hydrogen peroxide has shown that hydrogen peroxide–based creams are as effective as and often cheaper than traditional medications, and less likely to cause adverse side effects.

However, Bocci writes that because pharmaceutical companies have preferentially used creams with antibiotics with or without corticosteroids (far more expensive than hydrogen peroxide, not always effective, and possibly delaying cicatrization), there has been a lack of clinical interest in oxidative therapy. Patients suffering from painful skin problems tend to seek out the quickest relief possible, so they are less likely to volunteer for long-term clinical trials.[1] Yet despite these problems, scientific research has often testified to ozone's effectiveness.

For example, a "preliminary study" of sixty-five patients suffering from one or more of thirteen different skin diseases (including herpes zoster, herpes simplex, eczema, and pyoderma) at Russia's Dermatovenerological Dispensary in Nizhny Novgorod was reported by Dr. S. L. Krivatkin at the Eleventh World Ozone Congress in San Francisco in 1993.

Minor autohemotherapy with ozone was given at different doses and frequencies according to the patient's symptoms; some patients received ozone administered through the ozone bagging method as well. In addition to ozone, traditional medications were given to the nineteen patients suffering from acne, eczema, and alopecia (an abnormal baldness affecting different parts of the scalp).

The best results were reported among patients suffering from herpes zoster, who reported a total disappearance of symptoms with an 80 percent remission rate after six months. Twenty-five of the twenty-six patients with pyoderma (any pus-producing skin disease) experienced either complete remission or considerable improvement, with nineteen patients still in remission after six months. All sixteen patients with eczema either were completely cured or showed marked improvement, with a 50 percent remission rate after six months. At the end of his presentation, Dr. Krivatkin commented: "This preliminary research provides every reason to conclude that ozone therapy in practical dermatovenereology produces positive results due to its sufficient therapeutic efficacy, ease of use and safety."[2]

This study was later expanded to 351 patients with the following conditions: symptoms of acne and rosacea (60 patients); alopecia (17 patients); drug-related skin eruptions (3 patients); eczema (52 patients); herpes (70 patients); lichen planus (14 patients); neurodermatitis (22 patients); prurigo (2 patients); psoriasis (27 patients); psoriatic arthritis (8 patients); pyoderma (47 patients); scleroderma (4 patients); tinea pedis (15 patients); and venous leg ulcers (10 patients). Different forms of ozone therapy (such as autohemotherapy, ozone bagging, or intramuscular injection) were applied, depending on the symptoms being treated; in some cases, ozone therapy was complemented with traditional allopathic medications.

In his presentation at the Twelfth Ozone World Congress in Lille, France, two years later, Dr. Krivatkin and his colleagues reported that ozone therapy continued to be effective in treating skin diseases. Diseases that best responded to ozone therapies (i.e., ones for which the treatment most often brought about "complete recovery") included herpes, pyoderma, drug-related eruptions, and tinea pedis. "Considerable improvement" took place most often in patients with venous leg ulcers, lichen planus, alopecia, neurodermatitis, psoriasis, and eczema. "Improvement" was found mostly in patients suffering from acne, venous leg ulcers, and neurodermatitis, while some of the patients least responsive to ozone therapy suffered from lichen planus and alopecia. In some cases, therapeutic results were found to be roughly equal in more than one category. For example, six patients suffering from venous leg ulcers enjoyed "considerable improvement" while six showed "improvement." Dr. Krivatkin concluded: "Thus, ozone therapy is effective, almost universal, safe, inexpensive, easy to use and useful in out-patient dermatological practice."[3]

It's important to note that Dr. Krivatkin's research did not utilize applications of ozonated oil, which has been found to complement autohemotherapy and ozone bagging. Let's take a more focused look at how oxidative therapies have been used to treat specific skin conditions.

ACNE

Acne (acne vulgaris) has traditionally been treated with benzoyl peroxide (BP), but this medication has been found to cause dryness and mild skin irritation. A team of Italian researchers undertook a randomized clinical trial comparing benzoyl peroxide with a formulation of hydrogen peroxide stabilized (HPS) in a monoglyceride-based cream. During the eight-week trial, sixty patients diagnosed with acne vulgaris (both the inflammatory and noninflammatory type) were selected. Half were given BP, and half were treated with HPS to compare effectiveness and tolerability.

In comparison with baseline values, the percentage of reductions of the inflammatory type were 58 percent for HPS and 61 percent for BP; the tolerability score was 2.9 in the HPS group and 2.4 in the BP group. Two HPS patients (7 percent) and seven BP patients (23 percent) suffered mild to moderate local erythema (redness due to inflammation). While HPS proved to be statistically as effective as BP, it proved to cause far fewer adverse side effects.[4]

Fifteen years later, a randomized clinical trial involving fifty-two patients was performed by researchers at the famous Gemelli Polyclinic in Rome (and reported in the *British Journal of Dermatology*). The study confirmed the results of the earlier trial. In addition to the basic BP and

HPS cream, the drug adapalene was used. After eight weeks, researchers confirmed that "the combination of adapalene and HP [hydrogen peroxide] cream is an effective topical treatment regimen in mild to moderate AV [acne vulgaris]. This combination has shown a better tolerability profile in comparison with the combination of BP and adapalene."[5]

ALOPECIA

Alopecia is a rare disease where a person loses body hair, including that of the scalp. A study was carried out by Dr. E. Riva Sanseverino and colleagues from the Institute of Human Physiology at the University of Bologna in Italy in 1995 to study this problem. Forty-two patients suffering from androgenetic alopecia (alopecia that is genetic, usually involving moderate to severe loss of hair around the crown and temples in men and the crown in women) were studied both before and after they received cycles of sixteen treatments of major autohemotherapy at a dosage of 2,500 to 3,000 µg of ozone for each treatment. The researchers concluded that results "showed a marked improvement of the hair cycle."[6]

After reviewing this study, Dr. Bocci cautions, "This does not mean that alopecia was cured, so personally I doubt that we should propose this therapy. As a far simpler alternative, I would propose daily application of strongly ozonated water on the scalp for a couple of months."[7]

ATHLETE'S FOOT

Because of the warm and humid tropical climate, athlete's foot (epidermophytosis) is very common in Cuba. It is often resistant to medication and tends to return repeatedly. A study of one hundred patients was undertaken at the Pasteur Polyclinic in Havana, with half of the subjects applying ozonated sunflower oil three times a day to the infected area and the other half using traditional antifungal medications. Symptoms cleared up completely within ten to fifteen days for 96 percent of the patients using ozonated oil, while only 20 percent of the control group were cured after fifteen days.[8]

HERPES SIMPLEX

In addition to his pioneering research on the effects of medical ozone on hepatitis, Dr. Heinz Konrad of São Paulo, Brazil, is believed to have been the first physician to treat herpes with ozone, having shared his experience with other physicians for the first time in 1981. His second study with herpes involved twenty-eight patients suffering from different varieties of herpes simplex: twenty had genital herpes, four had cutaneous (skin) herpes, two had herpes labialis (herpes of the lips), and two suffered from herpes of the eye. Most had been treated unsuccessfully by other physicians. Dr. Konrad gave all patients 9 mg of ozone in the form of autohemotherapy twice a week. Most were given six treatments, although a few received up to nine. Their progress was monitored over a period of two and a half years.

The results of this second study, reported in 1982, were impressive, especially among the patients suffering from genital and cutaneous herpes. "Absolute success" was recorded in 85 percent of the patients with genital herpes; 15 percent reported partial improvement. All of the patients with cutaneous herpes recovered completely. Half of those with oral herpes and half with ophthalmic (eye) herpes recovered completely, while the other half experienced what Dr. Konrad called "questionable success."[9]

Dr. R. Matassi and his associates at the Division of Vascular Surgery at the Santa Corona Hospital in Milan, Italy, also studied the effects of ozone and oxygen on different varieties of herpes. In one study, they treated twenty-seven patients with herpes simplex labialis with intravenous injections of oxygen and ozone. All patients healed completely after a minimum of one and a maximum of five injections, with a recurrence in only three patients over the next five years. As is usual with ozone therapy, no adverse side effects were reported among any of the participants in the study.[10]

HERPES ZOSTER (SHINGLES)

Dr. Matassi and his colleagues also treated thirty patients diagnosed with herpes zoster at the Santa Corona Hospital in Milan, Italy. Herpes zoster is a very painful disease that often takes many weeks to treat. Many patients suffering from shingles have trouble sleeping, and some are known to have even attempted suicide to escape their intense discomfort.

In the Matassi study, the patients were treated daily with intravenous injections of oxygen and ozone, a practice now prohibited in Italy. All of the subjects experienced a complete remission of symptoms of skin lesions after a minimum of five and a maximum of twelve injections. In most cases, local redness disappeared after two to three days of treatment. However, five elderly patients with long-term herpes complained of pain up to two months after therapy, even though their observable symptoms disappeared.[11]

In a yearlong study sponsored by the Center for Medical-Surgical Research in Cuba, fifteen adults suffering from herpes zoster were treated daily with a combination of ozonated sunflower oil and intramuscular injections over the course of fifteen days. All patients noted marked improvement after only three applications, and by the end of treatment, all patients were judged symptom free. Follow-up inquiries a year later revealed no relapse of symptoms. The researchers concluded: "We can say that this study demonstrates the superiority of treating herpes zoster with ozone over traditional therapies. Its low cost, easy availability and simple application make it preferable to other methods."[12]

In his presentation at the 1983 Ozone World Congress in Washington, D.C., Dr. Konrad made the following observations in the treatment of herpes zoster with ozone therapy:

Those few patients I could treat from the very beginning of their herpes zoster experienced a relatively fast recovery. It never took longer than 6 to 8 weeks to get them well and stop the ozone therapy. However, those patients whom I could only treat after they had already had their herpes zoster for weeks or months, or even years, needed a much longer time to feel any better. . . . It seems, thus, of utmost importance, to treat a herpes zoster patient with ozone from the very beginning of his disease in order to have a chance of *complete* recovery.[13]

In 1995 Dr. Konrad presented a paper at the Twelfth Ozone World Congress in France detailing his seventeen years of experience in treating herpes patients with ozone. Of special interest were his findings about the ability of ozone therapy to reduce the "post-zoster neuralgia" pain of individuals suffering from herpes zoster:

8 percent of patients had pain that remained absolutely unchanged.
4 percent had pain that was "somewhat" (25 percent) reduced.
28 percent had pain that was "significantly" (50 percent) reduced.
14 percent had pain that was "mostly" (75 percent) eliminated.
46 percent of patients had pain that was totally (100 percent) eliminated.

Dr. Konrad recalled that the best results were achieved when ozone therapy was combined with the Huneke brothers' "neural therapy" methods introduced early in this century, and he stressed that speedier healing was seen in people who began ozone therapy in the earlier stages of the disease.[14]

HYPODERMATITIS

A randomized open study of 117 adults suffering from indurative hypodermatitis (a subcutaneous hardening of tissue) or localized lipodystrophy (atrophy of subcutaneous fat) was coordinated by researchers affiliated with the Institute of Pharmacology II at the University of Pavia in Italy. Participants were divided into two random groups. After careful examination and evaluation, one group of patients was given subcutaneous injections of ozone and oxygen according to established protocols once a week over a five-week period. Members of the control group were given treatments of Essaven gel, a conventional medication, three or more times a day for five weeks. At the end of the trial, both the physician and patient evaluated the efficacy of treatment in terms of "very good," "good," "fair," "poor," and "nil."

Overall, ozone treatments showed a much higher success rate than the gel treatments, as seen in the chart below.

Researchers concluded that "oxygen-ozone therapy applied within the limits and with the methods indicated in protocol, leads to a more rapid and more extensive remission of the major objective signs of the pathology (circumference of the affected part and skin temperature) as compared with conventional gel therapy."[15]

	Ozone (%)	Gel (%)
Physician evaluation of treatments		
Very Good	35.1	0.0
Good	59.5	7.5
Fair	5.4	10.0
Poor	0.0	52.5
Nil	0.0	30.0
Patient evaluation of treatments		
Very Good	33.8	0.0
Good	57.1	7.5
Fair	9.1	10.0
Poor	0.0	52.5
Nil	0.0	30.0

NEURODERMATITIS

A significant percentage of the patients seeking care at the Kief Clinic in Germany suffer from neurodermatitis. It is a chronic and disfiguring autoimmune disease that manifests as eczema, skin rashes, skin eruptions, and intense itching, causing severe physical and emotional distress. There are both genetic and emotional factors to this disease, and it affects people of all ages, from very young children to elderly adults. The symptoms of many of the patients who visit the Kief Clinic do not respond to traditional medical therapy, such as corticosteroids.

In a statistical study carried out at the clinic, 115 patients suffering from neurodermatitis were given autohomologous immunotherapy (AHIT) over a period of three months. Treatment consisted of injections and oral medication for the adults, while children were given oral AHIT only.

The results, published in the medical journal *Erfahrungsheilkunde* in 1989, were classified as follows: "full remission" was described as being totally free of symptoms until the study was published, two and a half years after treatment; "significantly improved" included greatly improved skin symptoms with a corresponding decrease or disappearance of itching; and "improvement" meant that skin conditions got better and/ or itching was relieved. Under these classifications, forty-three patients (37 percent) had full remissions, fifty subjects (44 percent) showed significant improvement, and thirteen patients (11 percent) improved. Seven of Dr. Kief's patients (6 percent) did not respond to therapy, while two (2 percent) experienced a worsening of symptoms over the long term.[16]

The results of a later study of 333 individuals with neurodermatitis (blindly selected from a total of 2,254) were reported by Dr. Kief in the March 1993 issue of *Erfahrungsheilkunde*. Patients with multiple symptoms, such as neurodermatitis and asthma, were included. Kief's findings were consistent with the earlier results regarding long-term remission. However, results demonstrated a temporary full remission of 65 to 67 percent, which represented an increase over earlier statistics.[17] Figure 19.1 shows "before" and "after" photos of two of Dr. Kief's patients.

IMPETIGO CONTAGIOSA

Impetigo contagiosa is an acute and contagious staphylococcal or streptococcal skin disease that includes the appearance of vesicles, pustules, and yellowish crusts. Researchers from the Department of

Figure 19.1. Two of Dr. Kief's patients with neurodermatitis, before and after receiving AHIT. (Photographs courtesy of Dr. Horst Kief.)

Dermatology at the General Hospital in Malmo, Sweden, undertook a double-blind clinical trial with 256 patients suffering from this condition. The trials were performed at forty-seven medical centers in Germany, Sweden, and the United Kingdom. Half of the patients (128) were given hydrogen peroxide cream (Microcid), and the other half (128) were treated with fusidic acid cream/gel (Fucidin).

During the three-week period of the trial, 72 percent of the patients treated with Microcid were healed, and 82 percent of the Fucidin group were healed, although the researchers claimed that this was not statistically significant. In addition, hemolytic streptococci were eliminated among patients receiving the hydrogen peroxide cream. Researchers concluded: "Microcid cream has been documented as a topical alternative to fusidic acid in the treatment of impetigo."[18]

LEPROSY

Scientists have known that ultraviolet A (UVA) rays from the sun are a poor inactivator of dangerous living cells like bacteria. Yet when combined with certain chemical creams applied to the skin, UVA rays (whether from the sun or a UVA lamp) can kill such cells. Dr. S. I. Ahmad, a researcher at the Department of Life Sciences at Nottingham Trent University in England, decided to compare various chemical creams (combined with UVA therapy) to see how effective they would be in treating skin infections related to leprosy *(Mycobacterium leprae),* a common and often disfiguring skin disease that affects millions of people globally. He found that not only was hydrogen peroxide cream cheaper to use than other creams (an important factor in treating patients in third-world countries), but "out of several agents we have tested, this [hydrogen peroxide cream] was found to be the most potent."[19]

A team of Brazilian researchers from the Physiotherapy Institute (Realengo Campus) and the School of Medicine at the Instituto Federal do Rio de Janeiro treated an eighty-year-old man diagnosed with five wounds on his left hand resulting from leprosy. The researchers utilized a high-frequency current using what they called a *sparks technique* to produce ozone. The researchers postulated that the electric field generated by the device and the passing of the current through the body can produce thermal effects (heat production). The ozone effect is due to the sparking produced by the electrical current passing through the electrode. They believed that the thermal effects contribute to peripheral vasodilation, increasing blood flow and oxygen delivery to the wound.

The patient's wound care protocol was limited to application of the high-frequency current. The patient received five applications on each ulcer per day, which varied in terms of the size of the lesions. The patient was treated once per week for a total of four weeks. Despite it being possible to measure the area at the end of the fifth treatment session, the ulcers were considered clinically healed because they showed complete skin closure with no drainage and no sign of infection. The researchers concluded:

> The ozone provided by a high-frequency device seemed to be useful in the treatment of ulcers contributing to the healing process. However, it is important to highlight that this intervention can be considered as adjuvant in skin damage treatment. We recommend that this modality be used in combination with self-care strategies, protective clothing, modified tools and footwear adaptation.[20]

WARTS

Warts are a common skin problem caused by any of numerous genotypes of the human papilloma virus. They are often treated by physicians through cutting, burning, or medication. Hydrogen peroxide is a little-known remedy for removing warts painlessly and permanently. The following treatment for warts with 30 percent hydrogen peroxide was described by the German physician Dr. M. Manok in the journal *Hautarzt:*

> One needs a sharp spoon, not to remove the wart, [but] rather to open the surface. One doesn't need to get to the root which would

cause it to bleed. . . . With an eyedropper, drop 1 drop of 30% H_2O_2 onto the opened surface and let it dry. After 2 or 3 days scrape off the dried layer and add another drop of H_2O_2. How many times depends on size of the wart. For middle-sized warts it will usually take 4 to 5 applications. Larger ones will take longer. With *Verrucae planea juvenilis,* the most it will take is 2 applications to have it disappear without a trace. Of special importance is, that the plantar wart, which is otherwise hard to remove, can be treated successfully that way. The pain stops mostly after the first or second application. So the patient shouldn't have trouble walking.[21]

VARICOSE ULCERS

Varicose ulcers are open sores in the extremities found primarily among individuals suffering from either diabetes mellitus or varicose veins. These ulcers often get infected and are difficult to treat. Scientists at the Pasteur Polyclinic in Havana, Cuba, wondered if the germicidal properties of ozonated oil could stimulate tissue regeneration among patients suffering from varicose ulcers. They chose 120 subjects with varicose ulcers. Half of the patients were treated with ozonated sunflower oil, and the other half (the control group) were given conventional topical medications.

All of the patients using the ozonated oil were completely cured within fifteen to thirty days, while the majority of the control group needed much more time. A few members of the control group had not recovered by the end of the study. In addition to its efficiency, the researchers noted that the patients receiving ozone therapy did not require hospitalization, since the oil could easily be applied at home.[22]

STEVENS-JOHNSON SYNDROME

Stevens-Johnson syndrome (SJS) is a life-threatening skin condition in which cell death causes the epidermis (the outer layer of the skin) to separate from the dermis (the thick layer of living tissue that lies below the epidemis, containing glands, capillaries, nerve endings and other structures). SJS is thought to arise from a disorder of the immune system. The immune reaction can be triggered by medications or infections, although genetic factors have also been associated with a predisposition to SJS.

Dr. Lamberto Re and colleagues from the Medinat SAS clinic and the National Institute of Health and Science on Aging in Ancona, Italy, reported a case of Stevens-Johnson syndrome treated with ozone therapy. The patient, a twenty-eight-year-old woman, had been diagnosed with SJS three months before admission to the Medinat clinic by her treating physician. The doctors at the clinic observed ulceration of the mouth, nose, and ear mucosa in varying grades of severity. Previous treatment with antiviral and anti-inflammatory drugs had been done without any apparent result.

The physicians at the clinic gave the patient a total of eight oxygen-ozone treatments via major autohemotherapy, with treatments administered every third day. They began with a first infusion of blood treated with low ozone doses followed by 7.5 grams of vitamin C. Doctors reported that after the first treatment the patient showed a sudden relief of symptoms and the ulcers disappeared. The treatment was repeated over the next several weeks to enable the patient to reach a stable condition. Follow-up exams over the next six months showed the complete healing of the patient.

The authors concluded: "The clinical observation described in this case report, suggests that oxidative therapy by mean of low ozone doses (ozone hormesis or ozohormesis) could be helpful and considered as a valid complement to the pharmacological assessment in conditions where immune system is weak or unbalanced."[23]

OZONE AND "SUPERBUGS"

Whether from diabetes, atherosclerosis, or aging, millions of individuals around the world suffer from skin problems that have degenerated into infected wounds. Many do not respond to commonly prescribed medications. Over the years, a number of clinical reports (some cited in this book) have shown that the daily application of ozonated oil can eliminate infection and promote healing of a variety of even the most drug-resistant skin infections.

A group of researchers from four departments at the University of Siena in Italy studied the antimicrobial effect of ozonated oil by testing in vitro four bacterial "superbug" species and one yeast without—or in the presence of—human serum, a product obtained from blood plasma after fibrinogen and other clotting factors have been removed.

The substances tested were *Staphylococcus aureus, Enterococcus faecalis, Pseudomonas aeruginosa, Escherichia coli,* and *Candida albicans.* Ozonated sesame oil was applied to the different pathogens in a laboratory setting and results were measured at one hour, three hours, and six hours after application.

The researchers observed:

> No viable bacteria were obtained only after six hours and at the maximum peroxide content of the ozonated oils, except in the case of the less amount of OSO [ozonated sesame oil] for *E. faecalis* that appeared to be the most resistant strain. Considering all the data, also *P. aeruginosa* and, to a lesser extent, *C. albicans* were quite resistant. On the contrary, *S. aureus* appeared to be the most sensitive one, with a sensible growth diminution since after the first hour with the minimum content of both ozonated oil and peroxide content. As regards *E. coli,* after three hours, a marked sensitivity to treatment has been observed, regardless of the amount of the ozonated oil.

The researchers suggested that a gentle and continuous removal of debris and exudate is an essential condition for the potent bactericidal effect of ozonated oils to take place, noting that even small amounts of human serum can inactivate ozone derivatives and protect bacteria. They concluded that when correctly applied, ozonated oil preparations can be very promising in treating a wide variety of skin and mucosal infections at low cost.[24]

20
Eye Diseases

As they have in other areas of scientific research, Polish investigators have explored the medical value of ozone therapy in treating a wide range of eye problems, including retinal pigment dystrophy, glaucomatous optic atrophy, optic neuritis, eye injuries, degenerative atrophic changes of the choroid, severe myopia, postinflammatory cases, other degenerative diseases, bacterial corneal ulcerations, and cases of unknown etiology. A 1992 article reported the preliminary general findings concerning 206 patients with eye problems. Autohemotherapy was performed on 174 patients; the remaining 32 patients ozone were given intra-arterial oxygen and ozone injections. The researchers observed an improvement in both visual acuity and the visual field. The report added: "Ozone therapy in these conditions seems to be favorable, especially when the pathological process is not extensive."[1]

However, the most exciting research in ozone therapy to treat eye diseases has taken place in Cuba. Over the past few years, Cuban scientists have pioneered research in developing treatment protocols for eye diseases with ozone therapy. Studies have been done to evaluate the beneficial effects of ozone for treating glaucoma, corneal ulcers, atrophy of the optic nerve, and diabetic retinopathy. Ozone was also studied as an adjunct to corneal transplant operations.

GLAUCOMA

Glaucoma is a serious disease that affects approximately 2 percent of adults over forty years of age. However, in some countries, up to 11 percent of adults can suffer from glaucoma, making it the third leading cause of blindness in the world. Cuban research to evaluate the therapeutic effectiveness of ozone to treat glaucoma was reported at the Twelfth World Congress of the International Ozone Association in 1995.

Conducted by scientists at both the National Center for Scientific Research and the Carlos J. Finlay Hospital in Havana, the study involved two hundred outpatients suffering from different stages of simple chronic glaucoma. Ninety percent of patients were over forty years of age. After undergoing visual acuity tests, visual field tests, slit lamp examination, fundoscopy, and visual evoked potentials tests, patients were divided into three random groups for fifteen daily treatments. The first group received ozone therapy (through rectal insufflation); the second received magnetotherapy; and the third received both ozone therapy and magnetotherapy. After the course of treatment, patients were subjected to the same battery of examinations as before.

Visual acuity results were basically similar among all groups, although those receiving ozone therapy alone scored several percentage points higher. Overall, 71 to 75 percent of patients showed "highly significant" improvement, while 25 to 29 percent showed "significant" improvement. However, visual field results showed that ozone therapy is more effective: 73 percent of patients receiving ozone therapy alone showed "highly significant" improvement, while 27 percent had "significant" improvement; 58 percent of those receiving magnetotherapy alone experienced "highly significant" improvement, while 42 percent showed "significant improvement"; and 67 percent of patients using combined therapies had "highly significant" improvement, while the remaining 33 percent experienced "significant" improvement.

Overall, the researchers found that best results were attained through ozone therapy alone. They also noted that a fifteen-treatment course of ozone therapy worked best with patients suffering from the earlier stages of the disease.[2]

OPTIC ATROPHY

Optic nerve dysfunction, or optic atrophy, is a leading cause of blindness in Cuba. A preliminary study with forty patients (sixty-seven eyes) was carried out at the Institute of Neurology and Neurosurgery in 1992. One treatment of major autohemotherapy with ozone was given every weekday for three weeks.

A number of standardized tests were administered before and after the course of treatment, including visual acuity, visual field by Goldmann perimetry, visual evoked potentials, and Pelli-Robson contrast sensitivity test (PRCST). The results were as follows:

Test	Percentage of patients improved
Visual Acuity	54.5
Visual Field	82.7
Visual Evoked Potentials	37.0
Pelli-Robson Contrast Sensitivity Test	85.7

While not all patients achieved a total cure with ozone therapy, the results of this preliminary study so impressed the head physician on the research team (which usually comprises chemists, physicians, and technicians) that she decided to treat all of her future patients suffering from optic atrophy with ozone, either alone or as an adjunct to other treatments.[3]

OPTIC NERVE DYSFUNCTION

A team of researchers at the Institute of Neurology and Neurosurgery in Havana investigated the healing potential of ozone therapy on patients diagnosed with optic nerve dysfunction.

Sixty patients with optic nerve dysfunction were given a total of fifteen autohemotherapy sessions over a three-week period. Ophthalmologic tests to determine visual acuity, visual field by Goldmann perimetry, visual evoked potentials, and PRCST were done before and after treatment.

The most positive findings were found in PRCST and visual field parameters, indicating improvement in 86 and 83 percent of patients, respectively. Visual acuity improved in 55 percent of the patients, while visual evoked potentials increased in 37 percent of patients. No improvement was found in patients diagnosed with Leber's optic atrophy.[4]

RETINAL MACULOPATHY

Retinal maculopathy is an eye disease affecting the muscles of the eye that often appears in one's later years. The effects of oxygen-ozone therapy on twenty patients affected by age-related degenerative maculopathy was studied by Dr. E. Riva Sanseverino and his colleagues at the University of Bologna in Italy. Before-and-after tests to determine visual acuity and eye fluorangiography were used to evaluate the efficacy of the therapy. Ozone was administered via major autohemotherapy at 1,500 to 2,000 µg/session over a four-month period. The results were very heartening: tests indicated that "the majority of patients showed an improvement of their ocular condition, suggesting continuation of this type of investigation on a larger group of people."[5]

RETINITIS PIGMENTOSA

One of the major successes of the Cuban medical system has been in treating retinitis pigmentosa, a chronic progressive disease involving atrophy of the optic nerve and widespread pigmentary changes of the retina. Blindness is often the result. The first major study was carried out at the Salvador Allende Hospital in Havana in 1985 with two hundred patients who had a range of tubular vision of 5 degrees or less. Believing that ozone might be able to help restore blood circulation to the capillaries of the retina, activate protective enzyme systems, and stimulate metabolism of oxygen, researchers gave the patients either major autohemotherapy or intramuscular treatments of ozone and oxygen daily for fifteen to twenty days, depending on the individual and the severity of symptoms. The patient was said to improve when the range of vision increased between 10 and 20 degrees.

The results were surprising. Of the 175 patients in the study who received autohemotherapy, 112 showed "notable improvement," 45 had "slight improvement," and 18 experienced "no progression of symptoms," meaning that although they did not get better, they also did not get worse. Of the twenty-five patients receiving intramuscular oxygen and ozone injections, twelve were notably improved, nine slightly improved, and four with no symptom progression. While a complete cure was not achieved, marked improvement took place in 89 percent of the patients and persisted for at least two years after treatment. Figure 20.1 on page 275 offers a view of one patient's visual range (in white) before and one year after ozone therapy was administered.[6]

A later study was carried out at several hospitals in the city of Holguin, Cuba, as part of a larger research project encompassing other ophthalmologic diseases. Eighty patients with nonsystemic stage I and stage II retinitis pigmentosa were given daily ozone therapy via rectal insufflation for a period of twenty days. Clinical evaluation was made every three months for one year after therapy.

A total of 75 percent realized clinical improvement in their visual acuity up to six months after treatment. However, after one year only 23 percent of patients maintained this improvement. Regarding visual field, 75 percent of the patients improved after treatment for up to nine months, but after a year, only 59 percent maintained their level of improvement. These results led the researchers to recommend that follow-up ozone treatments be scheduled every six months to maintain patient improvement.[7]

These results reflected the opinions of researchers who completed a ten-year study of twenty patients at the National Reference Center of Retinitis Pigmentosa of the Salvador Allende Hospital in Havana, who wrote: "The best results were achieved when ozone treatment is repeated, at least twice a year, among all these years, with improvement of 70% in the visual field and 42% in the visual acuity."[8]

By the beginning of 2007, an estimated eight thousand patients had been treated with ozone at Cuban hospitals for a variety of eye diseases. Ozone is given routinely to the majority of patients with retinitis pigmentosa, retinitis diabetica, keratitis, corneal ulcers, and other eye diseases, either alone or as an adjunct to traditional medical therapies. For retinitis pigmentosa patients, follow-up applications of ozone therapy are recommended twice a year.[9]

Other research is taking place in Russia. A study by Dr. V. V. Neroev and colleagues studied the effects of ozone therapy on patients with involutional central chorioretinal dystrophy, another disease involving retinal degeneration. They found that ozone leads to increased activity of neurons in the muscular region and better functional activity of the retinal peripheral segments. They concluded that ozone has "a positive influence on the dynamics of functional retinal activity" and recommended that ozone therapy be implemented with electroretinography monitoring.[10]

Not all researchers have had such positive results. Dr. Bocci found that after providing fourteen autohemotherapy treatments over a seven-week period to patients diagnosed with retinitis pigmentosa, there was only slight and occasional improvement.[11] However, he believes that ozone therapy could indeed be a useful complementary treatment for this and other eye diseases to do the following:

- Improve perfusion and cellular oxidation (by activating the body's erythrocyte function)
- Increase vasodilation through the release of nitric oxide and carbon monoxide
- Upregulate the enzymatic antioxidant system
- Induce and release cytokines and growth factors[12]

Figure 20.1. Diagram showing range of vision (in white) of patient
with retinitis pigmentosa before and after ozone therapy.
(From *Revista CENIC 20,* no. 1-2-3, 1989.)

AGE-RELATED MACULAR DEGENERATION

Age-related macular degeneration (ARMD) is an eye disease affecting approximately 25 percent of individuals over sixty-five years of age. The "dry" form of this disease comprises approximately 90 percent of cases and there is currently no cure. However, several clinical trials were carried out by scientists at the University of Siena in Italy, and it was found that ozone therapy can stop the progression of the disease while improving both the visual acuity and the well-being of the patient.

One trial was performed by Emma Borrelli, M.D., and her colleagues in the Department of Biotechnologies. They enrolled 140 dry ARMD patients from 2008 to 2011 with ages ranging from fifty-nine to eighty-two. A total of seventy patients underwent ozone therapy while the control group (also seventy patients) received multivitamin therapy. Ophthalmic examination was recorded for each eye at baseline and after six months and twelve months for both groups.

The results showed that patients receiving ozone therapy did far better than those who did not. At six months and twelve months, ozone treated eyes showed an average acuity change of −0.1 and of −0.2 logMAR respectively, while control group eyes had a change of 0.2 and of 0.3, respectively. As far as the best corrected visual acuity (BCVA) changes over time, at six months none of the eyes treated with ozone had a deterioration in BCVA of more than two lines. In the control group, 16 percent had eyes with more than two lines of loss, and 25 percent had more than three lines of loss ($P<0.05$). At six months, 4 percent of the treated group eyes had an improvement of 1 line compared to 0 percent of the control group patients. At twelve months, none of the treated group eyes showed a loss of more than three lines in BCVA. In the control group, 40 percent had a loss of more than two lines, and 38 percent lost more than three lines ($P<0.05$).

The researchers also found that plasma oxidative stress was significantly decreased after ozone treatment, confirming the role of antioxidant enzymes in the increase and the reduction of oxidative stress. In addition, patients receiving ozone therapy reported an improvement of their general condition, particularly in terms of increased efficacy, mental concentration, and memory as assessed by the National Eye Visual Function Questionnaire (NEI-VFQ) before and after the end of the study.

The researchers commented that ozone therapy appears to trigger a number of defense mechanisms against ischemic and neurotoxic injury of the eye, thus preventing the death of photoreceptors. They outlined the effects of ozone therapy on patients with ARMD:

1. Improvement of blood rheology (blood flow)
2. Improvement of the glycolytic pathways on erythrocytes (red blood cells that deliver oxygen); the increased concentration of ATP levels may facilitate a microrelease at hypoxic sites
3. Activation of chemicals that increase oxygen availability to hypoxic tissues
4. Vasodilation due to enhanced release of nitric oxide and prostacyclin (a vasodilator)
5. Release of growth factors from platelets
6. The upegulation of antioxidant enzymes, proteins and heme-oxygenase-1, an enzyme, which facilitate healing

The authors concluded: "The observation that visual acuity improves more rapidly in patients with an initial deficit than in almost blind patients strongly suggests that patients should be encouraged to start ozone therapy as early as possible. It appears obvious that the therapy minimizes the death of photoreceptors."[13]

21
Diseases of the Ear

HEARING LOSS

When I first visited Cuba in 1994, I was introduced to Ernesto Basabe, M.D., an ear, nose, and throat specialist. After meeting him at Cira Garcia Central Clinic in Havana, he took me to the Lina Odena Special School for children with hearing problems. At the time, he was working with thirty-four children suffering from sensoneural hearing loss, known as ototoxicity. Believing that improved circulation in the inner ear may improve hearing, Dr. Basabe decided to explore the value of ozone therapy to combat hearing loss in children.

Dr. Basabe and his colleagues divided the students into two random groups. One group received ozone therapy through rectal insufflation over a three-week period, while the other group was given insufflations of oxygen. Careful evaluations of both ears of each child (including audiometry, brainstem auditory evoked potentials, and psychopedagogical tests) were made before and after the therapy.

Of the children who received ozone (thirty-four ears), the "grave level" improved in twenty-three ears (68 percent) and the conversational level improved in nineteen ears (56 percent). In the "acute level," nine ears (26 percent) improved, but not significantly. Among those treated with oxygen (thirty-four ears), no improvement was noted. However, a one-year follow-up found that improvement tended to decrease in roughly half of the patients receiving ozone. For that reason, Dr. Basabe recommended follow-up ozone therapy within a year of the initial course of treatment.

The medical-psychopedagogical integration results showed that eleven (65 percent) of the children receiving ozone improved, while six (35 percent) remained the same. Two patients (12 percent) receiving oxygen showed improvement, while fifteen (88 percent) remained the same.

Although not a miracle cure, ozone therapy was found to both increase hearing levels and improve overall scholastic efficiency among many of the children receiving ozone therapy. While no adverse side effects were reported, it was among this group that one student, who happened to be suffering from chronic asthma, was completely cured of his symptoms, to the delight of his parents and teachers.[1]

BLOCKED EAR TUBE

Three percent hydrogen peroxide is a common home remedy for removing wax from the ear canal. A team of physicians at the Royal Ear Hospital in London compared the effectiveness of ear drops made from sodium bicarbonate with ear drops of hydrogen peroxide to clear a blocked tympostomy tube, which makes up part of the middle ear. The condition is often treated with surgical reventilation.

One hundred ten ears were studied in this randomized clinical trial. Patients were examined two weeks after treatment, and the physicians found both methods therapeutically effective. The physicians concluded that treatment with either hydrogen peroxide or sodium bicarbonate offers a great potential for cost savings if either of these conservative treatments is used effectively.[2]

EAR INFLAMMATION

A team of Russian researchers explored the effectiveness of therapeutic ozone in treating otitis media, or inflammation of the ear. Twenty-eight patients diagnosed with acute and chronic inflammatory diseases of the middle ear were selected for the study, with one group receiving ozone in the form of gas and ozonated solutions along with traditional medicines, and the other group given traditional medication only.

Based on visual examination, bacteriological tests of discharges from the middle ear cavity, and the number of washings needed before the purulent discharges disappeared, the doctors observed that patients receiving ozone therapy were cured an average of three to five days faster than those who received medication only. They concluded: "Ozone therapy is a beneficial adjuvant in combined treatment of otitis media."[3]

MÉNIÈRE'S DISEASE

A group of physicians at the Audiological and Vestibular Laboratory at E. Warminski's City Hospital in Poland undertook a study on ozone therapy in conjunction with pressure-pulse therapy to treat Ménière's disease. Named after the French ear specialist Prosper Ménière (1799–1862), the disease is a disorder of the membranous labyrinth of the inner ear. Patients with this problem experience recurrent attacks of dizziness, tinnitus (ringing in the ear), and hearing loss.

Fifteen patients diagnosed with Ménière's disease were chosen for this study; all had been experiencing symptoms for one to three years. Ozone therapy and pressure-pulse treatments were given for ten minutes every day for ten days. Although test results did not show statistically significant changes, researchers found that the subjective state of the patients clearly improved, primarily manifested by fewer and less severe attacks of tinnitus.[4]

SUPERGLUE REMOVAL

On occasion, strange accidents happen. An article written by Dr. R. Persaud of Guy's and St. Thomas' Hospital in London described the case of a female patient who self-administered Bostik superglue into her left ear (the article did not mention why she did this!) and came to the hospital for treatment. Many of us know that superglue tends to bond strongly to skin, which can present considerable problems in removing it. Dr. Persaud (who must be a very resourceful physician) decided to try hydrogen peroxide. He wrote: "The superglue was removed successfully, in the form of a cast, with warm 3 percent hydrogen peroxide without damaging the meatus or the tympanic membrane. The use of hydrogen peroxide to remove superglue from the ear has not been described previously."[5]

22
Other Health
Problems

The broad spectrum of application for oxidative therapies was discussed in a paper by Dr. Velio Bocci published in the *Journal of Biological Regulators and Homeostatic Agents*. In this paper, Dr. Bocci wrote that brief oxidative stress "appears safe, simple, inexpensive and amenable to be adjusted to different pathological states" and that ozone's ability to upregulate intracellular antioxidant enzymes can eventually inhibit the chronic oxidative stress responsible for degenerative disease and aging.[1] In this chapter, we'll explore how oxidative therapies have been found to impact a broad spectrum of other health problems and can perhaps can be part of a health maintenance program.

DUODENAL ULCER

At the General Calixto Garcia Hospital in Havana, Cuba, twenty patients suffering from duodenal ulcer were treated several times daily with ozonated water over the course of one month. Clinical studies revealed that 40 percent of the patients were totally healed by the end of treatment, 10 percent were in the final stages of scar formation, 25 percent of the patients had 50 percent scar formation, 5 percent experienced a 33 percent scar formation, and 20 percent had to discontinue the study due to intense pain.[2]

COLITIS

Before he developed his revolutionary intraperitoneal ozone delivery system to treat cancer and sepsis, Dr. Siegfried Schulz did experiments with ozone on Djungarian hamsters as a basis for treating antibiotic-induced colitis in humans, a disease that is extremely difficult to treat with other antibiotics. Many patients with severe colitis require colostomies, or the removal of the colon. While enterocolitis in hamsters cannot be compared with human colitis in its anatomical and clinical outcome, Dr. Schulz felt that the term *colitis*—based on his electron microscope results from the colons of hamsters—was justified. In addition, because this type of hamster is omnivorous, it is more relevant to humans than other animal species as an animal model for studying this disease.

After the hamsters were infected, one group was given the drug clindamycin, with 100 percent mortality after three days; the same mortality rate occurred when animals were treated with air and clindamycin. When oxygen and ozone were administered rectally in clindamycin-treated animals, 30 percent died within three days. But when ozone and oxygen were administered via both oral (through a tube inserted into the stomach) and rectal insufflation, all of the clindamycin-treated animals were alive after ten days.[3]

Dr. Schulz concluded that insufflation of ozone into the gastrointestinal tract significantly prevented the fatal outcome of lethal enterocolitis, and he believes that greater attention should be paid to the role of ozone in treating antibiotic-induced or antibiotic-resistant bacterial infections of the gastrointestinal tract like pseudomembranous colitis.[4]

ULCERATIVE COLITIS

Ulcerative colitis (UC) is a disease that causes inflammation and sores, called ulcers, in the lining of the rectum and colon. It is one of a group of diseases called inflammatory bowel disease (IBD). Several types of drugs can help control it. In severe cases, doctors must remove the colon.

A team of researchers from three major hospitals and research centers (the 303rd Hospital of the People's Liberation Army, the Research Center of Clinical Medicine, and Nanfeng Hospital at Southern Medical University) in China undertook a study to assess the therapeutic effect of ozone therapy combined with sulfasalazine delivered via a colon therapy system in the treatment of distal ulcerative colitis. Sulfasalazine is widely used by conventional medicine to treat IBD, including Crohn's disease and ulcerative colitis.

This randomized controlled clinical trial involved fifty-four patients diagnosed with mild to moderate active distal ulcerative colitis. They were randomly divided into three groups of eighteen patients per group. Each group was given a daily dose of 2 g of sulfasalazine. For those in the "colon therapy group" and "ozone therapy plus sulfasalazine therapy group," sulfasalazine was delivered daily via a specially designed colon therapy system, while the control group received sulfasalazine via retention enema only. Colonoscopies were performed to evaluate disease activity before treatment and at two weeks and four weeks after the beginning of treatment. In addition, biopsy samples were obtained at zero weeks and at four weeks for histological examination. (Histology is the study of the microscopic anatomy of cells and tissues of plants and animals.)

The researchers found that when compared with the colon therapy group and the control group, patients in the ozone therapy plus colon therapy group experienced faster alleviation of their clinical symptoms as well as a greater degree of histological improvement, especially four weeks after treatment began. In the paper, which was published in the *Journal of Southern Medical University,* the researchers observed that ozone therapy was inexpensive to use and that it produced no adverse side effects. They concluded: "Ozone therapy combined with sulfasalazine delivered via a colon therapy system is feasible and effective for treatment of ulcerative colitis."[5]

GASTROENTERITIS

Robert Mayer, M.D., a pediatrician in Miami, Florida, used medical ozone to treat children suffering from gastroenteritis, an inflammation of the stomach and intestinal tract. Nonbacterial diarrhea was a common symptom. A total of 2,757 children from one month to eighteen years of age were divided into two groups. Group 1 consisted of 1,931 children who were treated with oxygen and ozone through rectal insufflation. Of that total, 1,265 received one treatment, 583 were given two treatments, and 83 received three insufflations of ozone and oxygen. Group 2 was a control group of 825, which was in turn divided into three subgroups: subgroup A received a restricted diet only, subgroup B received rectal air insufflation, and subgroup C was given rectal oxygen insufflation.

Of the children receiving ozone therapy, 95 percent of the group receiving one treatment were cured in one day. Of the subjects receiving two treatments, 95 percent were cured in two days. All of the remaining patients receiving ozone were cured in three days. By contrast, all members of the control group recovered more slowly and persisted in their symptoms for up to six days.[6]

HUMORAL IMMUNE DEFICIENCY

A group of researchers at the Central Havana Pediatric Hospital sought to evaluate the effects of ozone therapy on children with humoral immune deficiency. Fifty-nine children between one and five years of age who had not responded to conventional immune-stimulating therapies were chosen for the study.

Clinical manifestations of patients were as follows:

Frequent recurrence of respiratory infections: 3 patients (5 percent)
Chronic adenoiditis and/or tonsillitis: 10 patients (17 percent)
Pneumonia: 22 patients (37 percent)
Asthma: 15 patients (25 percent)

Chronic diffuse middle otitis (ear infection): 9 patients (15 percent)

Sepsis: 1 patient (2 percent)

Immunoglobulins are proteins that are capable of acting as antibodies to protect the body from disease. All patients in the study were deficient in one or more immunoglobulins: forty-eight patients (81 percent) were deficient in gamma A (IgA), which helps protect mucosal surfaces from invading pathogens; eight (14 percent) were deficient in gamma M (IgM), which is formed in almost all the body's immune responses; and thirty (51 percent) were deficient in gamma G (IgG), the principal immunoglobulin found in human serum.

Immunological improvement was rated as "satisfactory" when immunological studies were normalized or were higher than reference values. It was rated "unsatisfactory" when the immunological parameters remained pathological. Clinical improvement was "satisfactory" when recurrent infectious episodes were relieved or eliminated, and "unsatisfactory" when infectious episodes continued or increased.

Ozone was administered via rectal insufflation at age-dependent doses in three different cycles. The first cycle included fifteen daily treatments over a three-week period, the second cycle included twelve sessions over six weeks, and the third cycle called for nine ozone insufflations over six weeks, with a break of fifteen days between cycles.

The results were impressive. Researchers found that humoral immunity levels increased while clinical improvements were achieved to a satisfactory level in all patients. In addition, pathological IgA, IgM, and IgG values were normalized within the first cycle of treatment. Finally, the researchers noted that the ozone therapy was well tolerated by all patients and no adverse side effects were present.[7]

JAUNDICE

Mechanical jaundice is a type of jaundice caused by obstruction of the biliary passages by tumor or gallstones. A group of Russian physicians wanted to see whether ozone, when used as an adjunct, could improve patient response to traditional therapy. After evaluating results from ninety patients whose mechanical jaundice was due to tumor, the researchers concluded: "Ozone therapy facilitates more rapid arrest of hepatic dysfunction and endogenous intoxification."[8]

MIGRAINE

Dr. S. A. Kotov conducted a randomized clinical trial to see whether ozone therapy can help relieve symptoms of migraine. Sixty-eight adult migraine sufferers were chosen for this study. Forty patients received eight or nine infusions of ozonated saline solution at a concentration of 1,200 µg/l, and a control group of twenty-eight received infusions of saline without ozone.

The intensity of headache, expressions of anxiety, state of vessels in the brain, and other biochemical indices were evaluated. Dr. Kotov found that there was a 25 percent overall improvement among the patients receiving ozone as compared to the controls. He concluded: "In 59% of the patients the attacks were absent during 3–5 months after ozone therapy, less intensity of headache was observed after their relapse. Improvements in the patients coincide with changes in biochemical parameters."[9]

REFRACTORY MIGRAINE

While the majority of headaches are caused by tension and do not require medical intervention, roughly 20 percent of the population experience incapacitating headaches that resist medical treatment. Refractory migraines are those that continue persistently despite aggressive attempts to manage them, including medical, behavioral, and alternative modes of treatment.

A novel study was undertaken by Dr. Bernardino Clavo and his colleagues at the Chronic Pain Unit, Research Unit, and the Departments of Radiation Oncology and Neurology at the Dr. Negrin University

Hospital, Las Palmas, Spain, along with Dr. Velio Bocci of the Department of Physiology at the University of Siena, Italy.

Five patients were chosen for this study. All had suffered from severe/persistent headache that did not respond to standard headache management (including 5-HT1 agonist triptan drugs). Patients were treated with ozone therapy in the form of major autohemotherapy. The procedure involved venous blood drawn into a sterile single-use glass bottle containing anticoagulant, gently mixed with an equal volume of an ozone-oxygen gas mixture, prefiltered through a sterile 0.20-μm filter, and slowly reinfused back into the donor patient via the antecubital vein in the arm.

Outcomes were measured by analgesia requirements, days of sick leave due to headache, number of headache events, and pain intensity according to the visual analogue scale (VAS). Outcomes were recorded at three time points: before ozone therapy, after ozone therapy, and before the last follow-up (mean: 64.6 to 36.8 months).

One month before ozone treatment began, the median number of severe headache episodes was twenty a month, with eighty reported episodes over six months before the ozone therapy began. One month after ozone therapy sessions concluded, zero events were reported. After six months, zero severe headache events were reported. The VAS scores also recorded a large decrease in headache pain in general. In the six-month period before the study, 60 percent of the patients had to take time off from work due to headache pain. In a follow-up five years after ozone therapy, patients reported no sick days due to headache pain. All patients stopped using triptan drugs, which are primarily used to treat migraine and cluster headaches.

The researchers concluded, "Ozone therapy decreased headache episodes and pain severity over a protracted period." They added, "This novel approach is effective and merits further research."[10]

PAIN RELIEF

In the AIDS trials undertaken by the Canadian Department of National Defence in 1990, the analgesic effects of ozone were discovered unexpectedly. According to Capt. Michael Shannon, M.D., who coordinated the study, "Inadvertently, we discovered that this particular type of therapy has an incredible effect, a very pronounced effect in managing pain. It has a very potent analgesic effect."[11]

I personally observed the analgesic effects of intravenous hydrogen peroxide on an individual who was suffering from a variety of serious AIDS-related symptoms and was given only a few weeks to live. Daily intravenous hydrogen peroxide administered at home appeared to relieve much of his discomfort, lift his spirits, facilitate sleep, and increase his overall energy level. Although the patient died, the quality of his final days was dramatically improved.

SICKLE CELL ANEMIA

Sickle cell anemia is a hereditary chronic form of anemia affecting primarily people of sub-Saharan descent. It is difficult to cure, and its symptoms include episodes of intense pain and fatigue. Believing that ozone could help those suffering from this disease, James Caplan of CAPMED/USA, a research organization, originally proposed that a study be done at the Philadelphia Children's Hospital, but he was rebuffed by hospital authorities. Knowing that Cuba has a large population of people of African origin, Caplan offered his proposal to scientists at Cuba's National Center for Scientific Research. The Cubans were glad to collaborate, and the study was undertaken in 1989 at the Salvador Allende Hospital with fifty-five adults.

A control group of twenty-five patients received fifteen conventional medical treatments for sickle cell anemia, while the other group underwent fifteen sessions of oxygen-ozone therapy via rectal insufflation. Some members of the second group also received topical applications of ozone to treat skin ulcers, while patients in the control group were given conventional skin medications.

The results showed that the average time for resolution of the sickle cell crisis among those treated with ozone was half that of the control group. In addition, the frequency and severity of painful crises among the patients receiving ozone diminished during the six-month follow-up, in comparison to members of the control group. Skin ulcers, which are common among sickle cell patients, completely disappeared among the patients receiving ozone. The results of this simple, low-cost therapy were so impressive that Cuba's Ministry of Public Health later approved ozone therapy as a standard treatment for sickle cell anemia throughout the country.[12]

Studies of sickle cell anemia were also undertaken by Dr. Bocci and colleagues in Italy. Dr. Bocci verified the validity of the Cuban studies and offered a possible treatment schedule for patients suffering from this disease and its common complications:

> After an initial cycle including 24 treatments in three months (twice weekly), the therapeutic effect can be maintained with three treatments per month. Upregulation of antioxidant enzymes and 2,3-diphosphoglycerate (2,3-DPG) is likely to occur during the first two months while rheological improvement (decrease of arterial pressure is the norm) due to NO^-/O_2^- rebalance may take two to three months.[13]

SINUSITIS

A team of Russian physicians undertook a randomized clinical trial to see whether ozone therapy was more effective in treating sinusitis than conventional therapy. A total of 102 patients diagnosed with chronic purulent rhinosinusitis were chosen for the study. Seventy-two received five to seven irrigations of the paranasal sinuses with an ozone-oxygen mixture, while thirty control patients received traditional treatment. After evaluating all of the participants in the trial, researchers found that 89 percent of the patients receiving ozone recovered an average of 4.3 days earlier than the controls.[14] Certainly, nasal irrigations with ozonated water offer the greatest level of safety, because this method prevents inhalation of ozone.

URINARY TRACT INFECTION

Urinary tract infection (UTI) has become a common health problem in developed countries, especially among patients who have undergone kidney transplants or are suffering from hypoglycemia, glycosuria, or neurogenic bladder. Urinary tract infections are normally treated with antibiotics. Yet given the expanding problem of multi-antibiotic resistant bacteria, scientists are searching for alternative and adjunct methods to deal with this problem.

Because ozone is known for its powerful antimicrobial properties against bacteria, spores, fungi, viruses, and protozoa, researchers at the Nephrology and Dialysis Unit at Sant'Anna Hospital in Como, Italy, investigated its possible usefulness in treating patients suffering from UTI.

Three female patients were chosen for this study. All had undergone kidney transplants and were suffering from one or more recurring urinary tract infections that did not respond to antibiotic therapy.

After urinary bladder catherization and urinary bladder emptying, a total of 100 to 150 centiliters (cc) of ozonated saline was prepared (ozone concentration: 50 μg/ml). The ozonated saline was then injected via a catheter into the urinary bladder and allowed to remain until the next voiding. The procedure was repeated at day one, day three, and every week thereafter until the patient's symptoms disappeared or urinary tests showed normalization.

The researchers found that the use of ozonated water allowed for a "substantial bacterial clearance and prolonged urinary discomforts relief." Although recognizing that this was a preliminary study with only three patients, they concluded: "In light of the emerging multidrug resistant bacteria strains and the need for alternative or adjunct antiseptic strategies, we believe that future studies should investigate and establish the best way to administer ozone, the safety, efficacy and long term outcomes of this cheap and commonly available drug for UTI management."[15]

23
Accidents, Injuries, and Wound Healing

One of the most serious threats in cases of burns, postoperative states, and wounds is infection, which can often lead to serious illness or death. Over the past few decades, ozone and hydrogen peroxide have been studied for their powerful antibacterial effects.

Traditional medical therapy often calls for the use of antibiotics. While effective for minor infections, they may not work against those bacteria that have natural or acquired resistance to drugs. Ozone and hydrogen peroxide may be useful because they are effective in killing drug-resistant bacteria with minimal side effects. Another important aspect is their low cost, which can make them especially useful in developing countries where antibiotics are often beyond the financial resources of many patients. That is probably why most of the studies we cite in this chapter were carried out in Cuba, Russia, and China.

BURNS

In a Cuban study of twenty-five patients suffering severe burns at the Calixto Garcia Hospital in Havana, ozone was given in the form of autohemotherapy over a course of ten days. Ozone normalized levels of immunoglobulin G and M, complement C4, and antithrombin III, three indicators of greater immune response. The researchers concluded that these results are due to the anti-inflammatory, immunoregulatory, and bactericidal qualities of ozone.[1]

A more recent study by doctors at the Third Municipal Hospital of Wuhan in China evaluated the role of ozonated solutions in disinfecting burn wounds. The researchers found that "all the bacteria tested were killed in vitro by ozone solution. In addition, when ozone solution was applied on burn wound[s], its clearance rate of bacteria was 94.7% and the clinical effective rate was 97.1%." They concluded: "Ozone is low in cost and high in effect which might be used as an agent for burn wound disinfection."[2]

The potential of post-burn treatments containing hydrogen peroxide was explored by Drs. Shamim Ahmad and O. G. Iranzo of the Department of Life Sciences at Nottingham Trent University in England in 2003. Noting that while ordinary antibiotics can be effective against minor infections, some pathogens, like *Pseudomonas aeruginosa,* are very resistant to even the strongest medications. In an article appearing in *Medical Hypotheses,* Drs. Ahmad and Iranzo wrote about the potential benefits of a combination of diluted hydrogen peroxide and ferrous sulfate:

> It should be particularly useful for the ubiquitous opportunistic pathogen like *Pseudomonas aeruginosa* known to be notoriously resistant to various antibiotics. This reactive oxygen species (ROS)-induced inactivation of bacterial skin infections may be of particular importance in Third World countries where the incidence of burns and post-burns infections by MDR [multiple drug resistant] bacteria (due to the indiscriminate use of antibiotics, lack of stringent safety regulations and proper hygiene) may be more prevalent and where cocktails of antibiotics may be less affordable.

The researchers added that this type of therapy could work not only to treat post-burn infections but also for other kinds of skin infections that are resistant to antibiotics.[3]

A group of researchers from the Dermatology Clinic of the Department of Clinical Medicine and Biotechnology at the Polytechnic University of Marche in Ancona, Italy, undertook an in vivo study to evaluate the effectiveness of ozonated oil on second-degree burns.

A total of thirty patients suffering from second-degree skin burns in the phase of re-epithelialization (the regrowth of skin over a wound) were included in this study. Each burn was divided in two symmetrical parts. One part was treated with an occlusive application of ozonated oil; the other part of the lesion was treated with a topical application of hyaluronic acid gel. Both medicines were applied once a day for twelve weeks. A clinical evaluation and an intra-vital video-capillaroscopy were performed on every patient at baseline, six weeks after, and twelve weeks after.

The researchers found that all of the treated burns improved regardless of the treatment used. Ozonated oil was found to be as effective as hyaluronic acid in improving erythema (superficial reddening of the skin, usually in patches, as a result of injury or irritation causing dilatation of the blood capillaries), tension, itching, and a burning sensation reported by patients. In addition, ozonated oil did not exert a specific anti-angiogenic effect (i.e., having to do with reducing the growth of new blood vessels) compared to hyaluronic acid. It also appeared to be more effective than hyaluronic acid in reducing post-lesional hyperpigmentation of the skin.

Reporting their findings in the journal *Burns,* the researchers concluded: "Ozonated oil, topically applied for 12 weeks, seems to be as effective as hyaluronic acid in reducing symptoms related to skin burns, but it could be more effective in preventing the post-lesional hyperpigmentation."[4]

POSTOPERATIVE CARE

A team of physicians from the Silesian Medical Academy in Katowice, Poland, explored the benefits of using ozone to reduce postoperative complications of rhinoplasty (plastic surgery of the nose). Forty-five patients were divided into two groups. Twenty-five were given intravenous ozone daily for three days prior to their operation and for three days after the rhinoplasty was performed. The other group of twenty patients did not receive ozone. The researchers reported that ozone therapy was very helpful, "resulting in a significant reduction in postoperative complications duration as compared with the control group."[5]

A Russian clinical trial involving fifty-eight patients suffering from postoperative diffuse peritonitis was carried out by Dr. E. P. Kudriavtsev and colleagues at a Moscow hospital. The study also involved forty experimental animals. One group received washings with ozonated solutions; the other group was given traditional therapy. Results showed ozone's "marked detoxicant effect that manifested with early decrease of ESR [erythrocyte sedimentation rate], leukocytosis, plasma concentration of bilirubin and medium sized molecules and microbes." The death rate in the group receiving ozone was 5.2 percent, while that of the controls was 16.6 percent.[6]

Ozonated Saline in Surgery

Many deep wounds require medical and especially surgical care. Unfortunately, infections often result from these procedures (including infections from contaminated medical hardware), leading doctors to explore adjunctive treatments to prevent and eliminate them.

A group of researchers at the AO Research Institute Davos in Switzerland studied the ability of ozonated saline solution to eradicate infections associated with deep wounds requiring extensive surgical and medical care. Specifically, the purpose of their study was to investigate the antibiofilm potential of ozonated saline against biofilms of *Staphylococcus aureus,* a microorganism (often referred to as a "superbug") that is often found in infected wounds. A biofilm is any group of microorganisms in which cells stick to each other on a surface and are thus more resistant to eradication.

The researchers used a custom-made bioreactor to grow *S. aureus* biofilms on discs of medical grade titanium alloy. An ozone generator was connected in-line and biofilms and planktonic bacteria (bacteria drifting in water) were exposed to ozonated saline. In tests against planktonic *S. aureus,* the researchers noted a 99 percent reduction in bacterial numbers within just fifteen minutes of exposure. They noted that *S. aureus* biofilms were significantly more resistant to ozonated saline, although complete eradication was eventually achieved within five hours. The researchers concluded, "Ozonated saline may be suitable as an adjuvant therapy to treat patients as an instillation fluid for wound irrigation and sterilisation."[7]

SEPSIS

Sepsis is a highly dangerous and often fatal form of blood poisoning that can occur after accidents or operations. At the Carlos J. Findlay Hospital in Havana, Cuba, the effectiveness of ozone therapy was studied in the intensive care unit on patients suffering from severe sepsis. It was found that ozone not only increased general oxygen transport to the tissues, circulatory system, and respiratory system, it also proved to be an effective germicide. The results of this study led the hospital administration to authorize ozone therapy for accident victims in the intensive care unit of the hospital whenever the risk of sepsis existed.[8]

Research has also been done on the effects of intraperitoneal ozone on sepsis. In 2006 an article by Dr. Siegfried Schulz and colleagues appeared in the peer-reviewed journal *Shock* reporting the ability of peritoneal ozone (along with piperacillin and tazobactam) to treat lethal sepsis. The researchers infected rats with bacterially induced severe peritonitis. One group was given doses of piperacillin/tazobactam alone, and all of them died. Another group was pretreated with intraperitoneal oxygen and ozone before infection, and the survival rate increased to 35 percent. A third group was both pretreated with oxygen-ozone and given the antibiotics, and the survival rate increased to 93 percent. While animal studies do not always apply to human subjects, the researchers concluded: "The preconditioning effect of O_3/O_2-PP [ozone-oxygen pneumoperitoneum] seems to support the biological effectiveness of TZP [tazobactam/piperacillin] by altering the immune status before and during the onset of sepsis. The combined therapy could be a simple, preoperative intervention for abdominal surgery to reduce postoperative morbidity and mortality."[9] These findings may also hold great promise in the treatment of humans suffering from severe bacterial infections, especially those resistant to drug therapy alone.

SNAKEBITE

In 1983 Robert A. Mayer, M.D., reported on the antitoxic effects of ozone and oxygen at the Sixth World Ozone Conference in Washington, D.C. After acquiring cobra venom from the Miami Serpentarium, Dr. Mayer injected the venom into two groups of mice. (No humans came forward to volunteer for this experiment!) One group was given the venom alone; the other group received an injection of cobra venom mixed with ozone gas. The control group died immediately, while the mice injected with venom and ozone showed no evidence of disease. In another test, rattlesnake venom was used with similar results.

Dr. Mayer also reported the case of a dog (not a laboratory animal) that was bitten by a rattlesnake in the leg. The dog was given two intravenous injections of ozone and oxygen, and similar injections were applied around the bite itself. Within thirty-six hours, the dog recovered completely, with no infections of the leg or lymph nodes appearing for the six months the dog was monitored.[10]

TRAUMA

An unusual study on the effects of ozone therapy on patients suffering from a variety of severe physical trauma was undertaken by researchers from the Center of Ozonotherapy in the intensive care unit at a hospital in Nizhny Novgorod in Russia. The researchers worked with sixteen pediatric patients (between twenty months and fourteen years of age) who were admitted to the emergency room for severe injuries caused by explosions, fires, carbon monoxide poisoning, bullet wounds, and car accidents. All patients suffered obvious damage to the skin, soft tissues, and/or bones.

Over a forty-eight-hour period, one or more types of ozone therapies were administered on a case-by-case basis. They included tiny amounts of ozone (2 to 5 µg/l) added to oxygen for therapeutic inhalation, ozonated sodium chloride solution given intravenously, major autohemotherapy administration, and ozonated water applied to wounds, either topically or poured in and then drained out. In cases of scalp wounds, open fractures, anaerobic infections, burns, and initial gangrene, ozone was administered through a plastic bag wrapped around the wound. At times, ozonated water or ozone gas was injected directly into bones. Burn victims were sometimes placed in a bathtub containing ozonated water for thirty to forty minutes in order to speed the healing of damaged tissues.

The researchers found that ozone accelerated the healing of wounds, reduced pain, and prevented necrosis of the tissues. They concluded that ozone therapy can be of significant value in trauma cases, especially in the treatment of patients with sepsis and anaerobic infections.

We mentioned earlier that ozone is generally not recommended for inhalation. However, the Russian researchers found that extremely small amounts of ozone mixed with pure oxygen can be both harmless and, in some cases, beneficial. It is now considered an accepted adjunct to other therapies in Russia.[11]

WOUND HEALING

An early study at the Baylor University Medical Center in Texas, reported in the *American Journal of Surgery,* analyzed the ability of intra-arterial hydrogen peroxide to heal wounds, especially those caused by radiation treatment for carcinomas. In the five cases discussed in the paper, the researchers found not only that the tumors in patients receiving hydrogen peroxide responded more rapidly to irradiation, but that the wounds healed at a much faster rate and with less scar formation than is normally expected. The researchers attributed this accelerated healing to regional superoxygenation with hydrogen peroxide. The patients participating in the study had been unresponsive to conventional modes of therapy in treating their wounds.

The article also reported how hydrogen peroxide helped speed the healing of other wounds, including a persistent skin ulcer (caused by previous irradiation); athlete's foot; stasis ulcers of the foot, leg, and jaw; varicose ulcers; diabetic ulcers; and a draining osteomyelitis (bone inflammation) of the tibia, all with significant success.[12]

A more recent study carried out in Moscow evaluated the effects of ozone therapy to enhance the effectiveness of antibiotics among patients suffering from face and neck injuries. Researchers reported: "Ozone therapy of wounds to the face and neck increased the sensitivity of microorganisms to antibiotics in 79% [of] cases."[13]

Diabetic Foot Ulcers

Diabetic foot ulcers are becoming increasingly common as the rate of diabetes increases around the world. Conventional treatment modalities are often of limited success in promoting complete wound closure. A study by researchers at the Diabetes Research Unit of the Wolfson Medical Center in Israel examined the efficacy of noninvasive ozone-oxygen therapy in the treatment of diabetic foot ulcers.

A total of sixty-one diabetes patients with a Wagner classification stage 2 or 3 ulcer or a stage 4 ulcer after debridement (debridement involves the removal of dead, damaged, or infected tissue to improve the healing potential of the remaining healthy tissue) of at least eight weeks in duration were included in this double-blind, randomized, placebo-controlled clinical trial. Patients received conventional medical treatment in combination with either ozone-oxygen treatment (thirty-two patients) or sham treatments (twenty-nine patients) for twelve weeks. After an additional twelve weeks, each patient's wound status was reexamined.

The researchers found that among the thirty-four subjects who completed the study (sixteen in the ozone group, eighteen in the placebo group), a significantly higher rate of complete wound closure was observed in the ozone group (81 percent versus 44 percent). In addition, the rate of total wound closure was 100 percent in the ozone group versus 50 percent in the placebo group.

The researchers concluded: "Among PP [per protocol] patients, ozone treatment in addition to conventional treatment was superior to conventional treatment alone in promoting the complete healing of diabetic foot ulcers."[14]

Buruli Ulcer

Buruli ulcer is caused by a germ—*Mycobacterium ulcerans*—that mainly affects the skin but can also affect the bone. Although this mycobacterium belongs to the same family as organisms that cause leprosy and tuberculosis, it is unique because it produces a toxin—mycolactone—that destroys tissue. Buruli ulcer has been reported in over thirty tropical countries, but countries in West and Central Africa—Benin, Cameroon, Côte d'Ivoire, Democratic Republic of the Congo, and Ghana—report the majority of cases. Over 2,200 cases were reported by the World Health Organization (WHO) in 2014. Approximately 80 percent of cases that are reported early respond well to antibiotics.[15]

The first reported case of treating Buruli ulcer with ozone was published in *BMJ Case Reports* by a team of physicians in Brescia, Italy, connected to InterMed Onlus, a charity that provides medical services in several countries in Africa. A sixteen-year-old female came to their clinic with an ulcer in the left arm. The patient had been diagnosed with Buruli ulcer and was treated for eight weeks with antibiotic therapy in accordance with WHO guidelines, without any clinically significant improvement in the ulcer site. The wound area was 60 square centimeters in size and was 0.5 centimeter deep. The ugly and discolored wound showed edema (excess of watery fluid), necrosis (death of body tissue), and exudate (a mass of cells and fluid that has seeped out of blood vessels or an organ, especially in cases of inflammation).

Oxygen-ozone treatments were applied through the ozone bagging method four times a week for two weeks. Each session lasted 20 minutes. The physicians reported that the ulcer improved after each application, with a progressive reduction of the wound area, continuous appearance of granulation tissue (new connective tissue and tiny blood vessels that form on the surfaces of a wound during the healing process), and skin recovery. There was also a parallel reduction of the edema, necrosis, and exudate beginning after the first ozone application. After the first week of treatment, the ulcer was clean and granulized, without any sign of infection. At the end of two weeks of treatment, the ulcer disappeared and granulation was present throughout the wound area. A histological examination after two weeks of treatment showed the absence of *Mycobacterium ulcerans*. At a six-month follow-up examination, the doctors found that the ulcer was completely healed.

The researchers plan to continue their investigation into this safe, cheap, and effective method for treating Buruli ulcer. They concluded: "The use of ozone to treat Buruli ulcer might become an effective and safe option if the outcome observed in our case is confirmed in a well-designed, randomised trial. Ozone preparation and its application could be a cheap and simple-to-be-used therapy in poor regions where recommended therapies, as antibiotics and surgery, are difficult to be administered."[16]

Canker Sore

Aphthous stomatitis (mouth ulcer) is a common condition affecting approximately 20 percent of the population. Known informally as "canker sore" in North America, this disease has no cure. In the West, canker sore discomfort is usually managed by different over-the-counter and prescription medications, while in India, more natural products like sesame oil are often used.

Researchers at the Drs. Sudha and Nageshwara Rao Siddartha Institute of Dental Sciences and Vishnu Dental College in India undertook a single-blind investigation to see if ozonated oil could treat this painful condition. They selected a total of thirty patients suffering from recurring canker sores and divided them into three groups. Patients in Group 1 were given ozonated oil, those in Group 2 were given sesame oil (a popular remedy in India that has been clinically shown to possess antimicrobial, anti-inflammatory, and analgesic properties), and patients in Group 3 were given distilled water, a placebo. Treatments were administered in the form of a cotton-tipped applicator with the patients not knowing what was being applied. Treatment response was assessed by measures of pain reduction and ulcer duration on the second day, fourth day, and sixth day of treatment.

The researchers found that the participants treated with ozonated oil showed significant reduction in ulcer size, erythema (redness of the skin), and also ulcer pain by the fourth day of evaluation when compared to patients who were given sesame oil or distilled water. On the sixth day, they found that the subjects treated with ozonated oil and sesame oil both showed significant reduction in ulcer size and erythema. No significant difference was observed in the placebo group when compared with other two groups during the six-day evaluation period. The researchers concluded:

> Ozonated oil and sesame oil both showed similar effectiveness in relieving the ulcer pain. Ozone with its wide variety of inherent properties has proven to be choice of treatment in completely relieving the ulcer pain and ulcer size when compared with that of its counter medication (i.e. sesame oil). Therefore the results obtained in the present study forecast ozone to be used as a novel treatment approach in recurrent aphthous ulcers. . . . Ozone provides a new path in recurrent aphthous ulcer treatment owing to its wide range of inherent properties which benefits the patient, with its cost effective and ease of use.[17]

24
Athletic Performance, Preventive Health, and Healthy Aging

A s we've seen in previous chapters, much research has been done on how oxygen therapies can help the body heal itself of a wide variety of disease conditions. Some of these studies have led researchers to believe that these therapies can also have value for healthy people, including athletes, who want to maintain their health and for people who want to stay young despite the number of their years. They want, to quote the adage, "to die young, but live as long as possible."

ATHLETIC PERFORMANCE

Ozone therapy has been viewed as an important factor in enhancing athletic performance—to such a great degree that Dr. Bocci warned against the use of ozone doping of athletes in *Oxygen-Ozone Therapy: A Critical Evaluation.*[1]

Ozone therapy can have many benefits for athletes. It not only enhances tissue oxygenation but also increases production of adenosine triphosphate, resulting in more energy and faster recovery. Ozone can also delay the onset of anaerobic fermentation of sugar in cells and reduce lactic acid buildup, thus helping prevent sore muscles and improving recovery time after physical exertion.

A study undertaken by Prof. M. Nabil Mawsouf involved two groups of female gymnasts at the Faculty of Physical Education at Helwan University in Egypt. Lactic acid measurements were taken before 10 minutes of intense exercise on an ergometric bicycle (with the heart rate reaching 160 beats per minute) and again after 20 minutes of rest. The same procedure was repeated on the second day for the test group, but instead of resting, the athletes underwent a 20-minute exposure to an ozone steam bath. This was repeated for six sessions over a two-month period. In addition, the gymnasts competed in rhythmic gymnastics (including jumps and leaps, balance, flexibility, turns and pivots, and waves) and were evaluated by three judges from the university both at the start of the study and after two months.

Results showed that lactic acid levels were approximately 66 percent lower in the group treated with ozone, both after a single session and over two months. In addition, the athletic performance scores increased by approximately 30 percent for those treated with ozone. Dr. Mawsouf concluded that ozone enhances athletic performance and decreases the recovery period.[2]

PREVENTIVE HEALTH

Much of today's mainstream medicine focuses on curing disease rather than maintaining good health. And while many physicians use oxygen therapies primarily for crisis care, some, like Dr. Frank Shallenberger, believe that occasional transient oxidative stress can do much to strengthen the body's natural immune defenses. As a result, the body is better able to fight off diseases related to viruses, bacteria, and fungi and resist degenerative diseases like arthritis, heart disease, and diabetes. Over time, this can help us enjoy longer and healthier lives. Much of the clinical research presented in this book can be viewed in the light of preventive health care, although the research itself was inspired by the quest to help cure disease.

At the present time, "disease care" is placing ever-increasing pressure on health insurance companies and national health care budgets. This ultimately has an impact on health care consumers, whether directly (through higher costs for medical care) or indirectly (through higher insurance premiums and taxes).

Oxygen therapies can offer an exciting new paradigm for helping us both achieve and maintain wellness. Though it is not very likely, I would love to see scientific research focus on the long-term benefits of oxygen therapies as part of a holistic program of preventive health and wellness care as opposed to merely curing disease symptoms. The chapters in part 3 will deal with complementary methods of preventive health and health maintenance in more detail.

HEALTHY AGING

A 2001 article in the London *Sunday Mirror* broke the news that Elizabeth, the Queen Mother, who was one hundred years old at the time, was receiving ozone therapy for health maintenance and rejuvenation. The article added that she had decided to try ozone at the suggestion of her grandson: "Prince Charles, whose interest in fringe treatments is well-known, suggested alternative medicine for his grandmother, who celebrated her centenary last August after a lifetime of mainly good health. She let slip the treatment to friends when they commented how good she looked."[3]

How can oxygen therapies assist in healthy aging? Prof. Shadia Bakarat of the Physiology Department at the Faculty of Medicine of Ain Shams University in Cairo developed an experimental protocol using a small dose of ozone administered via autohemotherapy (0.48 mg/kg of body weight at a concentration of 4 µg/ml) twice weekly for twelve weeks to female rats at both early and late stages of menopause. In her presentation at the First International Conference on Medical Ozone, held in Cairo in 2006, she concluded that medical ozone can play a more beneficial role than a swim training program in preventing alterations in microcirculation and the structure of muscular and visceral fat tissue. She also believes that ozone therapy at the late postmenopausal stage can improve altered mitochondrial density, collagen density, and vascular smooth muscle thickness. Specifically, it can do the following:

- Induce capillary vascular remodeling by promoting angiogenesis (the formation and differentiation of blood vessels). This not only prevents alteration of capillary density and muscle size but also reduces the alteration of mitochondrial density and collagen density.
- Promote tissue oxygenation and enhance the body's antioxidant enzyme capacity and antioxidant status.
- Enhance nitric oxide release.
- Promote vasoregulation.
- Increase antioxidant defense.[4]

Although Dr. Barakat's preliminary research on laboratory animals is promising, the role of oxygen therapies in human gerontology requires investigation. Given the generation of "baby boomers" who are reaching retirement age, perhaps the use of therapeutic ozone and hydrogen peroxide can hold much promise toward achieving a level of healthy aging that every individual wants and deserves.

25
Dentistry

It was mentioned earlier that one of the pioneers of oxidative therapies was a dentist. In 1932 ozonated water was first used as a mouth disinfectant by Dr. E. A. Fisch, a German dentist. Dr. Fisch also patented the first ozone delivery apparatus for dentistry, which he called Cytozon.[1] One of his patients was Austrian surgeon Erwin Payr, who immediately saw the therapeutic possibilities of ozone in medical therapy. Since that time ozone and hydrogen peroxide have been widely used in both dentistry and stomatology, a branch of medical therapy dealing with the mouth and its disorders. Hydrogen peroxide has been used in dentistry—either alone or in combination with salts—for more than seventy years. It has been found to help prevent plaque and gingivitis and is helpful in healing infections in the mouth and gums.[2]

Until recently ozone has been used in the dental office primarily as ozonated water. According to German dentist Fritz Kramer, writing in 1984, ozonated water can be effective in the following ways:

- As a powerful disinfectant
- In its ability to control bleeding
- In its ability to cleanse wounds in bones and soft tissue
- In speeding healing by improving the local supply of oxygen to the wound area

- In improving the metabolic processes related to healing by increasing temperature in the area of the wound

Dr. Kramer also points out that ozonated water can be used in a number of different applications:

- Mouth rinse (especially in cases of gingivitis, paradentosis, thrush, or stomatitis)
- Spray to cleanse the affected area and to disinfect oral mucosa and cavities and in general dental surgery
- Ozone-water jet to clean cavities of teeth being capped or receiving root canal therapy[3]

In 2013, a group of reserarchers at the University of São Paulo in Brazil undertook an in vitro study to compare the antimicrobial activity of three different concentrations of aqueous ozone on three standardized strains of bacteria: *Pseudomonas aeruginosa, Staphylococcus aureus,* and *Enterococcus faecalis.* The suspensions of bacteria were cultivated and spectrophotometrically adjusted to a final concentration of 4.46×108 CFU/ml.

The bacteria strains were then exposed to different solutions, which were divided into groups: Group 1—aqueous ozone, 2 µg/ml; Group 2—aqueous ozone, 5 µg/ml; Group 3—aqueous ozone, 8 µg/ml; and Group Control—bidistilled cold sterile water with no ozone. Although all three strains of bacteria exposed to the sterile water continued to thrive, the ozonated solutions were able to kill *Pseudomonas aeruginosa* and *Staphylococcus aureus.* Only the 8 µg/ml ozone solution concentration was able to eliminate *Enterococcus faecalis.* The researchers concluded: "According to the applied methodology, it was possible to conclude that the aqueous ozone in concentration of 8 µg/ml was the most efficient to eliminate the three evaluated bacteria."[4]

A 2012 article by Dr. Mansi Bansal and Dr. G. Gupta of the

Institute of Dental Studies and Technologies in India summarized the numerous applications and benefits of ozone therapy in dentistry, especially in the field of periodontics:

Goals of Ozone Therapy

1. Elimination of pathogens
2. Restoration of proper oxygen metabolism
3. Induction of a friendly ecologic environment
4. Increased circulation
5. Immune activation
6. Stimulation of the humoral antioxidant system

Uses in Dentistry

- Periodontology: gingivitis, periodontitis, peri-implantitis, surgical cuts, prophylaxis
- Dental and oral pathology: caries, enamel cracks, root canal treatment, tooth whitening, dentinal hypersensitivity, abscess, granuloma, fistulas, aphthae, herpes infection, stomatitis, candidiasis
- Surgery: implantation, replantation, extraction, wound healing, coagulopathy, prolonged bleeding
- Prosthodontics and restorative dentistry: stumps and crown disinfection, cavity disinfection
- Orthodontics and orthopedics: TMJ dysfunctions, trismus, relaxation, myoarthopathy

The authors noted that, in addition to ozonated water, the field has expanded to include the use of a mixture of ozone and oxygen in gaseous form. When compared to traditional medical modalities such as antibiotics and disinfectants, they concluded, ozone therapy is inexpensive, predictable, and conservative. Pointing out that ozone therapy is often a painless and minimally invasive procedure, the authors state that it is increasingly being favored by dentists and patients alike to treat a wide variety of dental problems. "The treatment is completely painless and increases the patients' acceptability and compliance with minimal adverse effects."[5]

On the following pages, we will explore some of the specific applications for oxidative therapies in the dentist's office.

DISEASES OF THE MOUTH

Three percent hydrogen peroxide has long been a popular and inexpensive mouthwash, taken either full strength or diluted in water. Today, a growing number of commercial toothpastes and mouthwashes containing hydrogen peroxide are available. Yet it was not until 1979 that a university-sponsored study was published in the *Journal of Clinical Periodontology* testifying to hydrogen peroxide's outstanding ability to retard the development of plaque and gingivitis, two of our most common dental problems.

Fourteen dental students at the Department of Periodontology at the University of Gothenburg in Sweden took part in this double-blind study. After a thorough dental examination, half of the students were given a mouthwash containing hydrogen peroxide, while the other group was given a placebo mouthwash. The students were told to rinse their mouths three times daily, after meals. Toothbrushing during this two-week trial was not permitted. Measurements of plaque and gingival "index scores" were performed after four, seven, and fourteen days of the trial. Bacteria from the mouth was microscopically examined and analyzed after the first and second weeks.

The results showed that the mouthwash containing hydrogen peroxide effectively prevented the colonization of a number of types of bacteria (including filaments, fusiforms, and motile and curved rods), as well as spirochetes in developing plaque. It also retarded plaque formation and "significantly retarded" gingivitis development. The researchers concluded: "It is suggested that H_2O_2 released by mouthwashes during rinsing may prevent or retard the colonization and multiplication of anaerobic bacteria."[6]

Over the past few years, most toothpaste manufacturers have been marketing toothpastes made with hydrogen peroxide. This led Dr. M. V. Marshall and his colleagues at Dermigen, a Texas-based biotech firm specializing in tissue-based toxicology and therapeutics, to review the safety of adding hydrogen peroxide to commercial toothpastes and report their findings in the September 1995 issue of the *Journal of Periodontology.*

The researchers found that daily exposure to the low levels of hydrogen peroxide present in dentifrices is much lower than that of bleaching agents that contain or produce high levels of hydrogen peroxide for an extended period of time. They also reviewed studies in which 3 percent hydrogen peroxide or less was used daily for up to six years. These studies showed occasional transitory irritant effects only in a small number of subjects with preexisting ulceration or when high levels of salt solutions were administered at the same time. The studies also pointed out that if mishandled, bleaching agents that employ or generate high levels of hydrogen peroxide or organic peroxides can produce localized oral toxicity following sustained exposure.

Dr. Marshall and his colleagues found that prolonged use of hydrogen peroxide decreased plaque and gingivitis. However, therapeutic delivery of hydrogen peroxide to prevent gum disease required professional cleaning at the dentist's office. They added, "Wound healing following gingival [gum] surgery was enhanced due to the antimicrobial effects of topically administered hydrogen peroxide. For most subjects, beneficial effects were seen with H_2O_2 levels above 1%."[7]

In former East Germany, a team of dental researchers investigated the germicidal value of hydrogen peroxide rinses in treating root canal patients suffering from osteitis, or bone inflammation. Thirty-two teeth with the diagnosis of periapical osteitis (established by clinical and radiological examinations) were subjected to irrigation with hydrogen peroxide, followed by bacteriological examinations. The timing of treatment termination depended solely upon clinical evaluation. The examination of smears taken before the last irrigation showed that twenty-six of the thirty-two root canals (81 percent) were germ free; in two cases, an anaerobic infection continued to persist, and in four cases, an aerobic infection was observed. Enterococci proved to be the most resistant bacteria to hydrogen peroxide.

The researchers pointed out, "The high percentage of root canals which were germ-free before the last irrigation testifies to the efficiency of hydrogen peroxide application for disinfecting root canals on the one hand, and demonstrates the good agreement between clinical and bacteriological findings on the other hand." They concluded, "The conservative treatment of periapical osteitis by means of root-canal disinfection with a hydrogen peroxide preparation and subsequent root-canal filling with a calcium peroxide paste is recommended."[8]

A team of dentists from the Department of Dental Specialties at the famous Mayo Clinic reported an unusual case of persistent local idiopathic gingivitis that had been resistant to previous oral hygiene measures in the *Journal of the American Dental Association*. They decided to try a product called Superoxol, a patented aqueous solution based on 35 percent hydrogen peroxide, with excellent results. The authors concluded: "This case illustrates a successful treatment measure for an uncommon clinical challenge."[9]

A Russian clinical study compared the effectiveness of ozone therapy to traditional therapy in treating patients with local sluggish pyoinflammatory diseases of the maxillofacial soft tissues, or tissues around the upper jaw. Thirty patients were given both general and local ozone therapy, while thirty-three patients received conventional treatment. The results showed that ozone "decreased the duration of treatment more than 2-fold due to antibacterial effect and stimulation of nonspecific and immunological activity." The researchers concluded: "Lack of obvious contraindications and selective activity and universal immunocorrective effect recommend ozone therapy to wide use in this patient population irrespective of the type of inflammatory reaction."[10]

A group of researchers at the Boston University Goldman School of Dental Medicine undertook a randomized clinical trial to determine the efficacy of a fluoridated hydrogen peroxide–based mouthwash to treat gingivitis and promote tooth whitening. Ninety-nine subjects were used for this six-month study, with approximately half of the subjects receiving the experimental rinse and the other group receiving a placebo.

Results showed that the Eastman interdental bleeding index, modified gingival index, and intensity of stain were "significantly" reduced in the test group (those receiving hydrogen peroxide), while only the Eastman interdental bleeding index score was significantly reduced in the control group. By the end of the study, the subjects receiving the test rinse were found to be six times more likely to show improvement in tooth color. The test mouthwash was found to be safe during the six-month period. The researchers concluded: "The results of this study indicate that the fluoridated hydrogen peroxide–based mouth rinse effectively whitens teeth and significantly reduces gingivitis."[11]

Oral Candida

Candida is one of the most common opportunistic infections of the mouth. For this reason, a study was undertaken by researchers at the Hitkarini Dental College and Hospital, in Jabalpur, Madhya Pradesh, India, to evaluate and compare the ability of ozonated water and topical clotrimazole in reducing the candidal species colony-forming unit (CFU) count in oral candidiasis. Clotrimazole is a popular medication primarily used to treat yeast infections of the vagina, mouth, and skin.

The study included forty candidiasis patients of both sexes between the ages of eighteen and sixty who were patients at the Hitkarini Dental College and Hospital's Department of Oral Medicine and Radiology. The patients were randomly assigned to two groups. One group received topical ozone therapy and the other received topical clotrimazole. Salivary candidal CFU counts were assessed during and after the treatments.

The researchers found that there was gradual but significant reduction in candidal CFU count in both groups. At the end of the treatment, candidal CFU count reduction in the ozone group (60.5 percent reduction) was greater than in the clotrimazole group (32.3 percent reduction). In the ozone group, the number of patients with candidiasis was reduced from fourteen (70 percent) to six (30 percent), whereas in the clotrimazole group that number dropped from thirteen (65 percent) to eight (40 percent). They concluded: "Ozone therapy was much more effective in reducing the patients with candidiasis to a state of carriers. These findings suggest that ozonated water might be useful to treat oral candidiasis."[12]

DENTAL CAVITY REVERSAL

Traditional dentistry has long employed the "drill and fill" approach to removing dental caries, which is often an uncomfortable and occasionally painful procedure for patients. Treated cavities frequently become decayed again. They then require additional drilling and filling, while in serious cases, the entire tooth is removed or a root canal and/or a crown is required.

One of the most exciting developments in ozone therapy involves the work of Dr. Edward Lynch, professor of restorative dentistry and gerodontology at the School of Dentistry in Belfast, Northern Ireland. He developed an innovative procedure to reverse tooth decay by applying ozone directly to the affected tooth.

Using a novel ozone delivery system (HealOzone, developed by KaVo, a German company, shown in figure 25.1), a ten-second application is given to the decayed tooth at a concentration of approximately 2,100 ppm. The ozone is delivered through a handheld device containing a disposable silicone cup that fits tightly around the tooth so that ozone cannot escape. After treatment, a suction mechanism draws out the gas to an ozone neutralizer that converts it into oxygen. This simple technique not only has been found to disinfect the cavity and remove dead tissue without drilling but actually promotes remineralization of the tooth itself!

Many clinical studies have evaluated this method of treatment, and a few of them will be cited here. In one study, Dr. Lynch and his research team found that after just ten seconds of ozone treatment, 99 percent of the tooth's microorganisms were eliminated and over 70 percent of the cavities either reversed or improved. Not a single lesion deteriorated. By contrast, 80 percent of the cavities among a control group deteriorated.[13]

Research done by Dr. Aylin Baysan of the School of Dentistry at the University of Birmingham in England and Dr. Lynch studied twenty-six patients with seventy primary root carious lesions (PRCLs). After ten or twenty seconds of treatment, the total number of microorganisms in the PRCLs was dramatically reduced. Out of the sixty-five PRCLs reviewed over five and a half months, thirty-three lesions had become hard, twenty-seven reversed to severity index 1 from severity index 2, and five lesions remained the same.[14] Figure 25.2 on page 316 shows the technique of applying the oxygen-ozone mixture.

Figure 25.1. The HealOzone unit (front view). (Photo courtesy of Dr. Julian Holmes.)

Figure 25.2. Applying oxygen-ozone to an infected tooth.
(Photo courtesy of Dr. Julian Holmes.)

Another randomized clinical study by Drs. Baysan and Lynch found that after twelve months of treatment with the HealOzone method, 47 percent of the root carious lesions reversed from severity index 1 to 0 (that is, hard) in the ozone group, while none of the lesions became hard in the control group. In addition, 52 percent of lesions reversed from severity index 2 to 1 in the ozone group, while only 11.6 percent of the control group experienced a similar reduction.[15]

A randomized controlled trial by Dr. Julian Holmes at the UK Smiles Dental Practice in England assessed the effects of this system on noncavitated leathery primary root carious lesions (PRCLs). Eighty-nine patients were chosen for this study, each with two of these lesions. The two lesions were randomly assigned for treatment with either ozone or air in a double-blind design; patients were evaluated after three, six, twelve, and eighteen months. Here are the results:

After three months: Among members of the ozone group, sixty-one PRCLs (69 percent) had become hard and none deteriorated, while among the controls, 4 percent had become worse. (Figure 25.3 on page 318 shows X-ray images comparing the effects of the treatment after three months.)

After six months: In the ozone group, seven PRCLs (8 percent) remained leathery and the remaining eighty-two (92 percent) remained hard; among the controls, ten PRCLs (11 percent) became worse and one had become hard.

After twelve months: Two subjects in the study had dropped out. Of the remaining eighty-seven participants, two PRCLs (2 percent) among the ozone group remained leathery, while eighty-five (98 percent) had hardened; among the controls, twenty-one PRCLs (24 percent) had progressed from leathery to soft, sixty-five (75 percent) were still leathery, and one (1 percent) remained hard.

After eighteen months: Among those treated with ozone, eighty-seven PRCLs (100 percent) were arrested, while in the control group, thirty-two lesions (37 percent) became soft, fifty-four (62 percent) remained leathery, and one became hard.

Dr. Holmes concluded: "Leathery non-cavitated primary root caries can be arrested non-operatively with ozone and remineralizing products. This treatment regime is an effective alternative to conventional 'drilling and filling.'"[16]

The future of this safe, effective, and noninvasive therapy is promising. Treating dental cavities with ozone requires no anesthesia, and uncomfortable drilling and filling can be avoided completely. In addition to treating dental cavities, this method could be used as an important part of preventive dentistry: treatments can be given to help avoid decay and strengthen teeth.

This method is now available in several European countries (including the United Kingdom and Germany) as well as Canada. At

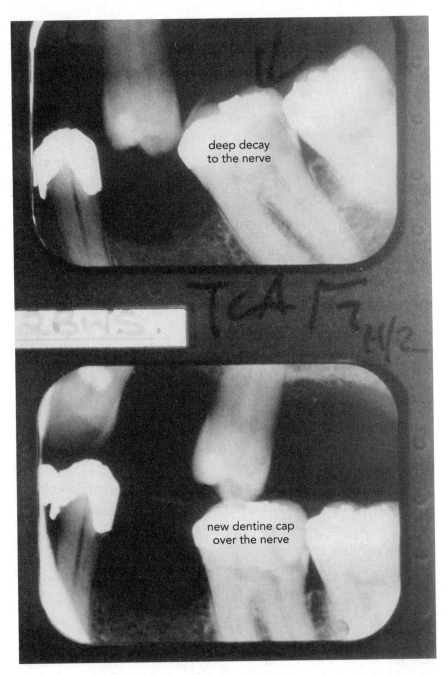

Figure 25.3. X-ray showing tooth before treatment and after three months. (Photo courtesy of Dr. Julian Holmes.)

the time of this writing, this ozone delivery device is being used by a growing number of dentists in the United States and has been welcomed by their patients. In an article in *Dentistry Today,* Dr. Russell Beggs, a dentist from California, wrote: "The ozone treatment has significant implications when dealing with new decay, recurrent decay, and an aging population. This is a new paradigm for dentistry."[17]

ROOT CANAL THERAPY

One of the major problems with root canal therapy (endodontics) is the danger of infection. While most practitioners feel that traditional means of disinfection are sufficient, some dentists have found that following endodontic therapy, some bacteria, fungi, and viruses remain in the multitude of the very small lateral canals and dentinal tubules that transverse the tooth root and communicate with the periodontal tissue.

The results of a cooperative study by researchers from three different dental schools in Portugal to determine if irrigation with sodium hypochlorite, chlorhexidine, and ozone gas, alone or in combination, was effective against *Enterococcus faecalis* and *Candida albicans* were reported in 2014. These two microorganisms often cause infections that can make root canal therapy unsuccessful. Sodium hypochlorite is frequently used as a bleaching or antibacterial agent, while chlorhexidine is often used as an active ingredient in mouthwash that reduces dental plaque and oral bacteria. Gaseous ozone was used in the study due to its well-known antibacterial action.

Using a total of 220 extracted teeth, researchers infected them with the two microorganisms. They found that sodium hypochlorite, chlorhexidine, and gaseous ozone alone were ineffective in completely eliminating the microorganisms. However, they found that a combination of chlorhexidine at 2 percent concentration followed by an application of ozone gas for twenty-four seconds brought about the complete elimination of both *Candida albicans* and *Enterococcus faecalis.* Flow cytometry—a technology used to analyze the physical and chemical characteristics of particles (such as cells) in a fluid as it passes through at least one laser—showed that ozone and chlorhexidine act differently, which could explain their synergic activity.

The researchers concluded: "This new disinfection protocol, combining irrigation with chlorhexidine at 2% and ozone gas for twenty-four seconds, may be advantageous when treating infected root canals."[18]

A 2013 study involving researchers from Yeditepe University and Istanbul University Capa in Turkey found that the application of topical ozone gas in recurrent doses is effective in killing the *Enterococcus faecalis* bacterium in root canals. They added that using ozone with sodium hypochlorate (NaOCL) was even more effective than ozone alone, totally eliminating *E. faecalis* biofilm in root canals. A biofilm is any group of microorganisms in which cells stick to each other on a surface, such as a tooth.[19]

Two American dentists, Philip Mollica and Robert E. Harris Jr., use ozone therapy in their practices and have trained over two thousand dentists in the use of ozone therapy over the years. In their article "Integrating Oxygen/Ozone Therapy into Your Practice," they outlined the three major stages of using oxygen and ozone in root canal therapy:

- Files are coated with ozonated olive oil for lubrication and disinfection.
- The canals are prepared, irrigated with ozonated water, and dried.
- The final step before filling each canal is slow insufflation with oxygen-ozone gas. The insufflation process allows the molecular oxygen-ozone to travel into the canals, lateral canals, and tubules. The molecular oxygen-ozone can travel through the tubules and kill the positively charged microbes and perform a true sterilization.[20]

POST-EXTRACTION PAIN

A joint study by researchers at the Department of Oral and Maxillofacial Surgery of the Faculty of Dentistry at both Bezmialem Vakif University and Istanbul University in Turkey evaluated the effects of ozone therapy on the management of pain, swelling, and spasm of the jaw muscles after the surgical extraction of impacted mandibular third molar teeth.

Sixty patients between eighteen and twenty-five years of age diagnosed with asymptomatic bilateral impacted mandibular third molars were selected for this study. The molar on one side of the mouth was extracted and ozone therapy was given (study side). The molar on the other side was extracted two weeks later and sham ozone therapy was given (negative control side).

The researchers found no differences between the two sides for mouth opening or swelling. However, they found that the degree of pain and the number of analgesic tablets taken was "significantly lower" for the study side.

Patients were all given the Oral Health Impact Profile (also known as the OHIP-14 questionnaire), which asks about the frequency of fourteen functional and psychosocial impacts that people have experienced as a result of problems with their teeth, mouth, or dentures. The researchers concluded: "This study showed ozone therapy to have a positive effect on OHIP-14 questionnaire results."[21]

ORAL MUCOSITIS IN DENTAL IMPLANTATION

Oral mucositis involves inflammation and ulceration that occur in the mouth. It is a common and often debilitating complication of cancer treatment but can also occur with dental implants.

A double-blind randomized controlled trial by researchers in the United Kingdom assessed the effect of subgingival ozone and/or hydrogen peroxide on the development of peri-implant mucositis. The term *subgingival* refers to the crevice between the gum margin and the neck or root of a tooth. Peri-implant diseases are inflammatory conditions affecting the soft and hard gum tissues around dental implants.

Twenty subjects (with a mean age of sixty) with a total of eighty implants (four implants each) were recruited for the study. First, a two-week pretrial phase took place to achieve healthy gums. Then, partial gum shields were constructed for the experimental area (i.e, around the four implants). Subjects were asked to refrain from brushing in that area by wearing the gum shield.

The following treatments were randomly applied for sixty seconds to implant sites on days zero, seven, and fourteen:

- oxygen and saline (0.9 percent NaCl) (control group)
- oxygen and hydrogen peroxide (3 percent)
- ozone and saline
- ozone and hydrogen peroxide

Plaque, gingival, and bleeding indices were recorded on days zero, seven, fourteen, and twenty-one. Significant differences were found among the treatments in plaque, modified gingival, and bleeding indices. Both the ozone + saline and ozone + hydrogen peroxide produced "optimum" gingival health scores and were considered equally effective. They were also the most effective in controlling bleeding (mean score = 0.05), while oxygen + saline was found to be the least effective (mean score = 0.56). The researchers concluded: "Ozone showed great potential for management of peri-implant mucositis."[22]

Writing in the *Journal of Natural Science, Biology and Medicine,* Dr. Rajiv Saini of the Department of Periodontology and Oral Implantology of the Rural Dental College in Maharasthra, India, stated: "Ozone therapy has been more beneficial than present conventional therapeutic modalities that follow a minimally invasive and conservative application to dental treatment. The exposition of molecular mechanisms of ozone further benefits practical function in dentistry."[23]

TEMPOROMANDIBULAR JOINT DYSFUNCTION

The temporomandibular joint acts like a hinge, connecting the jawbone to the skull. Dysfunction can lead to pain and discomfort, including jaw pain, difficulty chewing, and clicking and locking of the jaw joint.

Dr. William C. Domb, director of the Inland Institute of Aesthetic Dentistry in Upland, California, has incorporated ear insufflation of ozone to manage both sinusitis and temporomandibular joint dysfunction. In his article appearing in *Interventional Neuroradiology,* he writes, "Temporomandibular joint dysfunction has multifactorial origins and may sometimes be managed by joint injections. Muscle trigger points may also be areas where ozone placement can help with headache pain."[24]

Dentistry has probably become the most exciting area of research in ozone therapy today. Whether used as an oral disinfectant or in treating gum diseases and other mouth infections, dental cavity reversal, root canal therapy, dental implants, tooth whitening, or pain relief, a growing number of practitioners and patients consider ozone a safe, effective, and economical first choice.

26
Veterinary Medicine

Ozone and hydrogen peroxide have been used in veterinary medicine for over thirty years and have enjoyed a wide variety of applications. While most of us envision our local vet using ozone therapy on our cat or dog, perhaps the widest area of application is in agribusiness: ozone and hydrogen peroxide are already widely employed as disinfectants for washing equipment used in breeding facilities, wastewater treatment, and milk collection. In Russia, ozone has been used for decades to treat farm animals for a wide variety of diseases and to promote wound healing.

While carefully regulated by state and provincial licensing boards, veterinary medicine is not as tightly controlled as human medicine. As a result, holistic practitioners have somewhat more freedom to use nontraditional therapies like ozone or hydrogen peroxide in their practices, although much depends on laws of each state.

At least several dozen veterinarians (many of them members of the American Holistic Veterinary Medical Association) currently use ozone in the United States and Canada to treat both domestic animals, like cats and dogs, and farm animals for a wide range of health problems. In the United States at least, I've found that veterinarians who use oxidative therapies tend to be strong advocates of both natural and holistic approaches to health. Some, like Martin Goldstein, D.V.M., of New York (author of the acclaimed book *The Nature of Animal Healing*);

Judith Shoemaker, D.V.M., of Pennsylvania; Margo Roman, D.V.M., of Massachusetts; and Robert Smatt, D.V.M., of California, are respected leaders in their profession.

CLINICAL APPLICATIONS

In an article published in *IVC Journal,* an online publication devoted to integrative veterinary medicine, Dr. Margo Roman highlighted the major clinical applications of ozone therapy in veterinary medicine:

- Skin: wounds, especially degloving ones and deep abrasions; hot spots; pyodermas; allergic dermatitis; abscesses
- Pain relief
- Head trauma and spinal cord inflammation: ozone and oxygen go through the blood-brain barrier so it is an excellent way to aid treatment of any neurological issue
- Chronic and acute Lyme disease
- Mouth: stomatitis, gingivitis, abscesses; ozone therapy is ADA-approved for dental abscesses
- Cancer and autoimmune problems
- Ears: chronic and acute otitis from bacteria or yeast; aural hematomas
- Eyes: infections and allergic reactions
- Upper respiratory ailments
- Potentiates acupuncture, homeopathy, and chiropractic treatments as it brings more needed oxygen to the body
- Gastrointestinal tract: constipation, diarrhea, IBS (decreases inflammation)
- Equine infectious anemia

She also mentioned that antibiotics are more effective when ozone is used as an adjunct, thus potentially reducing the amount of antibiotics used in treatment. She adds that ozone therapy also increases the

Figure 26.1. Ozone therapy applications in veterinary medicine.
(Courtesy of Dr. Margo Roman.)

effectiveness of other natural modalities, like acupuncture, homeopathy, herbs, and chiropractic.[1]

In a response to her article, Kathy Backus, D.V.M., reported that ozone therapy also makes an excellent adjunct to biophotonic therapy, which utilizes the bactericidal properties of ultraviolet rays in healing. First developed in the 1920s by Dr. Emmitt K. Knott, biophotonic therapy is easily combined with ozone: A small amount of blood is withdrawn from the patient, mixed with saline, and treated with ozone gas. It is then reinfused past UV light and injected back into the patient. She found that this combination therapy, like ozone alone, improves immune response, helps fight bacteria and viruses, and promotes pain relief.[2]

A later article in the same journal by Dr. G. M. Buchoff focused on the use of injecting ozone and oxygen into joints to reduce joint pain and infection, primarily in dogs and cats. He wrote that ozone injected into joints can stop the pain/inflammation cycle in orthopedic surgery and joint trauma. As with humans, areas of trauma can also be covered with a plastic bag and an ozone gas and oxygen mixture pumped into it with a tube or large syringe (*ozone bagging*) to control pain and promote healing.[3]

DR. SMATT'S EXPERIENCE

In his monograph *The Use of Ozone and Oxygen Therapies in Veterinary Medicine,* Dr. Robert Smatt highlights a variety of methods used to treat his patients at the Genesee Bird and Pet Clinic in San Diego, California. Many of his methods are used by other veterinarians around the world to treat a wide range of health problems.

Major Autohemotherapy
Dr. Smatt, who treats a number of health problems with major autohemotherapy, spoke to me about his successful treatment of a dog suffering from cirrhosis. In his article about ozone applications, he writes:

> In dogs and cats, I often infuse the ozonated blood back into the patient by injecting it intraperitoneally instead of intravenously. This route of administration seems to be equally effective. This procedure is repeated every one to seven days depending upon the condition. This procedure should greatly enhance surgical healing and anesthesia recovery when done before and after surgery. In general, an obvious and immediate increase in vitality, appetite, and competitiveness is noted in people, dogs, cats, horses.[4]

Minor Autohemotherapy
Dr. Smatt has also found that his canine and feline patients respond well to minor autohemotherapy. He sometimes injects the blood and

ozone mixture via the intraperitoneal route, because the amount of blood injected can be much larger than through a muscle. In addition, he finds that the blood and gas can mix longer without danger of causing clotting problems.

Rectal Insufflation

Rectal insufflation is also widely used in veterinary practice. According to Dr. Smatt:

> Ozone should be retained for 40 minutes to be effective. We use rectal infusions for 80% of our small animal and equine patients, and could easily justify its use in 100% of all medical and surgical problems. It is very well tolerated (accepted by both animals and their human companions). Invariably there is an immediate increase in vitality and appetite after the first administration.
> Urinary bladder insufflation is used for bladder problems.[5]

Limb Bagging

As with humans, ozone bagging is used in veterinary medicine to treat infections and wounds. Dr. Smatt recommends using either a specially designed bag manufactured by Ozonosan or a normal plastic garbage bag. He wraps the bag with an elasticized bandage to expel air and to seal the top; the bandage is then removed and the bag is filled with oxygen and ozone. The gas is retained for 30 to 40 minutes, and treatments are scheduled one or two times per day.

Ozonated Water

Dr. Smatt recommends the use of ozonated water for drinking.

Ozonated Saline

Dr. Smatt believes that ozonated saline solution offers several advantages in veterinary practice. He finds that it can be used in the bladder, vagina, ears, rectum, and eyes and is able to irrigate large surface

Figures 26.2 and 26.3. Ozone bagging and ear insufflation
(Courtesy of Dr. Margo Roman.)

wounds with it, which increases healing rates. It can also be given intravenously. He reports that using ozonated saline solutions is an effective way to flush chronically infected nasal passages and sinuses in cats.

Oxygen-Ozone Injections

Like humans, domestic animals often suffer from painful joints. Dr. Smatt uses a method to treat his veterinary patients that is similar to the one Dr. Shallenberger uses to treat his human patients: a small amount of oxygen-ozone mixture is injected into the joint.

Dr. Smatt also administers oxygen-ozone injections to pressure points and to acupuncture points to relieve pain and promote healing. For example, he injects ozone gas in the "K 3, UB 60, Du 1, Ren 1, Ren 3, UB 40, UB 36, and the ba liao points," which he says works much better to control urinary incontinence than does the same treatment using vitamin B_{12}. Oxygen-ozone injections are also used to treat a variety of specific problems like spinal disc problems and even tumors, for which such treatment appears to be only partially successful.[6]

Inhalation of Ozone

In an interview in late 2005, Dr. Smatt told me about an ozone chamber he uses that allows his patients to breath oxygen and ozone that is bubbled through olive oil (we mentioned this method for humans in chapter 5). He finds that this method of treatment is very effective with small animals like birds, cats, and small dogs, and it is especially beneficial when treating infections. A normal treatment takes 20 minutes and is given once every day or once every other day for up to two weeks as needed.[7] This method could be of tremendous potential in treating birds suffering from avian influenza.

DR. GOLDSTEIN'S EXPERIENCE

Dr. Martin Goldstein, one of the country's best-known veterinarians, has treated animals at his Smith Ridge Veterinary Clinic in upstate New York for over twenty-five years. In *The Nature of Animal Healing,* Dr. Goldstein wrote extensively about his clinical experience with holistic therapies, commenting that ozone "often produces amazing turnarounds when conventional therapy fails." He followed this comment with a case history of Lucky, a shih tzu who was totally paralyzed by an inoperable spinal tumor in his neck. He was brought to Smith Ridge as a last resort (before euthanasia) after conventional therapy failed. After a careful examination, Dr. Goldstein administered intravenous vitamin C and ozone, put Lucky up for the night at the clinic, and the next morning found him walking. Two years later, Lucky was playing with his toys for the first time in eight years, and blood tests showed that the dog's immune system was actively handling his condition and that the cancer had ceased to be a factor in his health.[8]

Like Dr. Smatt, Goldstein and his colleagues have treated a wide variety of health problems with ozone therapy, including spinal problems and paralysis. Intravenous ozone is used, along with intravenous vitamin C, to treat canine distemper.[9] Ozonated oil is used topically to treat wounds and infections, as well as to relieve chronic ear problems.[10] In cases of severe or unresponsive liver problems (such as jaundice, hepatitis, and cirrhosis), Dr. Goldstein has used ozone as part of a holistic approach using intravenous and injectable vitamins and homeopathics.[11] Ozone therapy has also been utilized as part of a broad-scope treatment of spinal infarction or blood clot.[12]

However, Dr. Goldstein believes that ozone therapy (through direct injection into a tumor, intravenous ozone, or rectal insufflation, depending on the case) works especially well with different types of cancer. Commenting on bone cancer, Dr. Goldstein wrote: "With primary bone cancer, medically known as osteosarcoma, the only stories I could tell until about two years ago [1997] were unremittingly negative. The success I've had since then is due, I'm convinced, to the introduction of ozone therapy in treatment."[13]

SCIENTIFIC JOURNALS

Aside from reports of clinical experience with oxygen therapies by veterinary practitioners, there is little published research on the subject, especially in the United States. Like studies in human medicine, pharmaceutical companies often finance veterinary research by providing grants to researchers or by supporting programs in veterinary schools.

However, in addition to published human studies that involve the vivisection of laboratory animals, there are occasional reports in scientific journals about animals used in agribusiness, such as how ozone inhibits harmful spores in birds, published in the *Journal of Parasitology*,[14] or how autohemotherapy with ozone improves the immunological response in calves, published in the *Journal of Veterinary Medical Sciences*.[15] An article in *Poultry Science* by researchers at Texas A&M University explored how ozone, when applied to contaminated grain, can prevent aflatoxicosis in turkey poults,[16] while a Japanese study showed that ozone can be an effective way to treat acute clinical mastitis in dairy cows.[17]

In his book *Oxygen-Ozone Therapy: A Critical Evaluation,* Dr. Bocci surveyed a number of European veterinarians and reported that ozonated oil can be useful in getting rid of dog ticks, can be applied to the ear in cases of ear infection, and can be used to treat eye infections in low concentrations. He also mentioned that ozone applications can be useful for large animals before major surgery to strengthen them before the operation and to reduce the risk of postoperative infection.

Bocci also addressed rumors involving the illegal ozone doping of racehorses and dogs (either via autohemotherapy or rectal insufflation) in order to enhance their competitive performance.[18] In contrast to drugs used for doping, ozone cannot be detected after it is administered, so it is virtually impossible to prove that illegal doping ever took place.

OZONE, ANTIBIOTICS, AND *E. COLI*

A group of researchers at United Graduate School of Veterinary Medicine at Yamaguchi University in Japan noted that antibiotic therapy administered for treatment of gram-negative bacterial infections (such as mastitis)—especially among dairy cows—can exert a negative effect in the form of endotoxin shock. For this reason, they wanted to discover a sterilization method that releases less endotoxin than traditional antibiotics.

They undertook an in vitro study aimed to compare the amounts of endotoxin released from *Escherichia coli* exposed to antibiotics (aminobenzylpenicillin, kanamycin, oxytetracycline, sulfadimethoxine, and enrofloxacin) or ozone. The bacterial growth and amount of endotoxin released were measured at specific time points.

Compared with antibiotic treatment, they found that ozone sterilization induced a release of smaller amounts of endotoxin from the bacteria. In addition, they observed no major differences when ozone was used against the purified endotoxin. They concluded that compared with antibiotic treatment, ozone sterilization may release smaller amounts of endotoxin.

Noting the effectiveness of ozone therapy in treating mastitis among dairy cows (mastitis involves inflammation of the udder tissue and is the most common disease in dairy cattle), the researchers observed:

The high cure rate of acute mastitis in dairy cows is attributable to ozone's characteristic feature of inducing less release of endotoxin. The effects of ozone on immunity have been reported; ozone may downregulate the cytotoxic activity of immunocytes. Although we actually observed the effect of non-antibiotic (ozone) treatment, we cannot explain, based on the present study, whether the high cure rate is the result of less endotoxin release or whether there exists another reason. Considering that ozone induces release of smaller amounts of endotoxin and has no effect on endotoxin, ozone should be used as the first line of treatment for coliform mastitis to thereby, possibly, reduce mortality.[19]

SARS AND BIRD FLU?

Perhaps the most important contribution of oxidative therapies can be in treating animal-borne diseases that can be transferred to humans, such as SARS (severe acute respiratory syndrome), bird flu (avian influenza), and others that threaten to develop into human pandemics. Effective vaccines have not yet been developed for these diseases, which can potentially become resistant to antiviral or antibacterial drugs. As with other diseases among humans, contagious or not, mainstream medical and scientific researchers have been resistant to even *consider* the possibility that simple and inexpensive modalities such as oxidative therapies can be a viable solution to these serious global health threats.

Research urgently needs to be carried out to evaluate the effectiveness of ozone and hydrogen peroxide in helping prevent animal-borne diseases from spreading among animals, treating animals that may have been exposed to these pathogens, and treating people who may become infected.

PART THREE

A Holistic Protocol

Oxidative therapies are an integral part of a holistic approach to health. They assist the body in oxidating viruses and bacteria as well as weak and sick tissue cells so that stronger and healthier cells can take their place.

With the use of ozone and hydrogen peroxide by themselves having achieved important results (Cuban physicians, for example, often use ozone alone when treating patients), a growing number of oxidative practitioners have been looking toward the value of taking a holistic approach to health, one that teaches that in order to heal the patient, one must address the individual as a whole, including the physical body, mind, and spirit. According to Janet F. Quinn, Ph.D., R.N., in her essay "The Healing Arts in Modern Health Care":

> The Holistic Health perspective acknowledges the fundamental wholeness, unity and integrity of the individual in interaction with the environment. Body–mind–spirit are viewed as inseparable and interdependent dimensions of being. All behaviors, including health and illness, are manifestations of the life process of the whole person.[1]

Believing that all aspects of a person are interrelated and that each has an impact on all other aspects of one's being, holistic practitioners address issues like diet, nutrition, and exercise, as well as mental, emotional, and spiritual well-being. A good example of the holistic approach was formulated by John C. Pittman, M.D., who worked extensively with patients diagnosed with HIV and AIDS. An early advocate of oxidative therapies, Dr. Pittman created the following "Comprehensive HIV/AIDS Protocol," which is designed to assist in the healing of many aspects of the patient's being:

1. *Intravenous ozone:* Start with small amounts at low concentrations and increase gradually as tolerated on a near-daily basis.
2. *Intravenous hydrogen peroxide:* A dilute solution is given two or three times a week.
3. *Intravenous vitamin C:* 70 grams, along with other vitamins, minerals, and antiviral agents is given once or twice a week.
4. *EDTA chelation:* Chelation is performed using half the standard dose of EDTA [ethylenediaminetetraacetic acid], a synthetic amino acid. This involves a series of intravenous infusions of EDTA and various other substances.
5. *External oxygenation:* Devices spray hot ozonated water, followed by a bath with a high concentration of hydrogen peroxide.
6. *Hyperbaric oxygen chamber:* HBO therapy is used immediately following ozone infusion, whether by rectal insufflation or autohemotherapy.
7. *Metabolic and intestinal detoxification:* Three-day supplemented fast combined with intestinal cleanser and colonic irrigation.
8. *Raw and living food diet:* Includes green drinks and wheatgrass juice to stimulate enzyme pathways.
9. *Nutritional supplements:* Large quantities of antioxidants, sulfur-containing amino acids, specific immune-stimulating herbs, and hydrochloric acid are used to improve digestion.
10. *Exercise:* Daily aerobic exercise is used to elevate heart rate and improve oxygen delivery to tissues.[2]

In the following five chapters we examine a variety of natural approaches to health that can complement ozone and hydrogen peroxide therapy. Using material from a wide variety of sources—with special emphasis on the work of oxidative therapy practitioners—we will examine body cleansing, diet, nutrition, aerobic exercise and breathing, and mental, emotional, and spiritual well-being.

27
Body Cleansing

The body is perfectly designed to be a self-cleaning organism. It eliminates toxins efficiently through exhaling, sneezing, coughing, vomiting, moving the bowels, urinating, sweating, and the occasional formation of boils and pimples. In theory, the body should be able to eliminate all of the waste matter from normal metabolism as well as the toxic matter taken into the body through breathing, eating, and other contact with the environment.

Unfortunately, our modern lifestyles often make it difficult for the body to perform its natural functions efficiently. Lack of exercise, poor diet, overeating, smoking, environmental pollution, the high consumption of pesticides in food, and the stresses of daily life place unnatural burdens on the body, making the efficient elimination of toxins difficult. This is especially true if we are already ill, so that the body is further intoxicated by medications, radiation, or chemotherapy.

Hydrogen peroxide and ozone are powerful oxidizers. Although the dozens of studies cited in this book testify to their health-enhancing qualities, oxidative therapies can also cause problems: the accelerated oxidation of viruses, bacteria, fungi, diseased cells, and other substances the body no longer needs can bring about a toxic buildup in the body if it is not able to eliminate them efficiently.

Body cleansing can serve two main purposes. First, by helping the body to get rid of its toxic load, it enhances the body's ability to perform its normal functions of elimination more efficiently. Second, it prevents toxic overload, which can lead to discomfort and disease. Some body-cleansing techniques can easily be accomplished at home, while others require the guidance or assistance of a qualified health practitioner.

INTESTINAL CLEANSING

Intestinal cleansing is an important complement to oxidative therapies. Physicians like Frank Shallenberger often insist on intestinal cleansing regimens before they begin treating AIDS patients with ozone.

Advocates of intestinal cleansing maintain that over many years, toxic matter can accumulate in the colon and the small intestine. Impacted fecal matter and mucoid (defined by Robert Gray as "any slimy, sticky, gluelike substance originating in the body for the purpose of holding substances to be eliminated in suspension"[1] such as feces) tend to build up and pollute our inner environment through the intestine. Constipation has reached epidemic proportions in the industrialized nations, and problems like diverticulitis and spastic colon, as well as other health problems, may be due to a dirty, congested colon. Difficulty in assimilating nutrients, fatigue, and headaches may also be caused by a buildup of toxins in the intestines.

Dr. Horst Kief believes that when the colon is filled with excrement, ozone cannot reach all of the pathogenic flora residing in the intestine, especially the fungi that may have settled in between the intestinal villi and the crypts. For this reason, Dr. Kief recommends a thorough cleansing of the large intestine before ozone is administered through rectal insufflation. Furthermore, Dr. Kief feels that the insufflation properties are enhanced if the bowel cleansing is done with ozonated water.[2]

Safe, natural intestinal cleansing methods include the use of high-fiber psyllium husks and other natural substances like Kalenite, pectin, or agar. These can be found in any good natural foods store. Dozens of plants also help naturally loosen, soften, or dissolve impacted stools and mucoid matter in the intestines. According to *The Colon Health Handbook* (see the resources—appendix 2, page 444), they include aloe, barberry, bayberry bark, grapes, chickweed, goldenseal root, spirulina plankton, and yellow dock root.[3] Many can be taken as tea. It is also possible to buy commercial preparations (found in many health food stores) made up of a number of herbs that work synergistically to help cleanse the colon.

An enema is another natural method of cleansing the colon. There are many types of enemas, including coffee enemas, garlic and chlorophyll enemas, and enemas made with wheatgrass juice mixed with water. The idea is to get as much liquid into the higher sections of the colon as possible in order to receive maximum benefit. Chapters describing enemas are included in a number of books by living food advocate Ann Wigmore, including *Be Your Own Doctor,* as well as Mark Konlee's *Immune Restoration Handbook* (see appendix 2).

Colonic irrigation is a more intensive way to clean the large intestine. This type of cleansing is more than an enema; it involves circulating water through the colon under light pressure. The colonic debris is then carried out with the water. An important development in ozone therapy has been the design of colonic systems using ozonated water. One such system, codesigned by Actual Water Services and Ozone Services in Canada (see figure 27.1), utilizes a standard ozone generator and a specialized gravity-based water system. Practitioners and patients alike feel that colonics done with ozonated water are more effective than those done with ordinary tap water. In addition to introducing small amounts of therapeutic ozone into the colon, the water itself is completely free from the pathogens, heavy metals, and chemicals often found in municipal or well water. Disposable materials should always be used with this procedure, which is usually done by certified colon therapists. Many are members of the American Colon Therapy Association.

While painless and safe, many colon and intestinal cleansing meth-

Figure 27.1. Ozonated gravity-feed colon therapy system.
(Reprinted courtesy of Actual Water Services and Yanco Industries Ltd.)

ods can remove "friendly bacteria" from the intestine along with the impacted fecal matter and mucoid. For that reason, supplementing one's diet with acidophilus (found in any natural foods retailer) is recommended to restore a healthy level of intestinal flora.

JUICE THERAPY

The use of fresh fruit and vegetable juices has been recommended by naturopathic physicians for over sixty years. At the famous Gerson Clinic in Mexico, large amounts of fresh, raw juices have been an important component of a holistic cancer protocol for over fifty years.[4] Many people have also used fresh, natural juices as part of a holistic treatment of HIV/AIDS. Bottled or canned juices are considered to be of little value in a body-cleansing regimen, because processing and storage robs the juices of essential vitamins and enzymes that are important for healing.

In addition to providing concentrated amounts of easily digestible vitamins, minerals, and enzymes, many fruits and vegetables contain medicinal properties. Apples, for example, are mildly laxative, while carrots—in addition to being rich in the antioxidant beta-carotene—are natural purifiers that gently cleanse the intestine.

The juices that are most often recommended for intestinal cleansing are fresh carrot juice (either prepared alone or mixed with smaller amounts of celery, spinach, or beets) and fresh apple juice, which can be made with a few added carrots or lettuce leaves. Mark Konlee recommends a juice made of endive, parsley, Romaine lettuce, carrot tops, beet greens, and celery for people infected with HIV. One-half cup of cultured cabbage juice three times daily is also suggested to heal mucous membranes and help restore the viability of the gastrointestinal tract.[5]

Fruits and vegetables must be carefully washed before placing them in the juicer (many people wash them in a diluted hydrogen peroxide solution). Whenever possible, use organically grown produce, because it is grown without free radical–producing chemical pesticides and fertilizers. Organic produce often costs a bit more than ordinary produce, but it is worth the extra expense.

It is important that the juices be consumed as soon as possible after they are prepared. If fresh juices are a part of a body-cleansing regimen, drink as much as you comfortably can during the day. A quart or more daily is recommended for people dealing with a serious disease like cancer or AIDS. Fortunately, these juices are delicious and are easily tolerated by most people.

Some people decide to partake of a "juice fast" and drink nothing but fresh, raw juices for days at a time; others consume two to three large glasses of fresh juice every day in addition to their regular meals. If you are interested in fresh juices, consider investing in a good, reliable juicer. There are also a number of excellent books on juicing that contain recipes for a variety of health conditions. A few are listed in appendix 2, the resources section of this book.

FASTING

Therapeutic fasting is an ancient method of body purification that has been popular since biblical times. Although the human organism can live without air for only a few minutes and without water for days, it can go without eating for up to several months. Fasting—especially when combined with one of the methods of colon cleansing above—can enable the body to discharge years of accumulated toxins.

There are many different types of fasts. Some people ingest nothing but pure water during a fast, while others fast with vegetable broth, herbal teas, or certain fruits, such as grapes, alone. Fasts can last anywhere from one day to several weeks or more. While a simple juice-only fast lasting one day is safe for most individuals, fasting with only water or for longer periods than one day should only be undertaken under the supervision of a qualified health professional. Light exercise and deep, rhythmic breathing are often recommended with fasts; these techniques tend to make the fasting process much easier. As cravings for food often come up during fasting, it is good to avoid watching others eat during the fasting period. The famous Swiss naturopath Dr. Alfred Vogel offered the following sound advice on fasting in his book *The Nature Doctor:*

> During the fast it is necessary to maintain the normal rhythm of movement and take adequate rest. All extremes are harmful, so avoid them. For instance, do not spend your days on the couch or in bed in the mistaken belief that you must conserve your energy while not eating. On the other hand, do not engage in arduous sports or walks; it would do you no good. The balance of movement and rest during our fast will revive you, restoring vitality and giving you a new foundation for health and well-being.[6]

SKIN SCRUBBING

Everyone knows that the skin is our largest organ (sexual or otherwise), but most of us do not know that it is a primary way that toxins are eliminated from the body every day, mostly through sweating. Rubbing the skin with a skin scrubber (often made from a natural sponge known as a loofah or of a pad made of tightly woven rope) helps stimulate the skin and get rid of dead skin cells. Another good skin scrubber is a brush with bristles made of natural vegetable fibers. The preferred method is to brush your skin with long even strokes in the direction of your heart. Avoid brushing the face. Skin brushing is an invigorating experience and can be done gently but firmly. One skin brushing in the morning before your shower and at bedtime not only helps make the skin a more vital organ of elimination but is also pleasurable.

Dr. Juliane Sacher, of Frankfurt, Germany, offers the following suggestion to aid in both moisturizing the skin and facilitating the elimination of toxins through the skin: Take one cup of olive oil and heat it until a drop of water added to it will "burst" on contact. Let the oil cool to body temperature, and then rub it over the entire body. Wash off the oil and then rest. Although applying olive oil can be a great deal of fun (especially when done with a partner), Dr. Sacher recommends that it be done no more than twice a year.[7]

SAUNAS AND STEAM BATHS

Healers from around the world have long recommended the therapeutic use of steam baths and saunas. They have been an integral part of a healthy lifestyle among Russians, Scandinavians, Arabs, and Native Americans for hundreds, if not thousands, of years. My grandfather, who was a native of Odessa on the Black Sea, used to go to an old Russian *banya* on Manhattan's Lower East Side at least once a week and found it refreshing, relaxing, and invigorating.

Saunas and steam baths increase body metabolism. They make us sweat and enable the body to release toxins through the skin. They also disperse congestion, increase circulation, and help our immune system fight off diseases by raising body temperature. When combined with pure water, fresh juices, and skin scrubbing techniques, they can be especially effective in body cleansing.

We mentioned before that one of the most pleasant and least invasive ways to use ozone therapy is through the "steam bath" method, known technically as body ozone exposure or BOEX. This method utilizes a specially designed steam cabinet to accommodate an inflow of ozone gas, which mixes with the steam.

Contrary to popular belief, ozone is not "absorbed" by the skin. As the ozone touches the body, it dissolves in the superficial water film beneath the outer layer of the skin. It immediately reacts with the polyunsaturated fatty acids of the sebum (fatty lubricant matter secreted by sebaceous glands of the skin) to generate reactive oxygen species, hydrogen peroxide, and lipid oxidation products that promote healing.[8] The fact that the skin is warm and moist may facilitate this process. Special care is taken so that the subject does not breathe in the ozone gas while enjoying the steam bath: the space for the person's head and neck is padded with towels to avoid leakage, and a fan is placed behind the individual to prevent inhalation of gas. A typical bath can last from 10 to 15 minutes at 30 to 40 gamma of ozone (30 to 40 µg ozone/liter oxygen), which flows continually through the unit. This method is often used as a spa treatment for healthy people or to supplement other types of oxygen therapies. A typical steam cabinet costs from $2,000 to $3,000 without a generator, but an increasing number of health practitioners are using them and offering BOEX sessions at nominal cost to their patients.

As with all body-cleansing techniques, moderation is the key. Do not spend more time in a "hot room" than is comfortable. With practice, you will be able to remain inside for longer periods of time. Although most health clubs maintain high levels of cleanliness in their saunas and steam rooms, some do not. As a result, bacteria and mold tend to multiply. If you are suffering from an immune-related health problem, avoid saunas and steam rooms unless you are certain that they are regularly cleaned and disinfected. Persons suffering from high blood pressure, heart disease, or circulatory disease should consult a physician before using a steam room or sauna.

THE EXPERIENCE OF BODY CLEANSING: NOT ALWAYS PLEASANT

Most of us judge the process of body cleansing as "dirty" or "wrong." Diarrhea, for example, is an efficient way for the body to quickly free itself from substances that are toxic or irritating. While we often feel uncomfortable when we experience occasional diarrhea, it is essentially a normal function of a body striving for health.

Many of the techniques mentioned in this chapter enable the body to experience higher levels of cleansing through discharge. We may notice that our body odor is stronger, our urine may change its characteristic color, and bowel movements may be darker, stronger smelling, and more frequent than we are normally accustomed to. Some people may even experience nausea, weakness, fever, and headache. While it is useful to monitor these reactions to body cleansing, it is also important to respect the body's process of discharge. By carefully applying the principles of body cleansing as described in this chapter, such reactions should be minimal and temporary.

28

An Oxygenation Diet

Dietary considerations have often played a minor role in traditional medical therapy. Despite many clinical and laboratory findings showing that certain types of diets (especially those high in saturated fat, cholesterol, sugar, and salt) may contribute to a variety of degenerative diseases like cancer, atherosclerosis, hypertension, and diabetes, the mainstream medical community has always emphasized medications, radiation, and surgery to treat these health problems rather than looking to correct their underlying causes. It isn't that physicians don't care, but many simply do not have an adequate understanding of diet and nutrition to begin with. They receive minimal instruction about nutrition in medical school, which often totals six hours of class. Unless they decide to educate themselves about diet and nutrition after they graduate, many physicians know less about the subject than their patients.

This mind-set often exists regarding oxidative therapies. Many physicians view ozone and hydrogen peroxide as effective natural treatments that strengthen the body's immune system, alleviate symptoms, and keep them from reappearing. If a relapse occurs, additional oxidative treatments are recommended.

However, a growing number of oxidative practitioners feel that changes in diet and lifestyle are necessary in order to complement ozone or hydrogen peroxide and restore one's health for the long term. Although choosing the right foods for us is a highly personal matter and there is no one diet for everyone, this chapter will explore some of the components to several comprehensive nutritional programs that can complement oxidative therapies for most individuals. From time to time, references will be made to those suffering from specific health problems, such as cancer or AIDS.

Remember that the material provided in this chapter (like in all chapters in this section) is *for information only*. Consult a qualified professional for specific guidance regarding your personal dietary needs. An entire book could be devoted to the subject covered in this chapter. If you are interested in learning more about a specific approach to diet and nutrition, consult one or more of the diet books listed in appendix 2.

WHAT TO LOOK FOR

What kind of diet are we looking for? Ideally, we want to strive for a dietary program that will satisfy the following needs:

1. It will be low in elements that produce free radical damage, while being high in those that protect against and destroy free radicals.
2. It will provide adequate amounts of protein, carbohydrates, minerals, and fiber.
3. It will be low in fat, sugar, and salt.
4. It will provide additional oxygen to the body that will help oxygenate tissues and other body cells.

It was mentioned earlier that environmental pollutants are a major source of free radicals. Many of these pollutants come from what we eat and drink due to pesticide residues found in the food supply. According to the *Handbook of Pest Management in Agriculture,* the increase in pesticide use in the United States has jumped 3,300 percent since 1945.[1]

Unless we own our own private greenhouse and grow only organic fruits and vegetables, it is not easy to avoid pesticides and other pollutants completely. One way is to purchase only organically grown foods, which are free of persistent chemical fertilizers and pesticides. Although organic produce is somewhat more expensive than conventional produce, many feel that the long-term benefits are well worth the trouble.

The second way to reduce our consumption of pesticides and other free radical–producing substances is to eat as low as possible on the food chain. The food chain refers to the series of living things that are considered as being linked, with each thing feeding upon what is before it in a series. The higher up the food chain we go, the higher the levels of pesticide residues.

For example, when we ingest protein from the flesh of a chicken that has eaten grain sprayed with pesticides (or eat one of its eggs), we are consuming a far greater concentration of pesticides than if we were to consume the protein directly from the grain. While eggs and dairy products generally contain two-fifths the pesticide residues found in meat, vegetables and leafy vegetables contain only one-seventh as much. Fruits and legumes contain one-eighth, while grains and cereals have only one-twenty-fourth the pesticide residues found in meat.[2]

ANTIOXIDANT NUTRITION

Basically speaking, a good oxygenating diet consists of fresh, whole, and oxygen-rich foods that also provide an abundant amount of antioxidants such as beta-carotene, vitamin C, and vitamin E. Depending on their nature, these antioxidants will either protect cells from free radical damage or serve as scavengers to "mop up" excess free radicals in the body.

Beta-carotene
The best sources of beta-carotene include fresh carrots, leafy greens, squash (especially yellow squash such as pumpkin), yams, sweet potatoes, and broccoli. The best fruit sources include cantaloupes, apricots, and peaches. One of the best sources of all is nori, a seaweed that is used extensively in Japanese cuisine. Found in health food stores and Asian markets, it can easily be added to soups and stews. In her book

Good Health in a Toxic World: The Complete Guide to Fighting Free Radicals, Sara Shannon recommends two servings of beta-carotene-rich foods a day, with additional supplementation as needed.[3] We will examine nutritional supplements in detail in the following chapter.

Vitamin C

The best sources of vitamin C include citrus fruits (like oranges, tangerines, grapefruits, mandarin oranges, and lemons), tomatoes (technically a fruit), strawberries, leafy green vegetables, broccoli, brussels sprouts, green peppers, and acerola cherries. Three or more daily servings are recommended from this group, although many oxidative practitioners recommend additional supplementation.

Vitamin E

Cold-pressed and unrefined vegetable oils (such as canola, olive, safflower, and soy) are very high in vitamin E. Whole grains (including oatmeal and brown rice), dried beans and other legumes, and leafy green vegetables are good sources as well. Sara Shannon recommends a daily intake of three servings of leafy green vegetables, two servings of grains, and two teaspoons of unrefined vegetable oil. As with vitamin C, therapists working with oxidative therapies often recommend extra vitamin E.

B Vitamins

A number of vitamins make up the B vitamin family, including B_1 (thiamin), B_2 (riboflavin), B_3 (niacin), B_6 (pyridoxine), folacin (folic acid), and B_{12} (cyanocobalamin). Together, they are known as the vitamin B complex. The B vitamins are necessary to aid in the proper digestion and efficient utilization of carbohydrates, and they help break down proteins so they can be efficiently used by the body. They also aid body growth and help keep the nervous system in optimal condition, which is important in immunoregulation. Vitamin B complex has also been found to be an antioxidant cofactor, which means that the B vitamins play a supportive role in enabling the antioxidants listed above to work more effectively.

B vitamins are found primarily in grains, dried beans and peas, and seeds and nuts, especially oats, wheat germ, and peanuts. They are also found in brewer's yeast, a highly nutritious product available at many natural food stores. A varied diet including these foods will help preserve good health and can complement most oxidative treatment programs.

There are a number of other antioxidant cofactors, including the minerals selenium and zinc and the amino acid glutathione. Since many people have deficiencies in these substances, we will discuss them in the following chapter on vitamin and mineral supplements.

Antioxidant "Superfoods"

A team of researchers at the Department of Nutrition at the Institute of Basic Medical Sciences of the University of Oslo in Norway analyzed over 3,100 different foods and evaluated their antioxidant content, expressed as "mmol/100 g," or millimole (1/1000th of a gram) of antioxidant per 100 grams of food. Their findings were published in *Nutrition Journal* in 2010.

The Oslo researchers divided foods into different categories. Among the beverages, espresso coffee scored 12.6 mmol/100 g, followed by hibiscus tea (6.99), Lipton green tea (6.8), red wine (2.5), filter-brewed coffee (2.13), and pomegranate juice (2.1).

Among nuts and seeds, walnuts with pellicle—the thin skin or membrane surrounding the nutmeat—scored 21.9, followed by pecans with pellicle (8.5), sunflower seeds (6.4), and chestnuts with pellicle (4.7). Dark chocolate (70 to 99 percent cacao) samples averaged 10.9, while one popular 85 percent cacao bar from Switzerland scored 13.6.

Certain vegetables and fruits also scored high in antioxidant content, including dried apples (3.8), dried apricots (3.1), blue cauliflower (3.3), dried plums (3.2), curly kale (2.8), red and green chili peppers (2.4), red raspberries (2.3), and strawberries (2.16). Herbs and spices generally scored very high in antioxidant content, but most of us use them in small quantities. Those with the highest content included allspice, cloves, mint, oregano, rosemary, saffron, sage, and thyme.

It is important to remember that there are other nutritional criteria besides antioxidant content when choosing foods to eat. In addition to antioxidants, other phytochemicals in foods can help lower blood pressure, reduce cholesterol, regulate blood sugar, improve sleep, calm the nerves, and even help prevent cancer. One of my favorite books about the healing power of foods is *Healthy Foods* by George D. Pamplona-Roger, M.D. (see the resources—appendix 2, page 445).[4]

A NEW BASIC FOUR

In 1956 the famous "Basic Four" food guide was created by the U.S. Department of Agriculture (USDA), which set the standards for a healthy diet for Americans. Developed under the influence of the meat and dairy interests, it emphasized a high consumption of meat, eggs, and dairy products, which made up half of its four food groups. As consumers became more aware of the serious dangers of high-cholesterol and high-fat diets that resulted from following the Basic Four plan, it was later amended by the USDA's "Dietary Guidelines for Americans" of 1990, which expanded the four food groups to five. However, this plan, also influenced by the meat and dairy interests, still placed strong emphasis on an animal-based diet. This was later replaced by the "Food Guide Pyramid," which placed a somewhat stronger emphasis on plant foods. Although it represented an important departure from past recommendations, many progressive nutritionists felt that the Food Guide Pyramid did not go far enough.

A dietary plan that is most likely to complement the benefits of oxidative therapies is the little-known "New Four Food Groups," created by the Physicians Committee for Responsible Medicine (PCRM). First proposed in 1991, it is seen as an "optimal diet" that not only provides adequate nutrition but can actually help prevent many diet-related diseases like hypertension, cancer, and atherosclerosis. Like the original Basic Four food groups, the PCRM's food groups are easy to remember, but they emphasize plant foods rather than foods of animal origin. The plan features four primary food groups, with "optional" foods to be eaten sparingly.[5]

Group I: Whole Grains

This group includes bread, pasta, hot or cold cereal, millet, barley, bulgur, buckwheat, groats, and tortillas. These foods provide complex carbohydrates, protein, B vitamins, and zinc. Five or more servings are recommended daily from this group. A serving is considered to be one-half cup of cooked cereal, one ounce of dry cereal, or one slice of bread.

Group II: Vegetables

Group II includes dark green leafy vegetables like collards, kale, mustard greens, and turnip greens, as well as cruciferous vegetables, which include broccoli, cabbages, brussels sprouts, and cauliflower. These vegetables are generally good sources of a variety of vitamins (especially vitamin C and riboflavin), minerals (particularly calcium and iron), and dietary fiber, which is often lacking in standard diets. Dark yellow vegetables (including carrots, squash, sweet potatoes, and pumpkin) are also excellent sources of beta-carotene. Three or more daily servings (one cup raw or one-half cup cooked) from this group are recommended.

Group III: Legumes

Dried peas, beans, chickpeas, and lentils are good sources of protein, dietary fiber, iron, calcium, zinc, and B vitamins. Foods in this category also include textured soy protein, soy milk, tofu (soybean curd), and tempeh, made from fermented soybeans. One-half cup of cooked beans, four ounces of tofu or tempeh, or eight ounces of soy milk is considered a serving. Two to three servings from this group are recommended.

Group IV: Fruits

All fruits are recommended by the PCRM, to be eaten as close to their natural state as possible. Of special interest are citrus fruits, tomatoes, and strawberries (which are all good sources of vitamin C), as well as cantaloupes and apricots, which are high in beta-carotene. A minimum of three servings from this group are recommended daily. One medium piece of fruit, one-half cup of cooked fruit, or one-half cup of fresh fruit juice constitutes a serving.

Optional Foods

To the chagrin of the meat and dairy industries, the PCRM placed meat, fish, and dairy products (along with nuts, seeds, and oils) into the optional foods group to be used as condiments. While not banned, the committee felt that they should no longer serve as the focal point for the optimal American diet, as they did in the past. PCRM chairman Neal Bernard, M.D., called this plan "a modest proposal" that if adopted could have a profound impact on America's high incidence of heart disease and cancer. For more information about this organization, consult appendix 2 of this book.

DIETARY GUIDELINES FOR AMERICANS

Acknowledging that Americans were not only getting fatter but also becoming sicker, in 2005 the U.S. Department of Health and Human Services and the USDA finally proposed dietary guidelines that were much more in harmony with the above recommendations. The key recommendations for adults include the following:

- Consume a sufficient amount of fruits and vegetables while staying within energy needs. Two cups of fruit and 2½ cups of vegetables per day are recommended for a reference 2,000-calorie intake, with higher or lower amounts depending on the calorie level.
- Choose a variety of fruits and vegetables each day. In particular, select from all five vegetable subgroups (dark green, orange, legumes, starchy vegetables, and other vegetables) several times a week.

- Consume three or more ounce-equivalents of whole-grain products per day, with the rest of the recommended grains coming from enriched or whole-grain products. In general, at least half the grains should come from whole grains.
- Consume three cups per day of fat-free or low-fat milk or equivalent milk products.

The following guidelines are recommended for children and adolescents:

- Consume whole-grain products often; at least half the grains should be whole grains.
- Children two to eight years old should consume two cups per day of fat-free or low-fat milk or equivalent milk products. Children nine years of age and older should consume three cups per day of fat-free or low-fat milk or equivalent milk products.[6]

In January 2016 the Office of Disease Prevention and Health Promotion of the Department of Health and Human Services released *2015–2020 Dietary Guidelines for Americans*. While the full document is available online, the office's key recommendations include:

Consume a healthy eating pattern that accounts for all foods and beverages within an appropriate calorie level. A healthy eating pattern includes:

- A variety of vegetables from all of the subgroups—dark green, red and orange, legumes (beans and peas), starchy, and other
- Fruits, especially whole fruits
- Grains, at least half of which are whole grains
- Fat-free or low-fat dairy, including milk, yogurt, cheese, and/or fortified soy beverages
- A variety of protein foods, including seafood, lean meats and poultry, eggs, legumes (beans and peas), and nuts, seeds, and soy products
- Oils

A healthy eating pattern limits:

- Saturated fats and trans fats, added sugars, and sodium.

Key Recommendations that are quantitative are provided for several components of the diet that should be limited. These components are of particular public health concern in the United States, and the specified limits can help individuals achieve healthy eating patterns within calorie limits:

- Consume less than 10 percent of calories per day from added sugars
- Consume less than 10 percent of calories per day from saturated fats
- Consume less than 2,300 milligrams (mg) per day of sodium
- If alcohol is consumed, it should be consumed in moderation—up to one drink per day for women and up to two drinks per day for men—and only by adults of legal drinking age.[7]

WHAT OXIDATIVE HEALERS SUGGEST

A number of prominent individuals who have worked with oxidative therapies (and patients who have undergone these therapies) have offered sound dietary guidance as adjuncts to the therapeutic use of medical ozone and hydrogen peroxide. Although this book does not advocate any particular diet, they are worthy of consideration. Many complement each other extensively.

In his monograph *Protocol for the Intravenous Administration of Hydrogen Peroxide,* Dr. Charles H. Farr confines his dietary advice to the following suggestions:

Patients should be counseled to limit dietary fats and oils (all types) to approximately 20 to 25% of their total caloric intake. They should especially avoid heated, extracted and refined fats which are rich in lipid peroxide precursors of free radicals. Refined carbohydrates and simple sugars should be avoided and substituted with unrefined, complex starches containing adequate dietary fiber, obtained from whole grains, vegetables and whole fruit.[8]

In his book *The Oxygen Breakthrough,* Sheldon Saul Hendler, M.D., recommends an "ideal" diet to his patients that is very much in harmony with both the New Four Food Groups and Dr. Farr's recommendations. Dr. Hendler's "high-oxygen diet" includes the following:

- No more than 100 milligrams of cholesterol daily
- No more than 20 percent fat, with increased amounts of polyunsaturates and monosaturates and decreased amounts of saturates
- At least 65 percent carbohydrates, with emphasis on complex, unrefined carbohydrates
- 12 to 15 percent protein, with increased reliance on vegetable protein
- 50 to 60 grams of dietary fiber[9]

At the Hospital Santa Monica in Mexico, Dr. Kurt Donsbach offers the following modest food recommendations (along with friendly practical advice) to help patients achieve a higher level of health and well-being both at the hospital and after they return home.

1. Do eat a bowl of oatmeal or other whole-grain cereal every morning. (We shouldn't have to tell you to avoid white sugar and white flour products as much as possible.)
2. Do eat four cupfuls of vegetables daily—half raw and half cooked. It will surprise you how many vegetables really exist. Try them all.
3. Do eat one cupful of fruit daily, preferably raw unless unavailable.
4. Do eat only the following fats: butter, olive oil, peanut oil. *Margarine and unsaturated oils are the worst foods you can put into your body.* (Flaxseed oil, bottled in black and kept refrigerated, is the only exception—it can be used therapeutically at one tablespoon once or twice daily.)

5. Do reduce coffee consumption to one cup daily. Get in the herb tea habit.

6. Do eat your heaviest meals at breakfast and lunch [and have your] light meal at night. This is the hardest rule to follow for most people.

7. Do eat a minimum of five servings of chicken, fish, or turkey each week. You can have a serving of beef or pork occasionally. If you are a vegetarian by choice, eat seeds and nuts to supplement your diet. Eggs and dairy products may be used as desired.

8. Do not combine fruits or fruit juices with concentrated proteins (meats, dairy products, eggs). This will produce gas and discomfort.

9. Do eat whole grains, freshly baked breads, and rolls.

10. Do use a seasoning salt made up of potassium, sodium, calcium, magnesium, lysine, and kelp as your flavor enhancer.

11. Be positive and happy when you eat. Your digestive system will work better.[10]

THE "LIVESTRONG DIET"

According to an article published by the Livestrong Foundation, an organization founded by former cyclist Lance Armstrong devoted to helping cancer patients, there are several important ways that we can increase oxygen levels by the foods we eat.

Eat Iron-Rich Foods

Iron-deficient anemia occurs when diets have insufficient iron and leads to reduced levels of hemoglobin, the oxygen carrier in the blood. This can lead to a condition called *hypoxemia*. In addition to red meat, poultry, and seafood, iron-rich foods include dried beans and peas, such as chickpeas, green peas, lentils, and kidney, black, and lima beans; dark green leafy vegetables, such as spinach; dried fruit, such as raisins, cranberries, and apricots; peanut butter; tofu; brown rice; and iron-fortified cereals, whole-wheat breads, and pastas.

If you are getting your iron primarily from plant sources, try to combine the foods listed above (known as nonheme iron foods) with vitamin C to increase absorption of iron. Foods rich in Vitamin C include oranges, grapefruit, and other citrus fruits; broccoli; kiwi; leafy green vegetables (kale, collards, spinach); melons; peppers; strawberries and other berries; and tomatoes.

Eat More Fresh Fruits and Vegetables

Some health advocates believe that an acidic environment in the blood can lead to reduced levels of oxygen and increase the risk of certain cancers. The intake of alkaline water, along with fruits and vegetables rich in potassium and magnesium (such as bananas, potatoes, tomatoes, and green leafy vegetables), can help reduce acidity in the blood and increase oxygenation. Fruits and vegetables are also rich sources of antioxidants like vitamin C and vitamin E and can help protect the oxygen-carrying blood cells against the harmful effects of free radicals.

Go Low-Sodium

Diets low in sodium are believed to lead to increased oxygenation of the kidneys via the blood. Admittedly, reducing our sodium intake is a challenge, since so many of the foods we eat contain high amounts of sodium. Reducing our intake of prepared foods (especially instant noodles, soups, and sauces); smoked, salted, canned, cured, or precooked meats (including hot dogs, cold cuts, bacon, sausages, ham, and fish); frozen breaded meats and dinners, such as burritos and pizza; canned entrees, such as ravioli and chili; frozen entrees; salted nuts, popcorn, and seeds; canned and bottled spaghetti sauces; and canned beans and other vegetables with added salt can help. Limiting visits to restaurants (many restaurant meals are notoriously high in both calories and sodium) and preparing meals at home is another option. Generally speaking, a low-sodium diet aims to reduce sodium intake to less than 2,000 mg per day and includes a diet rich in fresh fruits and vegetables, beans, peas, legumes, and whole grains.[11]

THE MEDITERRANEAN DIET

The Mediterranean diet—which is high in fruits, vegetables, whole grains, and nuts and low in refined sugars, meats, and whole-fat dairy products—has been found to help maintain healthy lung function since at least 2007. According to a 2013 study at the University of Auckland published in the the *Journal of Asthma,* asthma patients who adopted the Mediterranean diet experienced both increased lung function and overall better quality of life.[12]

THE IMMUNE ENHANCEMENT DIET

The second edition of the *Immune Restoration Handbook* by Mark Konlee lists a number of "foods that heal." These foods are good for anyone who is involved in the healing process unless a physician prohibits their use. Many people fear that a health-oriented diet needs to be limited, but as we will see in the following diet plans, this need not be the case.

Vegetables

All vegetables are allowed on the immune enhancement diet except iceberg lettuce. Sprouts (including wheatgrass, red clover, radish, soy, and alfalfa), artichokes, asparagus, avocado, bamboo shoots, banana pepper, beet greens, beets, bok choy, Boston lettuce, broccoli, cabbage, carrots, cauliflower, celery, Chinese cabbage, collard greens, eggplant, endive, escarole, dandelion greens, garlic, green peas, green beans, jalapeno pepper, kale, kohlrabi, lamb's-quarter, leeks, okra, olives (green and ripe), onions, parsley, potatoes, pumpkin, radishes, red sweet peppers, rutabagas, sea kale, shallots, spinach, squash, sweet potatoes, Swiss chard, turnip greens, and turnips. Sauerkraut is also recommended.

Oil

Flaxseed oil (which can be mixed into yogurt or cottage cheese), olive oil, and hazelnut oil. These oils can be blended 50:50 with butter.

Seasonings and Spices

Paprika and crushed red pepper, seaweed (such as nori and kombu), hot peppers, apple cider vinegar, and thyme, as well as natural commercial seasoning mixtures like Spike or Bragg Liquid Aminos. Salt and black pepper are to be used in moderation.

Gluten-Free Grains

Rice (white or brown), rye crisp crackers, and products made with corn, quinoa, amaranth, buckwheat, millet, spelt, rye, kamut, or other gluten-free grains.

Fruit

Raw lemons, raw limes, grapefruit, raw pineapple, and unsweetened applesauce are recommended, while a maximum of one daily serving of all other fruits is suggested.

Sweeteners

Raw unfiltered honey, sucanat, raw cane sugar, brown sugar, date sugar, and blackstrap molasses are to be used in moderation.

Beverages

Reverse-osmosis filtered water, spring water, and mineral water are recommended over unfiltered municipal water. Green tea and black tea are good beverage choices if caffeinated drinks are required.[13]

THE RAW FOOD AND LIVING FOOD DIET

The legendary Ann Wigmore, D.D., N.D., was well known in the holistic community for her radical approach to helping people heal themselves of cancer, heart disease, candidiasis, diabetes, AIDS, and other "incurable" diseases through living foods eaten low on the food chain. Believing that raw, uncooked, fermented, and sprouted foods are easily digested, are free of chemical additives, and contain a minimum of pesticides,

"Dr. Ann" built her living food diet on fresh fruits and vegetables, seeds, grains, and nuts. Methods of preparation include juicing, sprouting, fermenting, and light blending. She believed that foods prepared in this way allow the body's cells to fully absorb the life force produced by the enzymes of live foods, many of which, by the way, contain hydrogen peroxide. Many living foods can be grown indoors as greens and as sprouts.

In her book *Overcoming AIDS,* Dr. Wigmore listed what she called "the most important foods for total health":

Greens: Sunflower, cabbage, buckwheat, dandelion, watercress, parsley, lamb's-quarter

Top of the ground vegetables: Corn, red pepper, celery, radish, zucchini, summer squash, mushrooms

Fermented foods: Cauliflower, beets, carrots, seed cheese, Rejuvelac (a drink made from sprouted wheat seeds; water is added to the seeds, and after several days, the water is drained out and consumed)

Fruits: Watermelon, peeled apples, peaches, figs, dates, avocado, tomato, bananas

Grains: Rye, millet, corn, wheat

Protein: Almonds, pine nuts, sunflower seeds

Sprouts: Alfalfa, fenugreek, mung bean, radish

Seaweed: Dulse[14]

Though this diet is admittedly unconventional, many holistic healers believe that it is probably the best diet to follow if one wants to make major changes in one's life as part of the healing process: live more simply, free the body of toxins, enhance the body's natural healing powers, and consume only the purest and freshest of foods. While some may feel that a total raw food diet is too extreme, certain aspects of her diet can easily become integrated into a personal diet plan. A number of Ann Wigmore's books (which include many "how-to" recipes), as well as the address of her healing center, are included in appendix 2 of this book.

29

Nutritional Supplements and Healing Herbs

In an ideal world, nutritional supplementation would not be necessary. We would be so in touch with our bodies that we would instinctively know what we need to eat and do so in the proper amounts. Our foods would be organically grown under ideal climatic conditions, they would be picked from the garden or orchard not far from home, and they would be eaten in their natural state within a few hours or days of harvesting.

Reality is different. For the most part, we have no idea what we should eat, let alone how much. Nearly all of our produce is harvested weeks before it is ripe, often transported over long distances (sometimes from around the world), and subject to days or weeks of storage, often in the presence of chemical additives. Many of our canned and packaged foods have essential vitamins, minerals, and enzymes refined out of them during processing. By the time they arrive at the dinner table, many of the foods we eat contain far less nutrition than they originally contained. For that reason, a growing number of nutritionists are recommending supplements to provide a "safety net" in order to avoid vitamin and mineral deficiencies and the diseases they can cause.

While the oxygen-rich diets described in the previous chapter (along with broad-spectrum daily multivitamin and mineral supplements containing ingredients with antioxidant activity) are designed to provide adequate nutrition under normal circumstances, people who are challenged by ill health often require additional elements that will help strengthen the immune system and optimize the benefits of the oxidative therapies.

This chapter is not a course in nutrition. Its purpose is to introduce and discuss some of the food supplements and herbs that are often used to enhance the benefits of oxidative therapies. While some references are made to mainstream nutritional publications, I also draw on the clinical experience of leading dietitians, physicians, and other practitioners who work with the nutritional aspects of healing. I hope that this chapter will inspire you to gain a more complete understanding of the role of vitamins and minerals in the healing process. In addition, a number of books that provide more extensive information are listed in appendix 2.

While supplements can be useful as daily addition to a good diet, they are often not recommended to be taken within several hours of a session of oxidative therapy, unless recommended by a physician. It is also important to remember that more is not always better. An excess of certain nutrients can depress immune function.

In the context of this book, a primary goal of nutritional supplementation is to provide adequate amounts of antioxidants to help scavenge excess free radicals and protect other cells from free radical damage. The three most important elements are beta-carotene, vitamin C, and vitamin E. For maximum benefit, it is important to take these antioxidants together because they produce synergistic effects; they work more effectively as a group than if they are taken alone.

As a general reference, table 29.1 (on page 366) is a listing of the current Reference Daily Intakes (RDIs, formerly known as Recommended Daily Allowances) for the major vitamins and minerals as determined by the U.S. Food and Drug Administration and the National Academy of Sciences. These estimates, which change from time to time, are based on the amount of nutrients necessary to prevent nutritional deficiencies in both children and adults. Many critics feel that the RDIs are far too low to help people achieve optimal health and that they should be used more as a guidepost for minimal nutrition rather than as a nutritional ideal.

BETA-CAROTENE

Beta-carotene is a precursor to vitamin A, which means that it must exist before vitamin A is formed. It promotes growth and wound healing and prevents night blindness and some diseases of the eye. It is also important for healthy skin and bones and helps maintain the well-being of the respiratory tract, the throat, and the bronchial region. It is found mostly in yellow and dark green leafy vegetables, especially yellow squash, spinach, carrots, and sweet potatoes, as well as in apricots and cantaloupes.

For a normal adult weighing 70 kg (154 pounds), the RDI as determined by the U.S. Food and Drug Administration is 900 μg of vitamin A, or 6 to 15 mg of beta-carotene. Much higher therapeutic amounts may be toxic to some individuals and should only be taken under a physician's supervision. In general, beta-carotene seems less liable to cause toxicity, as it is broken down by the body and cleaved into two molecules of vitamin A when needed.

VITAMIN C (ASCORBIC ACID)

Vitamin C is important in helping maintain healthy teeth and gums. It also supports the immune system and is viewed as a major factor in preventing colds and possibly other viral infections. Vitamin C is responsible for the health and maintenance of collagen in the teeth, bones, skin, capillaries, and connective tissue and aids in detoxifying the body of poisons. It helps the body use carbohydrates, fats, and protein and also has been found to strengthen blood vessel walls. Known as the "protector vitamin," vitamin C plays an essential role in protecting cells and preventing tissue damage from free radicals. For this reason, some feel that it helps prevent diseases associated with free radical damage, including heart disease and cancer. Vitamin C is found in citrus fruits, strawberries, kiwi fruit, tomatoes, acerola cherries, and many green vegetables, including peppers, broccoli, and cabbage.

The RDI of vitamin C is 90 mg for men and 75 mg for women,

Table 29.1. U.S. Reference Daily Intakes for Adults Nineteen Years of Age and Over

Vitamin A	900 µg
Vitamin C	90 mg for men/75 mg for women
Thiamin (vitamin B₁)	1.2 mg for men/1.1. mg for women
Riboflavin (vitamin B₂)	1.3 mg for men/1.1. mg for women
Niacin (vitamin B₃)	16 mg for men/14 mg for women
Pyridoxine (vitamin B₆)	1.3 mg
Cyanocobalamin (vitamin B₁₂)	2.4 µg
Vitamin D	5–10 mg
Vitamin E	15 mg
Phosphorus	700 mg
Potassium	4.7 g
Calcium	1,000 mg for men/1,300 mg for women
Magnesium	420 mg for men/320 mg for women
Iron	8 mg for men and women over age 50/ 18 mg for women under age 50
Iodine	150 µg
Zinc	11 mg for men/8 mg for women
Copper	900 µg
Folate	400 µg
Choline	550 mg for men/425 mg for women
Sodium	1.5 g
Chloride	2.3 g
Selenium	55 µg

Note: g = gram; mg = milligram (1/1,000 of a gram); µg = microgram (1/1,000 of a milligram).
Source: Food and Nutrition Board, Institute of Medicine, *Dietary Reference Intakes* (Washington, D.C.: National Academy Press, 2004).

which many practitioners believe is inadequate. To protect the body from free radical damage, a maintenance dose of 1,000 mg (1 g) of vitamin C is often recommended, while 1 to 3 grams a day is suggested for those with a serious disease like cancer or AIDS. Some physicians recommend even more. Dr. John C. Pittman's comprehensive HIV/AIDS protocol includes 70 grams of intravenous vitamin C (along with other vitamins, minerals, and antiviral agents) once or twice a week.[1]

Not all oxidative therapists agree with megadoses of vitamin C. Dr. Bocci believes that if a patient receiving oxidative therapies takes a daily multivitamin supplement including vitamin C, there is no need for additional vitamin C supplementation: "I do not see any need to take vitamin C after the AHT because if you take [a vitamin C supplement] every day you have practically a constant level. Moreover, at least 90 percent of oxidized Vitamin C is reduced and recycled back to effective Vitamin C within ten minutes." Yet with seriously ill "emergency" patients (i.e., those needing three or four autohemotherapy sessions daily), he suggests an IV supplementation of 500 mg of intravenous vitamin C between treatments.[2]

VITAMIN E

Because vitamin E promotes circulation and helps prevent blood clots, it has gotten much publicity for its role in helping to reduce the risk of heart disease. It is also important for the healing of wounds, burns, scars, and other skin problems and helps protect the body's store of vitamins A and D. As a powerful antioxidant, vitamin E is a scavenger of free radicals. It is found primarily in vegetable oils, nuts, green leafy vegetables, and fortified cereals.

A number of scientific studies have found that vitamin E can help reduce the risk of a variety of health problems, including heart disease[3] and certain types of cancer.[4] However, the scientific community is not in complete agreement, and further studies are being done.

The RDI for vitamin E is 15 mg (22.5 international units [IU]), although the Food and Nutrition Board of the Institute of Medicine has set an upper tolerable intake level (UL) for vitamin E at 1,000 mg (1,500 IU) for any form of supplementary alpha-tocopherol per day. Many holistic practitioners who work with oxidative therapies and progressive heart specialists who believe that vitamin E can reduce the risk of heart attack recommend between 400 and 800 IU daily. The natural form of d-alpha-tocopherol is more easily absorbed by the body. If you are taking an anticoagulant like Coumadin, do not take supplemental vitamin E because of its natural anticoagulant factor.

VITAMIN B₆

Vitamin B₆, or pyridoxine, is called an "antioxidant cofactor" because it synergizes with vitamins C and E and helps them work more effectively. This vitamin also plays an important role in converting fats, proteins, and carbohydrates into usable energy. It also is of importance to the thymus gland, which plays a major role in immunoregulation. The primary sources of vitamin B₆ include wheat germ, dried brewer's yeast, whole grains, lima beans, peanuts, bananas, cabbage, egg yolks, and meat.

The RDI for this vitamin is only 1.3 mg for adults, although many believe that up to 25 mg or more a day is valuable for people who are dealing with a health problem. Dr. Juliane Sacher recommends 20 to 60 milligrams a day for her AIDS/HIV-positive patients (her complete vitamin and mineral supplement protocol is included in table 29.2).

Nutritionists point out that all members of the B group of vitamins should be taken in proportionate amounts. For this reason, any supplements of vitamin B₆ should be taken as part of a general multivitamin or B-complex formula.

ALPHA-LIPOIC ACID

Like glutathione and coenzyme Q₁₀, alpha-lipoic acid (ALA) is informally known as a "factory installed" antioxidant, because it is produced by the body itself. ALA is believed to prevent and treat a wide variety

Table 29.2. Sacher Clinic Daily Nutritional Supplement Recommendations for People with HIV/AIDS

Vitamin A	5,000–10,000 IU
Beta-carotene	25–100 mg
Vitamin C	1–3 g
Vitamin E	400–1,200 IU
Vitamin B_6	20–60 mg
Vitamin B_{12}	25–100 µg
Folic acid	5–15 mg
Selenium	100–200 µg
Magnesium	500–2,000 mg
Calcium	500–2,000 mg
Potassium aspartate	500–1,200 mg
Zinc aspartate	50–100 mg
Copper gluconate	200–600 µg
N-acetyl-cysteine (an antioxidant)	300–1,200 mg

Dr. Sacher also recommends one to two tablets daily of ferrum phosphoricum D6, which is a special type of iron available in trace amounts, like many homeopathic remedies. She suggests that whenever iron is taken, antioxidants should be consumed as well.
Source: Vitamine, Mineralien und Spurenelemente bei HIV-Positiven und AIDS-Patienten (Frankfurt: Sacher Clinic, 1993). Reprinted courtesy of Dr. Juliane Sacher.

of degenerative diseases, including heart disease, stroke, diabetes, cataracts, Alzheimer's disease, Parkinson's disease, and declines in immunity, muscle strength, energy, and brain function. Recent scientific studies have shown that alpha-lipoic acid can help treat diabetic neuropathy[5] (German physicians currently prescribe ALA for long-term complications of diabetes), increase adenosine triphosphate (ATP) production and aortic blood flow,[6] and may help offer protection against atherosclerosis.[7]

Alpha-lipoic acid is widely found in plant and animal sources, and it is available in supplement form at vitamin shops and health food stores. Daily doses up to 600 mg have been well tolerated; however, due to lack of long-term safety findings among pregnant women and nursing mothers, these groups should avoid taking it unless they are under a doctor's supervision.

COENZYME Q$_{10}$

Coenzyme Q$_{10}$ is not a vitamin but an energy coenzyme that is essential for the production of ATP, or cellular energy. Coenzyme Q$_{10}$ has been the subject of much ongoing research. As an important antioxidant, it works with vitamin E to scavenge free radicals. It has been found to stimulate the immune system, promote cell growth, and protect cells from damage that can lead to cancer. It may also help reduce adverse side effects from traditional cancer treatments, like radiation and chemotherapy. Coenzyme Q$_{10}$ is often recommended for people challenged by diseases such as AIDS, cancer, heart disease, and chronic fatigue, as well as to help slow the aging process. Popular statin drugs may destroy coenzyme Q$_{10}$.

Coenzyme Q$_{10}$ is normally synthesized by the body, but it is believed that as people approach middle age, production of this coenzyme slows down. Although there is no RDI for this substance, a daily supplement of 10 to 30 mg is generally considered adequate; some holistic physicians recommend 100 to 200 mg a day for those at risk of heart disease or cancer. No serious side effects have been reported from people taking coenzyme Q$_{10}$, but those who wish to take more than 300 mg daily are advised to consult with a physician.

L-GLUTATHIONE

Glutathione (L-gamma-glutamyl-L-cysteinyl-glycine) is a powerful antioxidant and antitoxin. Naturally produced by the body, it has been found to be a cellular regulator and is important for cellular homeostasis and function. It helps protect the body against diverse free radical damage and other oxidative stressors. Glutathione participates directly in the neutralization of free radicals and reactive oxygen compounds and maintains exogenous antioxidants such as vitamins C and E in their reduced (active) forms. It also helps detoxify the body from impurities.

Parris M. Kidd, M.D., believes that glutathione holds promise for the management of conditions as diverse as Alzheimer's disease, atherosclerotic vascular degeneration, cataracts, lung insufficiencies, and Parkinson's disease.[8]

Glutathione is naturally found in meat and in many fresh fruits and vegetables. Oral glutathione supplements are available where natural foods and vitamins are sold, but they are difficult to absorb; intravenous infusions can be given in a doctor's office, but they only transiently increase plasma antioxidant capacity.

The best way to increase glutathione levels in the body is to take a supplement rich in cysteine, a precursor to glutathione. There are a number of cysteine-rich supplements available in vitamin stores, such as n-acetyl-cysteine (considered by Dr. Bocci the best source), bioactive whey protein, and Immunocal.

SELENIUM

Selenium is one of those "miracle" minerals believed to protect us from cancer, heart disease, and arthritis; counteract heavy metal toxicity; and even help slow down the aging process. An antioxidant and free radical scavenger, selenium synergizes with vitamin E in the body to mop up free radicals more effectively.

Studies have led scientists to believe that selenium may prevent or slow tumor growth, because certain breakdown products of selenium have been found to enhance immune cell activity and suppress development of blood vessels to the tumor. Studies are being carried out to determine if selenium can be effective against prostate cancer, heart disease, and arthritis. Selenium may also help patients infected with HIV.

The mineral is found primarily in Brazil nuts, seafood, meat, and vegetables (including corn, wheat, and soybeans), but its presence varies widely in soil. The RDI for selenium has been set by the Institute of Medicine of the National Academy of Sciences at 55 μg, with a UL of 400 μg for adults. Selenium toxicity is rare in the United States, but symptoms of toxicity include gastrointestinal upset, hair loss, white blotchy nails, garlic breath odor, fatigue, irritability, and mild nerve damage.

ZINC

Zinc is another important antioxidant mineral. It not only supports a healthy immune system but is essential for protein synthesis, carbon dioxide removal, wound healing, and maintenance of our sense of taste and smell, and it is needed for DNA synthesis. Zinc also supports normal growth and development during pregnancy, childhood, and adolescence and promotes and maintains cell membrane fluidity, which helps cells become more receptive to oxygen.

Like vitamin B6, zinc is needed by the thymus gland to manufacture T cells, so it is considered an important immune booster. This is one reason why many people take extra zinc supplements along with vitamin C when they feel a cold coming on.

Zinc is found primarily in whole grains, liver, seafood, sea vegetables, nuts, and carrots. The RDI for zinc is only 8 mg for adult females and 11 mg for adult males, and 40 mg daily has been set as the UL by the National Academy of Sciences. Intakes of 150 to 450 mg of zinc per day have been associated with low copper status, altered iron function, reduced immune function, and reduced levels of high-density lipoproteins (good cholesterol). Holistic practitioners recommend 50 mg daily for those who are challenged by disease or who wish to maintain their immune systems at a higher level of efficiency. Dr. Sacher recommends that zinc be taken in proportionate amounts with copper to achieve maximum benefit from both minerals.

VITAMINS DURING OZONE TREATMENT

Many people take various types of vitamin supplements when they are undergoing treatment with medical ozone or hydrogen peroxide.

Although taking vitamin supplements may be useful while undergoing conventional medical therapies, certain vitamins—specifically those with antioxidant properties like vitamins C and E—are not recommended.

The *Madrid Declaration on Ozone Therapy* was written with the primary intent of establishing safe and effective medical practices, determining scope of treatment, and introducing safe and effective ozone therapy protocols that are in accordance with the latest scientific research, while adapting to new medical developments and scientific findings. The Declaration included the following guidance to ozone practitioners in its section on the therapeutic uses of ozone:

> During the treatment with ozone [it] is necessary to suspend all the antioxidant supplements that contain vitamin C and vitamin E. The presence of these compounds in high concentrations in the blood interferes with the ozone's action as an oxidant agent and therefore the good course of the therapy. It is important to communicate to the patient that s/he must not consume excessive quantities of foods very rich in these vitamins. [Instead], the vitamins or antioxidants should be given before or after the ozone therapy but never during the treatment.[9]

HEALING FOODS AND HERBS

Several medicinal herbs have been used to complement oxidative therapies. While some are antioxidants, others strengthen the immune system and kill bacteria, viruses, and fungi. The herbs we include here are all easy to use and should not cause adverse side effects of any kind.

Astragalus

Astragalus is a Chinese medicinal herb. The dried root can be made into an important immune-strengthening tonic, and it has often been prescribed for diarrhea and general fatigue.

Studies are being carried out at many Chinese universities to scientifically determine the medicinal value of this herb. One study at the

Third People's Hospital in Hangzhou involved forty-two patients with congestive heart failure (CHF) who were treated with a 40 ml astragalus injection, while a control group of forty patients was given a placebo. After one month of treatment, the clinical heart function improvement rate increased by 26.2 percent and the total effective rate improved by 78.6 percent in the astragalus group. After six months, the improvement was 34.2 percent and 81.6 percent, respectively, leading the researchers to recommend astragalus for severe cases of CHF.[10] A recent clinical trial at Shandong University found that astragalus may help patients suffering from leukemia.[11] It is also considered of value for patients undergoing chemotherapy for cancer.

Astragalus is found through herb catalogs and at Asian herb stores. It can be used as a tea or added (whole) while cooking soups and stews. Astragalus should not be eaten but removed from the soup as you would remove bay leaves.

Echinacea

Echinacea (coneflower) root is known for its immune-enhancing qualities. Long popular among Native American healers, echinacea has been used to treat microbial and viral infections. While scientific opinion has often been divided about the usefulness of this herb, studies after 2000 have shown that echinacea can indeed strengthen the immune system[12] and play a role in healing recurrent respiratory disease.[13] A recent double-blind clinical trial at the University of Alberta in Canada showed a markedly reduced severity of cold symptoms among patients taking standardized echinacea extract when compared to the control group.[14]

Like vitamin C and zinc, echinacea is often recommended to counteract colds and flu. Echinacea is used by people infected with HIV to help strengthen their immune systems. There is some evidence that echinacea is best utilized as a short-term medicinal rather than taken continuously over months or years. Available in many natural foods stores and vitamin shops in capsule form and as a tincture, it can be added to water or juice. Echinacea root may also be prepared as a healing tea.

Garlic

Garlic has been used as a medicinal plant throughout Europe and Asia for centuries. In addition to containing a variety of essential vitamins and minerals, garlic is an important immune system strengthener. It acts on bacteria, viruses, and intestinal parasites and can be used as a preventive for many digestive and respiratory conditions. Garlic is also believed to help lower cholesterol and blood pressure and raise the level of high-density lipoproteins, which help guard against cardiovascular disease. A recent article by Ellen Tattleman, M.D., in *American Family Physician* described garlic's possible antihypertensive effects and reported that it may decrease platelet aggregation in blood vessels. The article especially praised garlic's proven ability to fight stomach and colon cancer.[15]

Many people make garlic an important part of their daily diets. Yet for those who are not fond of garlic's taste (let alone the aroma it can leave on the breath), powdered garlic supplements in capsule form—especially those made from aged garlic extract like Kyolic—are recommended instead. Dr. Tattleman wrote that one or two cloves of raw garlic a day is safe for adults and recommends a powdered supplement of no more than 300 mg taken two or three times a day. Garlic supplements should not be taken by those taking prescription anticoagulants.

Ginkgo Biloba

Ginkgo biloba is the oldest surviving tree species in the world. The leaves have been used by traditional Chinese herbalists to treat heart disease, circulatory problems, and lung disease for thousands of years. Since the mid-1990s, ginkgo has become the subject of extensive laboratory and clinical research in the West and has been studied in more than sixty-seven clinical trials and twenty observational studies and case reports.

An antioxidant, ginkgo has been found to lower cholesterol, relieve arthritis, and treat gastrointestinal ulcers. It also may play a role in relieving the symptoms of glaucoma,[16] attention deficit/hyperactivity disorder,[17] and early-onset Alzheimer's disease.[18] Numerous studies have been done to evaluate claims that ginkgo enhances memory, but they have been inconclusive. Ginkgo biloba extract is available in tablet or tincture form in many natural foods markets and in both Western and Chinese pharmacies.

Green Tea

Green tea has been a popular health drink in China, Korea, and Japan for almost five thousand years. Since the 1990s, it has attracted much media attention as an antioxidant and antibacterial and has been the subject (along with black tea) of numerous laboratory and clinical studies. Green tea has been found to help reduce the risks of heart disease (including atherosclerosis) and lower the risk of certain kinds of cancer, including breast, stomach, colorectal, bladder, and skin.[19] In addition to reducing the effects of low-density lipoprotein cholesterol, the catechins found in green tea have been shown to help people lose weight.[20]

Green tea, which contains caffeine, is easily found in almost any decent-sized supermarket, and finer grades can be found at Asian food stores and specialty tea shops. While "restaurant-grade" tea is inexpensive, finer grades can cost up to several hundred dollars a pound. Health-minded Chinese and Japanese people drink at least several small cups of this delicious tea daily. Green tea extract is also available in capsule form.

Pau D'arco

Pau d'arco comes from the inner bark of a tree found in Brazil. It is a popular antimicrobial, antiviral, antifungal, and antibacterial. Herbalists prescribe pau d'arco to help strengthen the immune system. Recent university studies have shown that pau d'arco also possesses significant anti-cancer properties (especially regarding lung[21] and prostate cancer[22]). It is available in many natural foods stores both as a tea and in capsule form.

30

Exercise and Breathing: Oxygenation and Oxidation

In this chapter, we will examine two very important complements to oxidative therapies: exercise and breathing. Not only do exercise and breathing offer the opportunity for oxygenation, but they can also increase oxidative stress. While transient oxidative stress can be good for our health, chronic oxidative stress due to years of intense exercise may lead to health problems and premature aging.

AEROBIC EXERCISE

Aerobic exercise provides increased oxidation and oxygenation to the entire body and can be an important part of a holistic approach to health. The term *aerobic* simply means "taking place in the presence of oxygen"; aerobic exercise encompasses any form of exercise that increases the amount of oxygen in the body while strengthening the heart and lungs.

Years ago exercise was rarely recommended for people who were sick. Patients with asthma, heart trouble, or cancer were advised to avoid physical exertion and rest as much as possible. While this may be appropriate for some individuals, a growing number of physicians have learned that most patients can safely participate in a wide variety of physical activities, including aerobic exercise.

Aerobic exercises appeal to many different tastes and are often fun to do. They encompass a wide range of activities from slight exertion to major physical challenge: walking, swimming, jogging, running, calisthenics, dancing, cycling, cross-country skiing, hiking, playing tennis, and martial arts such as tai chi, aikido, karate, and boxing. Aerobics can also include doing specific exercises (popularly known simply as "aerobics") and using exercise devices like stair climbers, rebounder-type trampolines, cross-country skiing devices, treadmills, rowing machines, and stationary bicycles.

According to *Physical Activity and Health: A Report by the Surgeon General,* the amount of energy used is roughly the same for the following exercises, moving from "less vigorous/more time" to "more vigorous/less time":

Washing and waxing a car for 45–60 minutes
Washing windows or floors for 45–60 minutes
Playing volleyball for 45 minutes
Playing touch football for 30–45 minutes
Gardening for 30–45 minutes
Wheeling self in wheelchair for 30–40 minutes
Walking 1.75 miles in 35 minutes (20 min/mile)
Playing basketball (shooting baskets) for 30 minutes
Bicycling 5 miles in 30 minutes
Dancing fast (social) for 30 minutes
Pushing a stroller 1.5 miles in 30 minutes
Raking leaves for 30 minutes
Walking 2 miles in 30 minutes (15 min/mile)
Doing water aerobics for 30 minutes
Swimming laps for 20 minutes

Playing wheelchair basketball for 20 minutes

Playing in a basketball game for 15–20 minutes

Bicycling 4 miles in 15 minutes

Jumping rope for 15 minutes

Running 1.5 miles in 15 minutes (10 min/mile)

Shoveling snow for 15 minutes

Stair walking for 15 minutes[1]

One of the most positive aspects of aerobic exercise is that we can adapt it to our physical condition and to the exercise goals we want to achieve: we can begin slowly, and then gradually build up to a workout that increases our heartbeat and breathing rate. Aerobic exercise can provide a number of important physical and psychological benefits. These benefits are synergistic, which means that they work together to provide optimum benefits.

Oxygenation

Through regular, moderate, aerobic exercise, the heart and circulatory system can deliver increased amounts of oxygen to the entire body. This increases the amount of oxygen delivered to all body cells and aids in the process of oxidation, which destroys cells that are sick and weak, replacing them with new stronger and healthier cells. When our blood is oxygenated, we feel lighter, healthier, and more alive. We feel more able to perform our tasks and confront the difficulties that sometimes present themselves in daily life.

Cardiovascular Fitness

Aerobic exercise also strengthens the heart and enables it to provide a reserve capacity of endurance when extra demands are placed on the body from time to time, especially if we have been dealing with illness. It also helps us recover our energy faster after physical or emotional burdens are placed on us.

Flexibility

Our bodies are designed to *move,* and regular aerobic exercise helps us achieve a full range of body motion. Because physical exercise (especially swimming and calisthenics) naturally causes us to move all of our joints, these joints will become more flexible, even if they weren't exercised much before. This not only enables us to use our bodies to the fullest but also decreases the chances of pulling or spraining our muscles. When used in conjunction with deep breathing, regular moderate exercise can also release tension in the chest, neck, and shoulders.

Strength and Endurance

Regular aerobic exercise helps build up our muscles and enables us to breathe easier. This brings about greater strength and endurance and simply allows us to get more out of life. Not only are we able to better accomplish our daily tasks, but we find we are able to enjoy certain activities we couldn't before. My ninety-year-old aunt is one such example. Years ago she didn't have the endurance to join her grandchildren in hiking a hilly nature trail in a park overlooking the Pacific Ocean. After going through two angioplasties to open up her arteries (and facing the threat of a coronary bypass operation if the second angioplasty didn't work), she decided to change her diet and take a walk every morning and every night near her home. After a year of brisk walking for two hours a day around the neighborhood, she discovered that she was able to join her family on the trail again for the first time in fifteen years.

A Positive Mental Attitude

As we saw in the last chapter, our state of mind can have a profound impact on our physical well-being. As part of a synergistic "benign cycle," aerobic exercise not only is good for the physical body but affects our minds as well. Moderate aerobic exercise helps us develop greater self-esteem, optimism, and the feeling that we are more able to do what we want to do. It also helps us gain a better self-image. After several weeks or months of regular aerobic exercise, we notice that we begin to look better: excess body fat tends to melt away, our posture improves, our complexion becomes clearer and healthier-looking, our eyes become brighter, and different muscles gradually develop, sometimes in places we never dreamed possible! Improved fitness and physique help us feel better about ourselves. This is especially important for people who are dealing with illness: regular aerobic exercise helps us move away from the image of being sick and toward a self-image of attractiveness, health, and vitality.

Oxidative Stress

It was mentioned earlier that cells continuously produce free radicals and reactive oxygen species (ROS) as part of metabolic processes. These free radicals are neutralized by the body's antioxidant defense system. This elaborate system consists of enzymes such as catalase, superoxide dismutase, glutathione peroxidase, and numerous nonenzymatic anti-oxidants, such as vitamin A, vitamin E, vitamin C, glutathione, ubiqui-none, and flavonoids.

Strenuous exercise—like intense aerobics or weightlifting—can pro-duce an imbalance between ROS and antioxidants, which is referred to as oxidative stress. Though more scientific research needs to be done, some physicians speculate that a short "spurt" of intense aerobic exercise may possibly bring about the type of beneficial transient oxidative stress produced by an ozone or hydrogen peroxide treatment, oxidizing harm-ful pathogens, delivering more oxygen to body tissues, and strengthening the immune system. The exact "dose" of aerobic exercise would naturally vary from person to person and would depend on his or her level of phys-ical fitness and conditioning. For a person enjoying a good level of physi-cal fitness, a relaxed 10-minute jog including a 1-minute run can produce a "spike" that can bring about such an oxidative event. A half-hour walk that includes a two-block (1-minute) run can do the trick as well.

The effects of long-term oxidative stress due to intense exercise are still not clear. Some researchers speculate that regular exercise brings about oxidative stress that can be linked to muscle damage.[2] Others show that oxidative stress can occur during intense exercise, but at the same time, exercise may enhance the ability of the body's antioxidant defense system to deal with the oxidative stress.[3] Others are not really sure. A recent article in *Sports Medicine* titled "Exercise-Induced Oxidative Stress: Myths, Realities and Physiological Relevance" highlighted the controversy:

> It remains unclear whether exercise-induced oxidative modifications have little significance, induce harmful oxidative damage, or are an integral part of redox regulation. It is clear that ROS play important roles in numerous physiological processes at rest; however, the detailed physiological functions of ROS in exercise remain to be elucidated.[4]

Nevertheless, there is little doubt that the benefits of regular exercise far outweigh the risks of chronic oxidative stress, let alone the health problems that occur when we don't exercise. According to a report by the surgeon general of the United States, regular exercise and physical activity can do the following:

- Reduce the risk of premature death
- Reduce the risk of developing and/or dying from heart disease
- Reduce high blood pressure or the risk of developing high blood pressure
- Reduce high cholesterol or the risk of developing high cholesterol
- Reduce the risk of developing colon cancer and breast cancer
- Reduce the risk of developing diabetes
- Reduce or maintain body weight or body fat
- Build and maintain healthy muscles, bones, and joints
- Reduce depression and anxiety
- Improve psychological well-being
- Enhance work, recreation, and sport performance[5]

In 2009 in an article in the journal *Circulation,* researchers at the Department of Cardiology at St. Olav's Hospital in Trondheim, Norway, described their study that highlighted the beneficial effects of intense aerobic exercise on heart patients.

A group of twenty-seven male patients who had previously suffered heart attacks participated in this study. Patients were randomly assigned to three groups. One group did high-intensity aerobic interval training (AIT) at 95 percent of peak heart rate, another did moderate continuous training (MCT) at 70 percent of peak heart rate, and the third group—the controls—received only standard advice regarding physical activity. Participants in the study continued to take their normal heart medications during the study. Members of the first two groups trained three times a week over a twelve-week period. The goal of the study was to compare training programs with moderate versus high exercise intensity with regard to variables associated with cardiovascular function and prognosis in patients with post-infarction heart failure.

Health-enhancing results were reported in both exercise groups but were greatest among subjects doing the more intense aerobic exercise (AIT). These included increased lung capacity, lower blood pressure, increased blood circulation, improved endothelial function (the endothelium is the thin layer of cells that lines the interior surface of blood vessels and lymphatic vessels), and *reverse* LV remodeling, which relates to beneficial changes in the size, shape, structure, and physiology of the heart. (Though a positive-sounding term, LV remodeling describes negative changes in the heart due to myocardial infarction or other types of heart disease.) In addition, the MacNew global score for quality of life in cardiovascular disease increased in both exercise groups. No changes occurred in the control group.

The researchers concluded: "Exercise intensity was an important factor for reversing LV remodeling and improving aerobic capacity, endothelial function, and quality of life in patients with postinfarction heart failure. These findings may have important implications for exercise training in rehabilitation programs and future studies."[6]

The benefits of intense, short-term exercise were recently reported by a team of researchers at the Sport and Exercise Sciences Research Institute of Ulster University in Northern Ireland who studied the effects of exercise intensity on post-exercise endothelial function and oxidative stress. Their goal was to measure endothelial function and oxidative stress immediately after, 90 minutes after, and three hours after exercise of varying intensities.

The researchers found that acute exercise at different intensities produced a variety of positive effects on oxidative stress and other blood measurements but did not appear to mediate changes in endothelial function. The researchers concluded: "A single bout of maximal exercise may be a more time efficient approach than traditional exercise based on physical activity guidelines and this may have important implications for future public health recommendations."[7]

Before You Exercise

Before beginning an aerobic exercise program, make sure you undergo a complete fitness assessment, especially if you have a history of heart disease or are undergoing treatment for a health problem. The assessment should include an electrocardiogram, a treadmill test, and other tests to determine lung function, strength, and flexibility. Even if you are enjoying good health, it is always a good idea to consult with your physician before undertaking any exercise program.

Proper warm-up before exercise is also important. Many people do stretching exercises before running or walking, which warm up the muscles gradually and help prepare the body for exercise. When your exercise session is complete, a cooling-down period of several minutes is also recommended.

Points to Keep in Mind

In the context of oxidative therapies, there are two additional points of caution worth noting. The whole idea behind aerobic exercise is to produce transient oxidative stress and to oxygenate the blood in order to achieve a higher level of health and well-being. For many people, jogging or running is a favorite aerobic exercise. Unfortunately, when we run or jog in a polluted environment, such as along city streets jammed with traffic, this type of exercise can be dangerous. As we breathe more frequently, fully, and deeply, we take in increased amounts of environmental pollutants (such as nitrogen monoxide, nitrogen dioxide, carbon monoxide, methane, sulfuric acid, and other noxious compounds that mix with ozone) that increase the number of free radicals in our bodies. In *The Oxygen Breakthrough,* Dr. Hendler cites a number of cases of runners suffering from a variety of diseases because they run in polluted areas.

Dr. Hendler also spoke about the dangers of excessive aerobic exercise. In his book, he cites cases of individuals (often marathon runners and triathlon athletes) who felt guilty unless they ran for hours each day, or who believed in exercising to the point of absolute exhaustion. Many of them became his patients because excess aerobic exercise depressed their immune systems (especially with regard to the production of antibodies and natural killer cells) and opened the door to a variety of health problems, including chronic fatigue syndrome, asthma, intestinal bleeding, allergies, and respiratory infections.[8] These health problems may be related to chronic oxidative stress in athletes who partake in intense physical activity several hours a day over long periods of time.

Moderation: The Key

This chapter stresses *moderate* exercise on a regular basis. Studies have found that weekend athletes—those who don't exercise regularly—tend to increase the number of free radicals in their bodies, while those who exercise regularly are able to easily get rid of them. In addition, by avoiding overexertion, we tend to enjoy our exercise more and are more likely to want to continue doing it.

Another problem we face when we begin an exercise program is an "all or nothing" attitude. Many of us feel that if we cannot run a mile, we shouldn't run at all. This not only makes exercise unpleasant, it sabotages many an exercise program. Again, modification is important at the start of an exercise program. Instead of running for a mile, you can cut down your run to a half mile. If you don't feel like running, take a brisk walk instead. Rather than spend 30 minutes on the stationary bicycle at full throttle, ride at half speed for 15 minutes. After several days, we can gradually build up to faster speeds and longer distances. Exercise instructors often suggest that it is better to begin an exercise regimen slowly and build up our level of activity by about 10 percent a week. They also suggest the importance of pacing ourselves: when we are on the running track, we can run for a while and then walk briskly. Or we can rest frequently during the exercise period when we feel that we need it. As we gradually build up our strength and endurance, we are better able to participate in longer periods of physical activity.

Exercise Should Be a Pleasure

In general, it is important to grow to like exercise, because if we enjoy what we are doing, we are more likely to continue with it. For this reason, we should choose an activity we enjoy doing. We can also enhance our enjoyment of exercise by choosing the right time or situation. For example, if you get lonely walking alone, do it with friends. If you don't like to walk outdoors, walk at the mall. Over the past few years, I have used a cross-country skiing machine at home. Sometimes I find it gets boring, so I play music, listen to a recorded book, or watch television while I exercise. I not only fulfill my need for exercise but also catch up on the morning news or enjoy new story plots.

How Much Exercise?

Many physicians recommend at least 30 minutes of exercise several days a week, although 30 minutes may be too long for people who are just beginning an exercise program or who are going through a period of healing. Ask your physician or exercise instructor how you can build up your exercise level gradually and safely.

BREATHING

Although all of us breathe, we are often not aware of the quality of our breathing. We tend to take partial, shallow breaths using only the upper part of the lungs, or we often hold our breath (especially when we are tense or nervous) without being conscious of it. When this type of breathing becomes habitual or chronic, we limit the amount of air that we take into our body, which impairs our body's ability to oxygenate the blood and other vital tissues.

Deep, rhythmic breathing is essential for proper oxygenation, and learning how to breathe in a way that involves both the upper and lower parts of the lungs has been viewed as vital by yogis for centuries. Perhaps the most important breath to learn is known as "the Yogi Complete Breath," first introduced by Yogi Ramacharaka to the West in the early part of the last century. He described performing this breath as follows:

> Stand or sit erect. Breathing through the nostrils, inhale steadily, first filling the lower part of the lungs, which is accompanied by bringing into play the diaphragm, while [distending] exerts a gentle pressure on the abdominal organs, pushing forward the front walls of the abdomen. Then fill the middle part of the lungs, pushing out the lower ribs, breastbone and chest. Then fill the higher portion of the lungs, protruding the upper chest, thus lifting the chest, including the upper six or seven pairs of ribs. In the final movement, the lower part of the abdomen will be slightly drawn in, which movement gives the lungs a support and also helps to fill the highest part of the lungs.

Yogi Ramacharaka also reminds us that this breath consists not of three distinct movements, but rather one continuous, fluid movement. He then recommends that we retain this breath for a couple of seconds and then exhale slowly, drawing in the abdomen slightly as the air leaves the lungs. He then suggests that we relax the chest and abdomen after the air is released.[9]

The Yogi Complete Breath can be done whenever we feel like it, although we may at first want to do this breath during a period of quiet contemplation or just before we begin our exercise program. Gradually, we can begin consciously breathing fully and deeply in more and more of our daily activities, until deep, rhythmic breathing becomes a normal part of our lives. In addition to Yogi Ramacharaka's classic work, many books about yoga offer instruction on deep, rhythmic breathing.

Limbic Breathing

Majid Ali, M.D., author of *Oxygen and Aging* and other books, recommends what he calls *limbic breathing* to allow more time for oxygen to pass from air sacs in the lungs to the capillaries in the lungs. The limbic system is a complex network of nerves in the brain that are connected to instinct and mood. Dr. Ali believes that limbic breathing reduces stress, promotes relaxation, and strengthens the immune system. He suggests that this breathing method can be practiced for several minutes a day, plus whenever we feel stressed, are upset, or need to relax.

- Sit in a comfortable chair with your hands on your lap. Let out your belly, which allows your diaphragm to press down on the abdominal cavity.
- Mentally count to four as you fill your lungs slowly through your nose, and then hold your breath for another count of four.
- Slowly exhale through your nose for a count of eight.
- Repeat this process until you feel comfortable with the rhythm.
- After some practice, extend the exhalation to a count of twelve, fourteen, and sixteen.[10]

Donald M. Epstein, the developer of network chiropractic, always points out, "Only living people breathe. Dead people don't." The more we breathe, the more alive we are. And the more we practice deep, rhythmic breathing, the more we partake of oxygen, the essence of life itself.

31
Emotions, Mind, and Spirit

Donald M. Epstein, D.C., author of *The Twelve Stages of Healing* and *Healing Myths, Healing Magic,* has often said that healing is "an inside job." He means that the most essential components to healing, such as life force, harmony, regeneration, and repair, are not given to us by others but come from within. Innate healing power is part of our birthright and is within reach of every one of us. In his essay "There Is No Cure for Healing," Dr. Epstein writes: "Healing is a process, not a magical event. Nothing new is added to your body or mind. . . . Nothing is taken out. Healing involves a greater experience of oneness, wholeness, and reconnection with all aspects of your being."[1]

Many of us have known people who experienced a health problem and, despite the finest medical care (and often a positive initial medical prognosis), got sicker and died. We have also seen people with life-threatening "terminal" diseases who were given up on by their doctors return from the brink of death to enjoy long, healthy, and productive lives. Most such cases are downplayed by members of the medical profession because they go against the dominant view that outside agents like drugs, radiation, and surgery are the determining factors in recovering one's health. The belief that healing primarily occurs from within is incomprehensible.

JOSÉ'S STORY

Fifteen years ago, my friend José was diagnosed with pancreatic cancer, which had spread to the liver. His physician, a prominent oncologist at a major Boston hospital, referred to José as "a sad case" to his colleagues and held out no hope for his recovery. He recommended surgery as the only way to prolong José's life.

José decided to return to his native Brazil, where he was examined by other oncologists at the hospital affiliated with Brazil's finest medical school. They confirmed the original diagnosis and, like the Boston doctor, held out no hope for his recovery. They offered him surgery, radiation, and chemotherapy, all of which were refused. José, a psychiatrist, had a medical degree and knew that these therapies would kill him. He decided instead to retreat to the countryside, where he embarked on a holistic path to healing that involved intense spiritual and psychological work, using a number of native healing plants. This led to important insights about his life, which brought about major changes in attitude, belief, behavior, and diet, all of which had a positive (and powerful) impact on his health.

When José returned to the hospital in Rio de Janeiro for a checkup six months later, a CT scan and other tests determined that the cancer had completely disappeared. His doctors were flabbergasted. Since they knew that nearly everyone with advanced pancreatic cancer dies within six months of the initial diagnosis, they simply could not accept evidence of a complete remission, let alone one taking place in the absence of traditional medical therapy. Although they were happy for José (who remained in excellent health for another eight years before dying of a heart attack), they announced that they must have erred in their original diagnosis and that he didn't have cancer after all! The idea of a complete recovery from pancreatic cancer through holistic healing was inconceivable to them.

MIND–BODY HEALING

The holistic view of healing teaches that human beings are more than just the physical body and that emotions, thoughts, attitudes, and spirituality play an essential role in healing. Rather than conform to the predominant medical view that there is "one cause" and "one cure" to disease, holism stresses that health and disease depend on a dynamic and often subtle interplay among the physical, emotional, mental, and spiritual aspects of our being, as well as our relationship to the environment in which we live. Larry Dossey, M.D., in his book *Space, Time & Medicine,* wrote: "For health is harmony, and harmony has no meaning without the fluid movement of interdependent parts. Like a stream that becomes stagnant when it ceases to flow, harmony and health turn into disease when stasis occurs. We return to the concept of the biodance, the endless streaming of the body-in-flux."[2]

During the past few years, an important new field called *psychoneuroimmunology* has come into being. It is concerned with identifying the links between the mind, the brain, and the immune system and how they communicate with each other. Researchers like Candace B. Pert, Ph.D., research professor in the Department of Physiology and Biophysics at Georgetown University Medical Center in Washington, D.C., have scientifically confirmed that our minds and feelings influence health, and our health has a powerful effect on the mind.

In her book *Good Health in a Toxic World,* Sara Shannon summarized the major findings of psychoneuroimmunology in understanding the interplay between mind–body healing:

1. Mind-directed, cell-enhancing chemicals communicate directly with the immune system.
2. Mental attitude and mood can alter the course of disease.
3. The mind can "will" changes in the body.
4. Stress-related hormones weaken the immune system.

5. Chemicals made by the immune system communicate with the brain.

6. The brain "talks" to the immune system, and the immune system "talks" to the brain.[3]

These discoveries reveal more emphatically than ever before that the way in which we view ourselves and life's situations can affect our immune response. For example, let's say that you are about to take a ride on the Cyclone, Coney Island's famous roller coaster. If you take this ride with a sense of dread and terror, your brain will produce a neurochemical called norepinephrine, which can contribute to the risk of high blood pressure, clogging of the arteries, and even heart attack. Fear, hopelessness, and the feeling that "nothing works" have also been linked to the production of neurochemicals that can lower immune response and promote the aging process.

However, you can view a ride on the Cyclone in another way: you can become excited at the prospect of the intense speed and look forward to the thrill of "letting go." You can scream with pleasure, marveling at the view of the ocean and the feeling of flight. As a result, your brain will produce endorphins and benzodiazepines, two neurochemicals that increase your overall sense of well-being. Other chemicals (known as neurotransmitters) created by positive feelings toward challenges strengthen your immune system, slow down the aging process, and protect you from cancer and a number of viruses.

While these different thoughts and emotions may have a temporary impact on health, chronic, repeated, and habitual thought and emotional patterns can have a far more profound, long-term impact on our well-being. Feelings of fear, hopelessness, worry, and worthlessness all affect our "body–mind" system, however subtle these effects may be. Critical attitudes, beliefs in negative outcomes, anger, resentment, and the belief (whether conscious or not) that "I have no control over my life" have been linked to a number of disease states, including cancer, ulcers, and heart disease.

Psychologist Thorwald Dethlefsen and physician Rüdiger Dahlke believe that symptoms are bodily expressions of psychological conflicts: "Symptoms are many and various, yet they are all expressions of one and the same event which we call 'illness,' and which always occurs within a person's consciousness. Just as the body cannot live without consciousness, so it cannot become 'ill' without consciousness either."[4] Dethlefsen and Dahlke's excellent book *The Healing Power of Illness* (see the resources—appendix 2, page 443) examines how understanding the symbolism of certain symptoms can lead us to transform these inner conflicts into power agents for healing and growth.

Stress and Distress

Researchers such as Hans Selye, M.D., have found that it is not necessarily the stresses of life that lead to disease, but rather *how we adapt to these stresses*. The ways in which we adapt are often based on our perspectives on ourselves and our life, many of which are learned from childhood. When a stressful incident occurs (whether the loss of a loved one, a difficult task, or a change in economic status), we tend to look at the problem through these old perspectives. If we are stuck in rigid, fixed perspectives about ourselves and the way that life "should be," we often find it far more difficult to deal with life's changing events. Instead of adapting to the situation and seeking practical solutions, we may instead feel hopeless, frustrated, and afraid. Rather than becoming a stimulus for action, the life challenge leads us to fear and paralysis.

In their classic *Getting Well Again*, Carl Simonton, M.D., Stephanie Matthews-Simonton, and James Creighton list a number of common psychological traits found in the cancer patients they encountered, which appeared to be precursors to their cancer diagnosis. These included the following:

- "Experiences in childhood result in decisions to be a certain kind of person." The Simontons believe that as children, we often adopt certain ways of thinking, feeling, and being. Some may be positive and some may be negative, but they result in a certain mind-set that is ingrained upon the personality.

- "The individual is rocked by a cluster of stressful life events." These events, such as the loss of a mate or a job or other position, place critical stress on the individual, which threatens personal identity.

- "These stresses create a problem with which the individual does not know how to deal." Very often, the stressful situation goes beyond our established ways of coping, and we feel a loss of control over our situation.

- "The individual sees no way of changing the rules about how he or she must act and so feels trapped and helpless to resolve the problem." We often feel incapable of resolving our problem, which often involves changing the way we view ourselves and the world. This causes us to feel helpless, hopeless, and victimized by outer circumstances.

- "The individual puts distance between himself or herself and the problem, becoming static, unchanging, rigid."[5] When this stage occurs, the individual feels that life no longer has any meaning and, despite outer appearances, feels resigned to his or her fate.

Oxidative Therapies and the Body–Mind

As tools for healing, ozone and hydrogen peroxide can have a powerful effect on our emotional well-being, largely due to their documented analgesic effects, described in an earlier chapter. Many people who have used oxidative therapies find that they feel less pain and are not as depressed as they were before. As they place less focus on feeling bad, they experience more energy, optimism, and emotional well-being.

Although the psychological benefits of ozone and hydrogen peroxide still need to be explored further, they can help provide valuable emotional respite from pain and discomfort that one needs to explore new avenues of growth, transformation, and healing in addition to the powerful effects they can have on the physical body.

Disease: A Wake-Up Call to Change

In the context of holistic healing, illness should never be viewed as a punishment or a failure. Instead, disease can be seen as the result of a lack of alignment among the physical, emotional, mental, and spiritual aspects of our being. Rather than being viewed as "bad" or "evil," symptoms are the body's way of telling us that something is wrong. They are a "wake-up call" that tells us that we need to change old attitudes, perspectives, and lifestyle habits that may have contributed to our health problem. To the degree that we are sensitive to our body's subtle messages, we can often deal with a problem before it becomes serious.

Life-threatening diseases like cancer and AIDS can play a special role in the transformative process. They challenge us to the very core of our being and can mobilize us—as cancer did for my friend José—to make major changes in personality, thinking, and lifestyle. According to Jason Serinus in *Psychoimmunity and the Healing Process*:

> A diagnosis of AIDS is not necessarily a death sentence; but transforming that diagnosis into an opportunity for healing demands a total commitment. Precisely because the disease is so insidious, it attacks people on the three levels of mind, body and spirit, it must be approached simultaneously on all three levels. The decision to live must be total, involving every thought, every cell, every habit and belief. . . . AIDS represents a real test of who one was and who one chooses to be.[6]

Illness forces us to make choices. Choices based on fear and other limited perspectives often lead to more suffering, whereas those based on knowledge and hope have often been found to lead to healing. These choices may involve seeking greater inner alignment and harmony, changing a destructive emotional or thought pattern, relinquishing resentment, letting go of childhood hurts, and coming to terms with other difficult aspects of one's past.

In their book *Living in Hope,* Cindy Mikluscak-Cooper, R.N., and

Emmett E. Miller, M.D., list some traits that long-term survivors with AIDS have in common. Many are similar to those of long-term cancer survivors. The ones appearing here are applicable to individuals suffering from all serious illness, whether it is life-threatening or not. These traits include the following:

- Having a sense of personal responsibility for their health and a sense that they can influence it
- Having a sense of purpose in life
- Finding new meaning in life as a result of the illness itself
- Having previously mastered a life-threatening illness or other life crisis
- Having accepted the reality of their diagnosis, yet refusing to believe that it is a death sentence
- Having an ability to communicate their concerns to others, including concerns regarding the illness itself
- Being assertive and having the ability to say "no"
- Having the ability to withdraw from involvements and to nurture themselves
- Being sensitive to their body and its needs[7]

Other common traits among long-term AIDS survivors are addressed in Scott J. Gregory's book *A Holistic Protocol for the Immune System*. Ten points in particular stand out, summarized as follows:

1. They had expectations of favorable results regarding their situation.
2. They took charge of their healing and took control of decisions that vitally affected their lives.
3. They developed a sense of humor and learned to laugh.
4. They developed compassion toward others.
5. They were patient in their expectations and did not expect to be healed overnight.

6. They changed their attitudes about themselves and developed a stronger self-image.
7. They realized that there was no one thing that could cure them and sought a combination of life-reinforcing factors and modalities.
8. They had no fear of death—or life.
9. They educated themselves in prevention and treatment.
10. They were fighters.[8]

While healing often leads to a marked improvement in our physical condition, this isn't always the case. Some people, for example, experience healing on psychological or spiritual levels, but physical healing may no longer be possible. Individuals may be too debilitated physically to survive, or they may have the deep realization that their life task is over.

Some years ago, I remember going to the hospital to visit an acquaintance with advanced AIDS who had a very difficult relationship with his father. An admiral in the Navy, the father never accepted the fact that his son was gay, and they hadn't spoken to each other in years. When he heard of his son's condition, the father rushed to his bedside and remained there for two months. During this time, a tremendous amount of healing occurred between father and son, which was often very moving for those of us who visited the hospital on a regular basis. By the time there appeared to be resolution in their relationship, the son finally decided to "let go" and die.

SELF-NURTURING

Although oxidative therapies and adjuncts like diet and body cleansing assist in the healing process, it is *we* who do the healing. We simply have to allow it to take place. An important component in the process is creating an environment that will facilitate the healing process in our lives. This is not unlike a farmer preparing the soil in expectation of an abundant crop. While the environment will differ according to our personal needs and life situation, it involves three often-overlooked aspects of ourselves: our emotional being, our mental being, and our spiritual being. The following pages offer a few ideas that can enhance self-nurturing on emotional, mental, and spiritual levels.

Keep in mind that the subject of this chapter easily deserves an entire book. Although the small amount of information provided can help lay the groundwork for healing on all levels, the potentials for healing are limitless, can be adapted to our individual needs, and can be mobilized—in different ways—by everyone.

Nurturing the Emotional Self

Our emotions play an important role in health and disease. Positive feelings produce neurochemicals that strengthen the immune system; negative, repressed, or distorted emotions can decrease immune response and open the door to a variety of health problems. This is why emotional well-being is an important aspect of healing. Rather than try to repress, deny, or control our emotions, we need to nourish and guide them so that they can help us become integrated and whole.

Emotional nurturing can involve creating a support system. This may take the form of being with others who support our healing process, such as relatives or friends. At times, we may need to distance ourselves from those who are not supportive or let them become more aware of our needs and how they might assist us in a positive way. We can also join an organized support group made up of people dealing with health problems similar to our own. Hospitals and social service organizations often can suggest groups that meet locally. The importance of having a support system of this kind cannot be underestimated, especially if one is challenged by a life-threatening disease.

Beauty is also important in emotional healing. Surrounding ourselves with beautiful paintings and prints or having a vase of fresh flowers in our bedroom or living room is a wonderful healing gift. Working in the garden, taking a walk in the woods, or sitting by a lake or stream helps stabilize our emotions and gets us more in touch with our natural rhythms. Visit an art museum, watch an inspiring movie, or listen to uplifting music. The possibilities are only limited by our imaginations.

Accepting all of our feelings (including sexual feelings) can be a powerful act of healing. Expressing anger, grief, frustration, and sadness is not always as easy in our culture as the expression of joy, excitement, and affection. Like a river whose current is obstructed, emotions that are blocked tend to become polluted and harmful, as by their very nature emotions are to be experienced and expressed. Long-term repression of emotions has long been viewed as a factor in a number of common diseases, including cancer, stroke, and heart attack. It probably contributes to less dramatic diseases as well, such as depression and chronic fatigue. This is why we need to reclaim our emotions and allow them to be expressed in nondestructive ways. Candace B. Pert writes in *Molecules of Emotion:*

> I believe *all* emotions are healthy, because emotions are what unite the mind and the body. Anger, fear, and sadness, the so-called negative emotions, are as healthy as peace, courage and joy. To repress these emotions and not let them flow freely is to set up a dis-integrity in the system, causing it to act at cross-purposes rather than as a unified whole. The stress this creates, which takes the form of blockages and insufficient flow of peptide signals to maintain function at a cellular level, is what sets up the weakened conditions that can lead to disease. All honest emotions are positive emotions.[9]

Through meditation, dynamic exercise, or different forms of body-oriented modalities such as bioenergetics, network chiropractic, and Zero Balancing, we can learn to accept our human emotions and channel them into more positive areas of expression.

Many people find that helping others can be a healing emotional gift to everyone involved. Volunteering in a hospital, tutoring a child, or cleaning up a neighborhood park can provide intense satisfaction and the feeling that we are being useful. These types of activities take us "out of ourselves"—we place less emphasis on our own problems and become more involved in our community.

Another important component of emotional nurturing is humor. In his book *Anatomy of an Illness,* Norman Cousins wrote about how 10 minutes of belly laughter at frequent intervals (he watched Marx brothers movies and old *Candid Camera* television shows) helped him overcome a life-threatening disease.[10]

Karen Shultz wrote about the healing aspects of hearty, sincere laughter in the anthology *The Essence of Healing:*

1. Exercise the muscles of the lungs, diaphragm, abdomen, chest, and shoulders, stimulating the circulatory system and exercising the breathing muscles
2. Increase the oxygen in your blood
3. Become profoundly self-relaxed—after laughing, the pulse rate, heartbeat, and blood pressure drop below normal and the skeletal muscles become deeply relaxed, indicating reduced stress
4. Control pain by increasing production of endorphins, the body's natural pain killers[11]

Another often-overlooked yet very pleasurable form of emotional nourishment is "hug therapy." Dr. David Bresler of the University of California at Los Angeles Pain Control Unit prescribes a minimum of four hugs a day for men and women to relieve stress and emotional tension.

Perhaps most importantly, we need to heal old emotional wounds from the past. Making peace with others, which can include forgiving those who have hurt us, asking forgiveness from those we have hurt, letting go of resentment, and especially forgiving ourselves, is essential to this process. The books of Louise Hay (see the resources—appendix 2, page 444) offer valuable tools to these aspects of emotional healing. Twelve-step programs such as Alcoholics Anonymous, psychotherapy, body-oriented therapies like bioenergetics and Core Energetics, Pre-Cognitive Re-Education, neurolinguistic programming, yoga, meditation, breathwork, network chiropractic, Zero Balancing, and books like *The Twelve Stages of Healing* and *Healing Myths, Healing Magic* (listed in appendix 2) can all facilitate the process of emotional healing.

Nurturing the Mind

At this point in human history, we have access to more information than ever before. While access to information can be valuable, the unrelenting amount of gossip, sensationalism, superficial ideas, and negative, fear-producing concepts from advertising, news reports, and politics is a type of "mental pollution" that many of us can do without. They dull our mental awareness, keep us living on the periphery, and inhibit our innate healing capacity.

Of particular concern is the constant barrage of negative reports concerning death and disease. Despite Louis Pasteur's advice that "the microbe is nothing; the soil is everything" (meaning that a healthy body will not provide fertile soil for germs to cause disease), news reports and magazine articles often focus on an ever-increasing number of outside agents that will give us cancer, tuberculosis, AIDS, and a myriad of other diseases. This creates a mental environment of fear and hopelessness.

Unless we throw out our radio and television and decide to avoid reading the news or going online, we probably cannot escape this onslaught. Yet we can avoid much of this negative information through our powers of discernment and discrimination. We can also choose not to "hook into" initial reports on certain diseases, understanding that many are the result of a limited approach and partial understandings. For example, in the early 1980s, we were told that AIDS was a terminal disease. After it was found that many patients remained alive and productive five to ten years after their original diagnosis, the media decided that it wasn't necessarily a terminal disease after all. In 2003, SARS (severe acute respiratory syndrome) was touted as a disease that would kill millions, but fewer than eight hundred people died.

More recently, the bird flu "pandemic" was touted as a disease that would kill millions of Americans. While not minimizing the dangers of avian influenza, instilling fear as a way to deal with disease is counterproductive. According to Dr. Marc Siegel, a practicing internist and associate professor of medicine at the New York University School of Medicine, "If anything is contagious right now, it's judgment clouded by fear."[12] Instead of a bird flu pandemic, we have a fear pandemic. History and logic dictate that the best way to fight off bacterial and viral diseases is with commonsense prevention techniques coupled with a strong immune system.

Questioning is an important aspect of mental healing. As children, a lot of us formed certain ideas about ourselves, our talents, and our tasks in life. We also created ideas about other people and the world in which we live. While many of those ideas may have been useful at one time, they may not be useful now. The image that "my older brother is mean and will beat me up" may have been true when we were five, but at age fifty, this is no longer the case. The old idea that "I'm no good at art" may reflect a bad experience in a second-grade art class that still stops us from experiencing our innate creativity as an adult. For this reason, we need to question whether an old concept is still valid and whether it can be changed. As a result, we expand our perspectives, which can bring us new opportunities for understanding and personal growth.

A common negative image is believing that because a friend or relative has died of a certain disease, we will also. While we may be genetically predisposed to certain health problems, this does not mean that they will manifest as symptoms. A friend once put it to me this way: "Just because my father had cancer doesn't mean that I will. I don't think like him, eat like him, or live like him. We are different people." In addition, we need to be aware that the body that we have now is not the same one we had five or ten years ago, because every cell of the body is in the process of dying and others are being regenerated constantly. The health of future cells, and therefore the future health of our entire body and mind, is dependent on how we live, eat, and think in the present. As members of the human race, we have become imbued with beliefs or myths that often prevent the healing process; we need to create other beliefs that facilitate healing.

In his breakthrough book *Healing Myths, Healing Magic,* Dr. Donald Epstein focuses on social myths ("healing means understanding what went wrong or who did what to me"), biomedical myths ("healing takes time"), religious myths ("disease is a punishment for my sins"), and new-age myths ("I must understand my feelings to heal") and suggests alternative ways to help us reclaim our innate ability to heal. He wrote:

> Every culture "sleeps" within its own mythology. If we wish to awaken from our sleep, we must be willing to evaluate the way we are programmed to experience our world, our circumstances, and ourselves. Then we may choose our own stories of the world we live in, and the way in which we will live in it. When we awaken from our sleep and question the stories given to us by our authority figures, we may choose to continue with those stories, or we can create new stories that work even better for us. Choosing our own stories can be a liberating, life-transforming, and empowering experience.[13]

The Great Epidemic

Negative thinking has become epidemic in our world. During the course of every day, each of us may be the source of hundreds of negative thoughts concerning impending disasters (large and small). We may also worry about negative outcomes; create images of being undeserving or unworthy of good things in life; hold on to ideas about being rejected, offended, or betrayed; and exaggerate notions of the importance of everyday aches and pains. Thought is a powerful creative force; thinking helps create the world in which we live. Given that billions of people are out there creating those negative thoughts, it should be no wonder that we live in a world that is violent, polluted, unhappy, and in great need of healing.

Negative thinking is a totally useless activity. It is anchored in the past and projected into the future, avoiding the truth of the present moment that is the only reality. By becoming aware of creating negative thoughts, we begin to stop contributing to the storehouse of negative thinking in the world.

There are many good books and courses available on positive thinking. Yet simply becoming more aware of our negative thinking and understanding how harmful it is for ourselves and others helps us gradually discover that our thought patterns can change. Even a simple affirmation like, "Today I will only have positive thoughts" every time we catch ourselves engaging in negative thinking can help transform a negative pattern into one that supports the healing process, if only for a moment.

Books that educate and empower us in our healing journey are powerful sources of mental nurturing as well. Some of the books included in appendix 2 provide that type of support and show how we can recover and maintain our health. In addition, inspirational readings from holy books, twelve-step meditation books, and stories about the healing journeys of others can inspire us and help create positive thoughts. Understanding the hidden meaning of fairy tales, studying books of ancient wisdom, and learning about the holistic healing practices of both traditional and modern cultures are also ways to enhance mental nurturing. Remember, however, that nurturing the mind should not be done at the expense of the emotions. Both need to be nurtured together in order to achieve harmonious fulfillment in our life.

Creative Visualization

Creative visualization is often used in healing. There are a number of excellent books dealing with visualization available in bookstores and libraries. Louise Hay outlines the three basic parts of a positive visualization, which anyone can adapt to their individual needs:

1. An image of the problem or pain or dis-ease, or the dis-eased part of the body
2. An image of a positive force eliminating this problem
3. An image of the body being rebuilt to perfect health, then seeing the body move through life with ease and energy[14]

Positive visualization can incorporate literal images, symbolic images related to treatment, or abstract images. One universal image is a source of bright, white healing light; we can imagine it shining around (and through) every aspect of our being. A powerful tool to use for this type of creative visualization is the "Divine Light Invocation Mantra" taught by Swami Sivananda Radha:

> *I am created by Divine Light*
> *I am sustained by Divine Light*
> *I am protected by Divine Light*
> *I am surrounded by Divine Light*
> *I am ever growing into Divine Light.*[15]

Some people may wish to visualize being healed by Jesus Christ or the Healing Buddha; others may wish to incorporate saints, yogis, angels, or other spiritual beings in their healing visualizations.

Finally, mental healing involves becoming aware of what is really important to us. Possessions, prestige, money in the bank, and a country club membership may be nice to have, but many people facing serious illness soon realize that those material things are not as important as they once thought. Good relationships, inner peace, connection with a Higher (or Deeper) Power, and a sense of purpose in life often move to the foreground during a healing crisis.

One of the benefits of illness is that it brings us into reality. We begin to discern the true from the false, and the essence from the superficial. We begin to see the kind of life we truly want to have and often come upon the methods needed to achieve it.

Spiritual Nurturing

Spirituality is often believed to have little impact on healing by physicians, yet it can provide the foundation for deep healing to take place. People know the source of spirituality by many names: God, Allah, the Inner Light, Organizing Wisdom, the Divine Teacher. Whatever label we choose to give that Source, spirituality involves tapping into the deeper levels of our being where inner wisdom and love can be found. As we connect to this love-wisdom, we are able to create a greater sense of harmony and alignment among all aspects of our being, allowing the healing process to occur.

If we participate in self-nurturing on the emotional and mental levels, spiritual nurturing is a natural result, because all are interconnected and interrelated. However, there are a number of specific ways to enhance healing through spiritual means that can be both inspiring and empowering.

Many of us engage in spiritual nurturing on special occasions, such as when we go to our house of worship or when we are experiencing a crisis. Although this is important, many teachers have stressed the importance of becoming aware of the sacred in everyday life. This involves not only understanding the spiritual component in daily challenges and viewing our immediate situation in the context of a greater or deeper reality, but also learning how to see the sacred in the world around us, including other people, animals, and nature.

Trees and flowers are an often-overlooked source of spiritual nourishment in our modern, industrialized world. Yet many of our ancestors—like members of indigenous and traditional cultures today—long appreciated the healing power of trees and used them for healing all levels of their being. In addition to their beauty, trees are strong, graceful, adaptable, and deeply grounded in what Native Americans call the "Earth Mother." By developing a close relationship with trees (many of us, in fact, had a "favorite tree" as a child), we can share their natural qualities.

There are many ways to commune with trees: resting under their shade, standing or leaning against their trunks, and even hugging trees can open us to a source of earth energy we rarely experience. In my book *The Deva Handbook* (Destiny Books, 1998), I included more detailed information about the spiritual and healing aspects of trees and other nature forms, and how we can partake of them.

Another powerful yet often-disregarded natural source of spiritual nourishment are flowers. Although most of us like flowers, we do not take the time to appreciate them. Flowers offer strength, grace, color, pattern, and dazzling beauty. Flowers have a lot to teach us about life. A wildflower growing (and thriving) in a crack in the sidewalk shows us how we can survive and thrive even under the most difficult circumstances. A new flower can reveal the beauty exhibited by openness and vulnerability. A flower in full bloom can tell us the value of giving fully of ourselves without holding back or being concerned about what others might say. A dying flower can reveal the grace and understanding of accepting death as a natural part of our life cycle.

Finally, prayer can be a powerful force in healing. It is an expression of yearning from deep within our being to realize our connection with the Source of all life. Prayer acknowledges our union with this Source, which is both outside of us and deep within. Prayer has been likened to our sending off "radio waves" of goodness into the world and beyond.

Prayers may take many forms. They may involve repeating a sacred word or phrase, they may be prayers for healing of self or a loved one, or we may articulate a prayer as a special blessing to the world. The following Buddhist prayer is especially beautiful:

> *May all people and all forms of life be surrounded with Infinite*
> *Love and Compassion. Particularly do we send forth loving*
> *thoughts to those in suffering and sorrow, to all those in doubt*
> *and ignorance, to all who are striving to attain the truth, and*
> *to those whose feet are standing close to the great change we call*
> *death, we send forth oceans of Love, Wisdom, and Compassion.*

Whenever we pray, we open ourselves to the possibility of deep healing blessing. It is a humble act that is grounded in our desire to realize our oneness and wholeness. This is, in effect, the essential goal of healing.

The Future of
Oxygen Therapies

Oxygen therapies have become far better known than ever before. More people have heard about them, more practitioners have decided to use ozone and hydrogen peroxide in their practice, and scientific research has moved forward in a wide area of study and practical application. At the same time, the "maturing" of this medical specialty has created important challenges for the future that need to be addressed.

I am writing this chapter as an objective journalist who (aside from earning royalties on sales of my book) has no business connections whatsoever with the world of oxidative therapies. While I know physicians and ozone suppliers—and many have provided material for inclusion in this book—I do *not* earn commissions from the sale of hydrogen peroxide, ozone-related devices, or oxygen supplements; represent any manufacturer of ozone generators; or receive referral fees or free treatments from any oxidative practitioner. My goals in this conclusion are to offer my perspective on the most viable opportunities in the field of oxidative therapies and to share suggestions and constructive criticism about the state of the profession today. While some may not agree with my ideas, they are offered in the spirit of good faith with the hope that they can be explored, debated, and perhaps acted upon.

POISED FOR ACCEPTANCE

By 2016, oxygen therapies—and ozone therapy in particular—had achieved wider mainstream acceptance as a scientifically based, clinically measurable health care modality. Several major developments have helped create this new and exciting paradigm.

The Bocci Breakthrough

The breakthrough research findings by Dr. Velio Bocci explained for the first time how hydrogen peroxide and ozone actually work therapeutically. In addition to putting to rest the long-held and pervasive belief that ozone is harmful to the body under all circumstances, Dr. Bocci identified a complex series of cascading chemical reactions that strengthen the immune system and assist the body's own self-healing. By reacting with blood components, ozone generates a number of chemical messengers responsible for activating important biological functions: oxygen delivery, immune activation, release of hormones, and induction of antioxidant enzymes. It also may mobilize endogenous stem cells, which can promote the regeneration of ischemic tissues.

Ozone Produced by the Body Itself

The 2002 discovery that ozone is actually produced by the human body to help fight disease and infection by scientists at the Scripps Institute in California reveals that ozone is not merely a foreign element that can affect the human body in different ways. Like hydrogen peroxide, it plays an important role in the body's own self-healing process.

Tooth Repair and Regeneration

The recent discovery that ozone therapy can not only repair decayed teeth but actually stimulate the regeneration of the tooth itself has been called a major breakthrough in dentistry. In contrast to the traditional "drill and fill" method, this new technique—which is simple, safe, and cost-effective—will forever change the face of dentistry and can have a powerful impact on dental health for decades to come. It is currently approved for use in several European countries (including Germany and Great Britain) but is still awaiting approval in North America.

New Delivery Systems

The development of new and more efficient delivery systems for ozone has far-reaching clinical possibilities. Of special note is the intraperitoneal application technique, developed by Dr. Siegfried Shulz at the Philipps-Universität in Germany. If results on humans are as promising as those on mice and rabbits, intraperitoneal ozone could play a major role in the treatment of a wide variety of cancers and other health problems.

A Better Way to Say "No" to Drugs

The frightening rise in both addiction and adverse side effects from the growing plethora of prescription medications has become a major concern of physicians and health care consumers. The big pharmaceutical companies' close ties with the federal government (and $235,107,261 spent by the pharmaceutical/health products industry on lobbying in the United States during 2015 alone),[1] physicians on the payroll of drug companies, and unbridled advertising in medical journals, consumer magazines, television, radio, and the Internet have led us to use more medications to treat more and more health problems: "A pill for every ill and a potion for every emotion." Many people take a dozen different medications or more a day. Many consumers have little idea how these various drugs may interact with each other and often suffer from additional health problems as a result.

These concerns have led health care consumers to look for less expensive, more general, and more low-tech alternatives to medication such as herbal remedies, acupuncture, chiropractic, hydrotherapy, bodywork, and homeopathy. Because many of these modalities are not covered by health insurance, consumers often pay for these therapies out of their own pocket. Oxidative therapies have become a recognized part of these so-called alternative therapies, and they are being embraced by a growing number of health care consumers.

An Alternative to Fight Drug-Resistant Microbes

In addition to opening up possibilities for addiction and adverse side effects, many modern drugs (especially antibiotics) have not only become ineffective against drug-resistant bacteria and viruses but are actually helping create new strains of "superbugs" that don't respond to traditional medicines. Ozone and hydrogen peroxide can help fight these superbugs, because oxidation kills them indiscriminately. They also help the body's immune system fight disease better. That's why ozone, for example, has been found to be effective against such a wide variety of pathogens, including flu viruses, HIV, *E. coli,* MRSA, and anthrax.

It was mentioned before that the main reason why these therapies have not been used to their potential is that there is no financial incentive for physicians and pharmaceutical companies to implement them. In addition, many people adhere to old beliefs that ozone and hydrogen peroxide are toxic no matter how they are used. Despite these problems, some feel that therapeutic ozone and hydrogen peroxide are finally coming into their own. Long ignored and misunderstood, oxidative therapies are beginning to be viewed in a new and more promising light by both patients and physicians. Hopefully, this will lead to more serious study and eventual recognition by mainstream physicians and government health agencies around the world.

The Madrid Declaration on Ozone Therapy

The *Madrid Declaration on Ozone Therapy* is the first consensus document in the history of the global ozone therapy. It is considered to be the only ozone therapy document that is not only truly international in scope but also the most authoritative document of its type.

The initiative of the Declaration was launched with the primary intent of establishing safe and effective medical practices, determining scope of treatment, and introducing safe and effective ozone therapy protocols that are in accordance with the latest scientific research, while adapting to new medical developments and scientific findings. It should be studied by every practitioner of oxygen therapies.

The document was approved at the International Meeting of Schools of Ozone Therapy organized by AEPROMO (the Spanish Association of Medical Professionals in Ozone Therapy) at the Royal National Academy of Medicine in Madrid, which took place on June 3 and 4, 2010.

AEPROMO took the initiative to write the initial document, and the draft was submitted to the twenty-two participating speakers and teachers at the international meeting along with the presidents of the participating scientific associations. The road to achieve consensus was a long one: it took four months and involved a total of seventeen drafts before the Declaration was finally approved.

The result is a dense scientific document that is seventeen pages long. It includes a section on therapeutic ranges for the use of ozone, which is the summary of the scientific research and clinical practice of ozone therapy conducted in various countries around the world.

By 2015, a total of thirty-eight ozone therapy national associations and international federations of Africa, America, Asia, and Europe had signed the *Madrid Declaration on Ozone Therapy*, as has the International Medical Ozone Federation (IMEOF) and all of its fourteen member groups.

While the official versions of this document are in Spanish and English, the *Madrid Declaration on Ozone Therapy* can also be read in the following languages: Arabic, Finnish, German, Italian, Japanese, Portuguese, Romanian, Russian, and Turkish.

The *Madrid Declaration on Ozone Therapy* is considered the primary reference and working document of the International Scientific Committee of Ozone Therapy (ISCO3). This organization has taken on the responsibility to introduce modifications whenever necessary, with the goal to update and modify the Declaration as needed. To purchase the latest hard or digital copy of the Declaration, visit http://isco3.org.

THE CHALLENGES AHEAD

Although several developments in the field of oxygen therapy point to greater acceptance and wider utilization by the health care practitioners, there are still several major obstacles.

Oxygen Therapies as "Experimental": A Two-Edged Sword

A growing number of U.S. states and Canadian provinces allow practitioners to use ozone and hydrogen peroxide as experimental treatments. This has been good news for health care consumers, who demand freedom to choose the types of health care modalities they feel are best for them. Physicians who offered these therapies in the past were branded as criminals; this is no longer the case. Many pioneers in oxidative therapy have had their offices subjected to search, had their finances targeted by overzealous tax agents, had their telephones tapped, were thrown into jail on often bogus charges, or were otherwise harassed by the Federal Bureau of Investigation and other government agencies.

Rather than have to travel to Europe or Cuba, health care consumers can now seek out a physician closer to home. However, patients are often required to sign a paper agreeing that their treatment is "experimental," which basically absolves the physician of any responsibility if the treatment fails or causes additional health problems. The only exception is in cases of outright fraud or gross negligence.

This situation not only allows the state and provincial medical boards to avoid taking responsibility but permits unscrupulous or poorly trained practitioners to use oxidative therapies more as a way to make money than to actually cure patients. Since many individuals turn to oxidative therapies as a last resort after traditional therapies have failed them, they are more likely to become victimized.

Such was the case for several parents in Georgia who sent their autistic children to an oxidative physician who claimed to be a specialist in treating autism (he actually shared the same name as a world-renowned expert in the field). The doctor charged more than $40,000 to treat each of the children and was eventually sued for malpractice and fraud by the parents of one of them. He was placed on probation by the state medical board and eventually decided to retire.

It almost goes without saying that unethical conduct or any form of malpractice can do more harm to the future of oxidative therapies than anything that opponents of these therapies can inflict. Making false promises or otherwise misleading patients, overcharging for treatments, or having unqualified people administer therapy should never occur. Although mainstream medicine is not without its crooks and frauds, practitioners of oxidative therapies need to be especially diligent and maintain the highest standards of professional behavior. If not, the future of these therapies in North America is bleak indeed.

The Need for Oversight

We mentioned earlier that in Europe (especially Germany, Italy, Switzerland, Russia, and Poland) and in Cuba, oxidative therapies make up part of the medical mainstream. While regulations vary from country to country, physicians are offered graduate-level courses in oxidative therapy at an accredited institute. If they satisfy the requirements laid down by the government of a recognized professional organization (such as the Medical Society for the Use of Ozone in Prevention and Therapy in Germany, the Swiss Medical Society for Ozone and Oxygen Therapies, or the National Center for Scientific Research in Cuba), they become certified to practice. These organizations not only set standards for education and training but also provide valuable oversight of how these therapies are used. They also serve as centers for the exchange of information among practitioners and offer ongoing seminars in physician education.

In North America, such organizations simply did not exist. Dr. Charles H. Farr and others founded the International Bio-Oxidative Medical Foundation, which later became the International Oxidative Medicine Association (IOMA). The association's goals included practitioner education, setting professional standards, and exchanging information, but it became inactive after Dr. Farr's death. A handful of oxidative practitioners, including Frank Shallenberger, M.D., went to Germany to become certified in ozone therapy; others received certification from IOMA.

Founded in 2010 by Dr. Shallenberger, the American Academy of Ozonotherapy (AAO) is an organization of health professionals dedicated to establishing standards for the art and science of ozone therapy, educating the public and other health professionals about the many uses of ozone therapy in medicine, and promoting research in the field. The AAO is presently the only professional academy dedicated to ozone therapy in the United States. AAO is affiliated with the International Medical Ozone Federation and adheres to the standards endorsed by the IMEOF as described in the Madrid Declaration, mentioned above.

I've found that many people who are drawn to oxidative therapies are individualistic, eclectic, and opinionated. These qualities, though useful for engaging in a pioneering field like oxidative therapies, have kept members of the profession from achieving a unified sense of purpose. There needs to be more cooperation, less rivalry, and a greater sense of community among oxidative practitioners and their patients. They need to come to consensus on accepted procedures and agree to collectively explore new ones. Like health professionals in other fields, they must communicate with each other and share information. This is why a professional organization is so needed at this time.

Finding a Competent Healer

Books on oxygen therapies by authors such as Ed McCabe, William Campbell Douglass, or myself have inspired some practitioners to enter the field of oxidative therapies. Others may have read a more scientific book by Dr. Viebahn-Haensler or Dr. Bocci and may feel they are ready to practice oxidative therapy without going through the proper instruction and training. They may have taken a few weekend seminars and decided that they are ready to hang out a shingle as an oxidative therapist. While such seminars can be of tremendous value, they are no substitute for graduate-level training with specific criteria and professional evaluation. One of the few organizations in North America offering such training is the American Academy of Ozonotherapy. According to Den Rasplicka, the founder of Ozone Services (a Canadian manufacturer of ozone generators and related equipment):

> We strongly believe that Ozone Therapies belong in the hands of well-trained and educated LICENSED MEDICAL PROFESSIONALS with extensive formal medical training. Good training in Biochemistry is an essential part for understanding the biochemical actions and reactions triggered by ozone, and this knowledge directly contributes to overall understanding of utilization of Ozone as a therapeutic agent.[2]

The uneven (and sometimes minimal) training of oxidative practitioners is a major concern. Very often, readers ask to be referred to a good practitioner near their home, and I am frequently at a loss to do so. While there are lists of practitioners posted on various oxygen-related sites on the Internet, it is impossible to know if they are competent, honest, or even qualified to practice. Some have only minimal knowledge of human physiology and the biochemistry of ozone and hydrogen peroxide. Because there is no required certification of oxidative physicians in North America, it is difficult to know if a practitioner is knowledgeable or competent unless we can verify his or her training.

As with finding a good mainstream practitioner, word of mouth can be helpful. Patients can also ask how, when, and where a physician was trained. One good source for finding a well-trained oxidative practitioner is the American Academy of Ozonotherapy website (see appendix 2), which lists practitioners who have completed its rigorous Ozone Certification Course.

Universal standards of practitioner training and certification in North America have lagged far behind recent scientific discoveries. This situation must change if oxidative therapies are to achieve the respect in the scientific community that they deserve.

Always Safe?

In the four editions of this book, I've written about the relative safety of therapeutic ozone and hydrogen peroxide when used according to established medical protocols. Flooding the body with ozone, hydrogen peroxide, or even oxygen can bring about chronic oxidative stress. This can not only render the treatments ineffective but can actually depress immune system function. In some cases, repeated overdoses of ozone or hydrogen peroxide can lead to serious illness or even death. Yet unless it is determined that a person was exposed to a lethal amount of ozone in his or her air or is burned by drinking undiluted 35 percent hydrogen peroxide, ozone or hydrogen peroxide will not be directly linked to the final result.

A similar dynamic concerns AIDS; no one actually dies of AIDS. People die from an opportunistic infection like *Pneumocystis jiroveci* pneumonia, lymphoma, or a yeast infection or may suffer a heart attack or other problem. Their death certificate will say that they died of pneumonia or cancer, but not from AIDS.

By the same token, if a person receives excessive amounts of hydrogen peroxide or ozone, especially over the long term, any resulting health problem often cannot be directly traced to a botched or ineffective procedure. An embolism occurring after an intravenous injection of ozone is not directly caused by the ozone, but by oxygen. Illness, death, or incapacity due to chronic oxidative stress brought about by overdoses of ozone or hydrogen peroxide will probably never be traced directly to these therapies. Like deaths from overdoses or adverse interactions of prescribed medications, they are usually unrecognized, overlooked, or covered up.

This is why leaders in the field of oxidative therapies implore practitioners to carefully study human physiology and become experts in the biochemical properties of ozone and hydrogen peroxide. They are also told to adopt the most conservative protocols possible ("start low, go slow") when treating patients.

Exact Calibration

Another of the challenges facing oxidative therapists, especially those who use ozone, is the need to have carefully calibrated generators that produce precise amounts of ozone. Over time, many generators lose their ability to produce correct amounts of ozone; they may produce too little or too much, no matter what level of concentration is set on the dial. According to Den Rasplicka, "Therapeutic ozone levels frequently used in a medical office can be easily 100,000 to 500,000 times higher than ozone levels we can find in nature even under the most favorable 'ozone producing' conditions."[3]

This doesn't mean that you have to buy a generator from Ozone Services (although Ozone Services does calibrate ozone generators, including those manufactured by other companies), but it highlights the need for every medical office to have good monitoring equipment to ensure that exact ozone dosages are produced. In addition, every generator should be equipped with an aspirator and ozone destructor unit, as well as an ozone analyzer that has warning lights and a sound alarm to alert the practitioner if contamination occurs.

Double Blind, Double Bind

The introduction to part 2 addressed both the benefits and the difficulties of double-blind testing. While I personally feel that double-blind studies can be useful, they are both complicated and expensive to perform.

Critics of oxidative therapies in the medical and scientific communities complain that few double-blind studies have been done with oxidative therapies, but it is almost impossible for oxidative researchers to obtain funding from the government, universities, or private foundations, let alone pharmaceutical companies who will never profit from them. As a result, researchers often must pay for the studies out of their own pockets, which is almost never the case with mainstream medical research.

I am continually amazed that oxidative therapies have made up part of the medical mainstream in many European countries and in Cuba for many years, yet they are still viewed as experimental in North America. The medical literature is replete with responsible and well-researched articles that testify to the safety and effectiveness of these therapies in a wide range of medical applications. Government funding is essential, and it's time to demand it.

The fact that these therapies have not been objectively studied and evaluated—let alone approved—by the U.S. Food and Drug Administration (FDA) is a slap in the face to health care consumers who need access to inexpensive, safe, and effective methods to prevent disease and improve their health. To continually neglect a promising healing modality—especially one that is accepted in other countries and already used on millions of patients—is nothing short of criminal.

Over the years, the government has responded to demands for change, albeit reluctantly. Pressure from consumers has finally brought about new FDA dietary recommendations and has made non-Western modalities like acupuncture legally accepted in the United States. Can pressure from health care consumers who demand FDA evaluation and approval of oxidative therapies produce similar results?

APPENDIX 1

Oxygen Products, Services, and Applications

This appendix will explore some of the growing variety of products, services, and applications related to oxygen therapy that have become available to the general public over the past few years. The intent is not to promote or endorse any particular products or applications but to explore their uses and value to the consumer.

OZONE GENERATORS

It was mentioned before that ozone is artificially produced by passing an electrical charge through a specially built condenser containing oxygen. There are a number of different types of ozone generators available commercially as either portable or medical office models (see figure A.1):

Ultraviolet (UV) ozone generators are less expensive than other types; however, the need to change the UV bulb approximately every 10,000 hours can drive up the cost of the equipment over time. Output of ozone is low and is not constant due to deterioration of the UV bulb. The regulation of ozone production is only possible by airflow.

When nitrogen in the air (air is made up of approximately 80 percent nitrogen) is exposed to a high-voltage discharge (including that made by most ozone generators), it will react with oxygen and form small amounts of NOx, or nitrogen oxides, a group of nitrogen and oxygen chemical compounds, including nitrous oxide (N_2O) and nitric oxide (NO). From this group of chemical compounds, we also find the highly toxic nitrogen dioxide NO_2, which is derived by oxidation of nitric oxide. This gas is highly toxic to the lungs and is used in the production of nitric acid.

However, when ozone is created from pure oxygen and discharged into the air, it does not react with nitrogen. Ultraviolet systems with a wavelength of 194 nm and shorter will produce ozone but no NOx, even if air (as opposed to pure oxygen) is used as the feed gas.

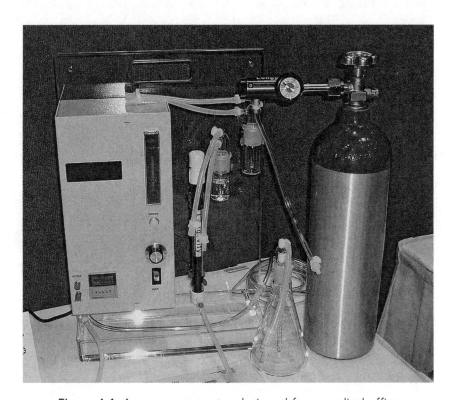

Figure A.1. An ozone generator designed for a medical office.
(Photograph by Nathaniel Altman.)

Cold plasma machines represent the middle range in both cost and ozone output. They do not require replacement of the ozone-producing cell, and their ozone output can be maintained at a constant level. The regulation of ozone production is only possible by airflow. However, when air is used as a feed gas, it can produce NOx.

Corona discharge generators cost more than the other systems and provide the highest output of ozone. Output is constant and one does not need to periodically replace the cell. Ozone production can be regulated by airflow and/or by changing the high-voltage discharge (voltage or frequency). Like the cold plasma machines, corona discharge generators will produce NOx when air is used as feed gas.

Corona discharge generators are also referred to as "hot spark"–type ozone generators. However, with the availability of high-quality dielectric materials and semiconductors, properly designed corona discharge generators produce far less heat than their ancestors. Over the past few years, they have become popular for a wide variety of applications due to their high ozone output and the possibility to regulate ozone output independently from airflow.

The quality of ozone generators varies considerably. For this reason, the *Madrid Declaration on Ozone Therapy* and individual organizations like the American Academy of Ozonotherapy (AAO) have published guidelines for the selection and use of ozone generators. The AAO recommends:

- All ozone generators for human or animal (in office or at home) use must bear a safety approval sticker such as ETL, CSA, UL, or QAI.
- No generator for human or animal use (in office or at home) must be constructed of any substances that come into contact with ozone other than quartz glass, Kynar, Teflon, or silicone. This includes all other materials such as ceramic, other plastics, aluminum, and steel.

The AAO has also published guidelines concerning components of ozone generators used for medicine, dentistry, and scientific research. They were divided into "necessary," "recommendable," and "optional." The necessary guidelines include:

1. High-quality solid state electronics with high voltage protection against spikes in power lines

2. The use of a double-walled quartz electrode to ensure consistency of ozone output concentrations

3. All materials in contact with the ozone gas must be 100 percent ozone resistant

4. Certification by an independent testing body [such as CE, ETL, CSA, UL, QAI, TUV] for electrical quality, fire safety and proof of professional manufacturing

5. The ozone generator must use purified oxygen as the feed gas. (The AAO specifies generators that were originally designed to use purified oxygen rather than those that were altered after manufacture)

6. A full range of ozone output concentrations must be available

7. A safe method of destroying "offgassing" ozone must be provided[1]

AIR PURIFIERS

Many people have become interested in commercial air purifiers that generate ozone. Manufacturers often claim that these ozone generators provide additional oxygen for breathing while killing bacteria, fungi, molds, yeasts, and dust mites. They are also supposed to remove harmful contaminants from the air, such as cigarette smoke and other airborne toxins.

The use of these machines is controversial. Many scientists believe that inhaling ozone in any amount is harmful to one's health, although there is some question regarding what constitutes a harmful concentration. As mentioned earlier, Russian physicians have introduced therapeutic ozone into the lungs of critically ill patients without adverse reactions. Many lay advocates of oxidative therapies believe that using ozone generators to purify the air is both safe and effective. One such machine was used to purify the air in the exhibition area at a conference on oxidative therapies I attended several years ago.

There are a number of points to consider when using an air purifier that generates ozone. Den Rasplicka, an engineer and the founder of Ozone Services (see appendix 2), points out that electronic equipment, such as computers, television sets, CD players, and VCRs, is sensitive to ozone. Ozone can enter air vents or cooling ducts and may damage delicate components. In addition, some components have printed circuit boards that lack a solder mask, which is a protective layer over the traces on the board. These traces can suffer from oxidation caused by ozone. Ozone can also oxidize drive belts in CD players, because these belts are made with rubber or latex and oxidize easily.

Rasplicka also advises that there are two ways to deal with household odors with ozone. The air alone can be treated with very low levels of ozone, or one can treat the source of the odor with heavy, prolonged periods of ozonation. When the second option is chosen, the area to be ozonated should be carefully prepared before treatment; sensitive electronic components like television sets, VCRs, CD players, and computers—as well as paintings and plants—should be removed before treating the room.

Some people are very sensitive to even small amounts of nitrogen dioxide (NO_2). In general, healthy people will not have any problems with an air purifier in the room. However, Rasplicka notes that people who are sick (or those with severely depressed immune systems) are sensitive to it. The two major symptoms that show that one is sensitive to NO_2 are sudden, severe headache and dizziness. Individuals who are sensitive to even extremely low concentrations of nitrogen dioxide will not be able to be present when the air purification unit is running. For these people, rooms treated by ozone air purifiers will have to be unoccupied and properly ventilated after treatment. The benefit of the treatment is not so much that the ambient air is purified with ozone but that the walls, ceilings, carpeting, bedding, and upholstery (which serve as a breeding ground for airborne bacteria, noxious gases, dust mite feces, mildew, mold, and other allergens and irritants) are purified.[2]

Although properly designed air purifiers will emit safe amounts of ozone, it is important to be aware of ozone levels in the ambient air in parts per million (ppm). A concentration of 0.001 to 0.12 ppm is typically found in the natural atmosphere. These levels of concentration vary with altitude, atmospheric conditions, and locale; 0.070 ppm is the level of the primary and secondary air quality standards set by the U.S. Environmental Protection Agency in 2015.[3] A limit of 0.040 ppm is said to be the maximum set by the Canadian Standards Association for devices designed for household use, while 0.050 ppm is the maximum allowable ozone concentration recommended by the American Society of Heating, Refrigerating and Air Conditioning Engineers in an air-conditioned and ventilated space. As of 2016, the U.S. Food and Drug Administration set a maximum output level of 0.05 ppm for indoor ozone generators.[4]

Ozone levels can be monitored. There is a new generation of ozone air purifiers that have a built-in ozone level sensor to help determine the amount of ozone in the air. However, an alternative low-cost option for monitoring or assessing ambient ozone levels present is ozone test strips, which are used in the same way as standard pH test strips. More sophisticated ozone testers, monitors, and controllers are also available but are often expensive.

Although more research needs to be done in studying ozone generation and air purification, a growing number of hospitals, hotels, restaurants, and offices are moving toward ozone, even to the extent of installing large permanent ozone generation systems in their buildings. A 1996 article in the *New Hampshire Business Review* described the benefits of purifying air with ozone:

Ozone is a fast-acting cleaning and oxidizing agent. Ozone eliminates office odors by chemically neutralizing them, not covering them up with another, albeit more pleasant, smell. Ozone helps rid the air of many common causes of inhaled allergies, and it kills mold, mildew, spores and pollen. Ozone also kills bacteria and many viruses and airborne diseases. This makes your office a healthier and more pleasant workplace and helps eliminate sick building syndrome.[5]

OZONATED WATER

Ozonation is an important method of purifying water used by thousands of municipalities around the world to remove impurities and pathogens from drinking water. A growing number of individuals have decided to ozonate their own drinking water for both disinfection and therapeutic reasons. While drinking ozonated water is a good idea, such applications require specific concentrations of ozone. In addition, ozonated water has a definite "shelf life," after which it will lose its therapeutic value.

Scientists view ozone application in water in terms of oxygen reduction potential (ORP), which is measured in mV (millivolts of DC). The following chart offers a general idea of levels of ORP needed for different ozone applications:

200–400 ORP: Cooling towers and aquaculture
400–600 ORP: Hot tubs, swimming pools, general water treatment applications
600–800 ORP: Water disinfection
800 ORP and up: Water sterilization
900 ORP and up: Water with residual ozone levels able to deliver a therapeutic effect[6]

Ozone tends to decompose in water over time. The shelf life of ozonated water depends not only on elapsed time after ozonation but on the type of container in which it is stored. Figure A.2 (on page 428) shows the shelf life of ozonated water in three types of containers: a 1,500 ml glass chamber that is 2.5 inches in diameter and 23 feet high; a 1,000 ml glass container 4 inches in diameter and 6 inches high; and a 1,000 ml plastic container 4 inches in diameter and 6 inches high. These figures were determined through laboratory analysis by Den Rasplicka of Ozone Services and were kindly provided by him.

Ozonated Water for Swimming Pools and Hot Tubs

Many companies install ozone equipment for swimming pools and hot tubs instead of using large amounts of chlorine, which has been linked to cancer and is harmful to the environment. Ozone is readily absorbed in water, can have therapeutic value to those who use the pool or spa, and is environmentally friendly. In addition, ozone is more efficient at neutralizing bacteria, fungi, parasites, toxic chemicals, and other water-borne contaminants: while chlorine slowly seeps into the cell wall of the contaminants, ozone ruptures the cell wall and shatters the molecular bonds of the complex chains of the contaminants, destroying them quickly and completely. In addition, less chemical exposure to spa or pool equipment can result in less maintenance, and the need for bromine floaters, chlorine, water clarifiers, and other chemicals is virtually eliminated.

There are few downsides to using ozone purification systems. Some have reported that water bugs and frogs, who rarely appear in chlorinated water, are attracted to pools and hot tubs cleaned by ozone. While a minor nuisance, it makes one realize that chlorine and other chemicals in the water create an environment that is not amenable to living beings. In addition, ozone in standard dosages for swimming pools (400–475 ORP) does not kill algae, although a dose higher than 500 ORP will.

Not all pool or hot tub filtering systems are designed to work with ozone gas purification; a knowledgeable spa contractor can determine how your system can be reconfigured, if necessary. As with any water purification system, make sure that you purchase ozone generators for pool or spa use from a reputable dealer who has extensive experience with ozone purification systems.

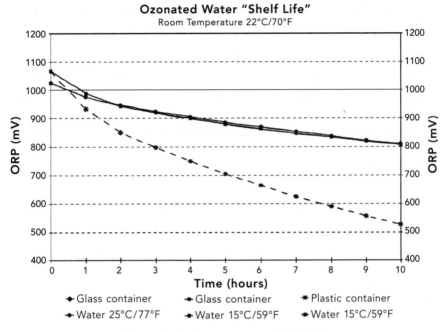

Figure A.2. Ozonated water shelf life.
(Reprinted courtesy of Ozone Services.)

What about hydrogen peroxide in pools and hot tubs? While utilizing 35 percent hydrogen peroxide in a swimming pool on a regular basis can be expensive, adding food-grade hydrogen peroxide to the water in a hot tub is both safe and practical. Den Rasplicka recommends that concentrations of 35 percent hydrogen peroxide should be 50 to 80 ppm concentration. Food-grade hydrogen peroxide is available in gallon (and larger) containers from dozens of sources, including vendors of agricultural supplies. Test strips to measure hydrogen peroxide concentrations are available commercially as well.

THE OXYGEN BAR

Another development has been the appearance of the "oxygen bar." The first one in North America (the O₂ Spa Bar) opened in Toronto, Canada, in 1996,[6] and others are sprouting up in trendy neighborhoods in many other cities, including Vancouver, New York, Los Angeles, and Detroit. Modeled in part after the "air stations" located in polluted downtown areas of Tokyo and Beijing, where oxygen is dispensed to beleaguered clients through a vending machine, oxygen bars offer a relaxing environment with comfortable seating, soft music, and healthy refreshments.

In addition to offering respite from the physical and psychological stresses of city life, these spas offer clients supplemental oxygen (in the form of 99.9 percent pure medical-grade oxygen) administered through the nostrils for about 20 to 30 minutes. While receiving their spa treatment, clients may listen to music, read, or watch a video with a cup of herbal tea. Proponents of supplemental oxygen point out that it is used therapeutically to treat more than a dozen health complaints, including migraines and cluster headaches. They also mention that supplemental oxygen can be beneficial to healthy people as well.

As can be expected, skeptics abound. They point out that there is no clinical evidence that supplemental oxygen is of value to healthy people and that overuse can be hazardous to health. However, the owners of oxygen bars generally make no therapeutic claims for oxygen, so that they can avoid being accused of practicing medicine without a license. The basic pitch is one of comfort and renewal. According to a publicity notice for an oxygen bar in New York City:

> Now imagine yourself sitting on a soft leather reclining chair in a beautiful cozy room with a couple of friends, listening to relaxing music, breathing pure, cool oxygen from a small, comfortable plastic tube under your nose. After a short time, when finished, most will walk out feeling relaxed, rested, awake and refreshed, ready to go out to the gym or to party. They've improved their health and leave feeling great.[8]

OXYGENATED BOTTLED WATERS

Commercial oxygenated water producers claim that their beverage, with approximately seven times more oxygen than is found in ordinary water, provides increased endurance, improved athletic performance, and an overall energy boost. Using patented technology, extra oxygen (approximately 70 milligrams per liter) is added to ordinary purified water. The reputed energy boost is due to the increased amount of oxygen in the blood.

As is the case for oxygen spas, skeptics find claims about oxygenated water hard to swallow. They question whether the intestine is able to absorb extra oxygen from oxygen-enriched water; proponents of oxygenated water claim that the patented process facilitates oxygen absorption through the colon. I have tried oxygenated water (marketed under the label O_2 Water) and found it both thirst-quenching and better-tasting than other types of bottled water. Despite the manufacturer's claims that athletes have improved their performance after drinking this water, I did not experience the promised extra boost of energy after drinking it.

OXYGENATION PRODUCTS

A growing number of oxidative and oxygenation products, including oxygen-saturated skin creams, stabilized oxygen dietary supplements, skin sprays, and colon cleansers, are becoming available to the general public through mail-order companies and health food stores. Some of the most popular have been marketed as food supplements and have gone by trademarked names like Cellfood, Liquid Life, Oxygen for Life, Chelo Zone, Oxy-Gen, Colo Zone, OxyBliss, OxyCleanse, Bioxy Cleanse, Oxy Aloe, SuperOxy, Homozone, and OxyToddy. Some have been promoted by writers and lecturers on oxygen therapies, who receive a commission on sales.* Some of the products claim to contain small amounts of hydrogen peroxide but are far more palatable than drops of food-grade hydrogen peroxide in a glass of water. Many users have reported that these products provide added energy and have helped

---

*I am not, and have never been, affiliated with any company that manufactures or sells these products, nor have I ever sold any such products through articles, advertisements, or public presentations.

them maintain good health; some even claim that these products have helped them overcome disease when traditional allopathic medications had failed them.

Even within the oxygen therapy community, these products have their critics. They point out that many commercial oxidative and oxygenation products are expensive and are sold through high-pressure multilevel marketing techniques, where a person sells the product to a customer and then contracts the customer to sell the product to others at a commission. In addition to commissions on direct sales, the original seller (now a distributor) earns a commission on sales made by the customers he or she recruits. While such marketing methods are not illegal, the quest for high commissions can lead to high-pressure sales tactics and exaggerated health claims. Many of these products are hyped to be the "latest" and the "best," only to disappear into oblivion soon afterward.

With the possible exceptions of ozonated oil, 35 percent food-grade hydrogen peroxide (diluted in water and taken internally or added to bathwater), Heritage's Oxy Aloe, and Dr. Donsbach's SuperOxy and Oxy-Gen products (which are made with magnesium peroxide), most products focus on increasing *oxygenation* as opposed to *oxidation*. Some skeptics point out that a session of deep yogic breathing or a five-minute aerobic workout would oxygenate the body more efficiently (and at lower cost) than the use of commercial oxygenation products.

Another criticism regarding these products is that they have not undergone rigorous laboratory and clinical trials to verify their safety and effectiveness. This is a valid concern that also applies to the plethora of vitamins, mineral supplements, and herbal preparations that have flooded the health care marketplace. This does not mean that these products are neither safe nor effective; indeed, some of them have been available for years and many people swear by them. However, until objective laboratory and clinical evidence is made available to the consumer, perhaps the best yardstick is to carefully examine health claims with common sense. In addition, consider using a product through recommendation of people you trust who have already tried it and who hopefully do not have a financial stake in the product.

HYDROGEN PEROXIDE IN THE KITCHEN AND GARDEN

It was mentioned earlier that 35 percent hydrogen peroxide diluted in water can be used for bathing and as a skin spray. Many have discovered that it can also be helpful in both the kitchen and the garden. The following practical suggestions have been gleaned from a variety of sources.

To make 12 ounces of 3 percent hydrogen peroxide solution using 35 percent food-grade hydrogen peroxide, mix 1 ounce of 35 percent hydrogen peroxide into 11 ounces of distilled water. If you spill food-grade hydrogen peroxide on your skin, rinse immediately with warm water and avoid contact with the eyes. When you store hydrogen peroxide in the refrigerator, clearly mark the container so you do not mistake it for water.

To clean vegetables and fruit, add 4 ounces of your 3 percent hydrogen peroxide mixture to a sink filled with cold water. Wash the vegetables thoroughly, rinse, and drain. Either consume the vegetables immediately or pat them dry and store them in the refrigerator. Another method involves spraying the fruits and vegetables with the 3 percent mixture of hydrogen peroxide. Rinse with cold water and drain. This process is said to prolong freshness.

To wash dishes in an automatic dishwasher, add 2 ounces of 3 percent hydrogen peroxide to your regular washing formula. You can also keep a spray bottle of your hydrogen peroxide solution in the kitchen to be sprayed on countertops and appliances. It will disinfect surfaces and will also give the kitchen a clean, fresh smell. This process can also be used to freshen the refrigerator and children's lunch boxes.

Some farmers are reported to have used hydrogen peroxide on their crops. To foliar-feed crops, add 16 ounces of 35 percent hydrogen peroxide to 20 gallons of water. Spray on plants early in the morning, while the plant pores are open. This should be enough to spray 1 acre of crops.

To facilitate seed germination, add 1 ounce of 3 percent hydrogen peroxide to a pint of distilled water. Soak the seeds for 8 hours. This method is reputed to increase the rate of seed germination by 30 percent.

To make a plant insecticide, mix 8 ounces or more of 3 percent hydrogen peroxide with 1 gallon of water and 8 ounces of molasses or white sugar. It has been found that blackstrap molasses works better than sugar. It seems to allow the mixture to better adhere to the plant.

To increase the growth of plants, add 1 ounce of 3 percent hydrogen peroxide to a quart of water (or add 16 drops of 35 percent hydrogen peroxide to a quart of water). Water or mist plants with this solution. Good results can even be obtained from adding just a tablespoonful of 3 percent hydrogen peroxide to a gallon of water. Farmers are also watering the ground around fruit trees with a solution made by adding 6 to 8 ounces of 3 percent hydrogen peroxide to a gallon of water; this can also be used as a spray. To increase the longevity of cut flowers, add a few drops of 3 percent hydrogen peroxide per cup of water to the vase.

Tropical fish enthusiasts have found that adding a maximum of 1 ounce of 35 percent food-grade hydrogen peroxide to 20 gallons of water will help disinfect the aquarium water and reduce fungal growth on fish.

APPENDIX 2

Resources

The field of oxidative therapies is an ever-changing one. In the past few years there has been an amazing growth of websites that offer oxygen therapy–related products like ozone generators, food-grade hydrogen peroxide, oxygen supplements, books, and periodicals. Here is a short list (which is by no means comprehensive) of these resources. I have listed the entries in each category (except for books, which are listed alphabetically) starting with the entries I have personally found most helpful.

DATABASES

The Oxygen Prescription

www.oxygenprescription.com

The author's official website for this book. Includes basic information, news, articles, and links related to *The New Oxygen Prescription* and oxygen therapies in general.

Oxygen Healing Therapies

www.oxygenhealingtherapies.com

A website containing information about different aspects of oxygen therapies, including Frank Shallenberger's course schedule and a list of practitioners who have attended his seminars. Note: This site is not affiliated with Nathaniel Altman or the book *Oxygen Healing Therapies*.

The International Scientific Committee of Ozone Therapy (ISCO3)

www.zotero.org/groups/isco3_ozone

The ISCO3 maintains an online library of all medical and scientific articles about ozone therapy published throughout the world. See its listing on page 435.

ORGANIZATIONS

International Medical Ozone Federation (IMEOF)

http://imeof.org

The IMEOF is an international organization of ozone researchers and health professionals, with national affiliates around the world. Holds conferences, publishes articles and books, and makes the *Madrid Declaration on Ozone Therapy* available to the public.

The International Scientific Committee of Ozone Therapy (ISCO3)

www.isco3.org

The ISCO3 is an independent board of researchers and practitioners from national and international associations or federations of ozone therapy, as well as representatives of companies that manufacture ozone generators and equipment. The ISCO3 publishes the *Madrid Declaration of Ozone Therapy,* containing information about the scientific basis and therapeutic applications of ozone as well as protocols for administering ozone therapy. The ISCO3 also publishes scientific documents related to ozone therapy and organizes conferences for professionals.

American Academy of Ozonotherapy (AAO)

http://aaot.us

Founded in 2010, the AAO is an organization of health professionals dedicated to establishing standards for the art and science of ozone therapy, educating the public and other health professionals about its many uses in medicine, and promoting research. The AAO sponsors practitioner training and certification, coordinates research projects, and holds annual meetings. It offers a listing of ozone practitioners in the United States and abroad through its website. The AAO is the only professional academy dedicated to ozone therapy in the United States.

International Ozone Association (IOA)

IOA Pan American Group (PAG)

www.ioa-pag.org/

c/o Southern Nevada Water Authority

PO Box 97075

Las Vegas, NV 89193

Tel: (480) 529-3787

Fax: (480) 533-3080

European African Asian Australian Group
www.ioa-ea3g.org

Nippon Islands Group (Japan)
www.j-ozone.org

Founded in 1973, the IOA is a nonprofit educational and scientific organization dedicated to the collection and dissemination of information on, and the promotion of research in, any and all aspects of ozone and related oxygen species technologies. The IOA sponsors seminars and international conferences on medical ozone.

European Cooperation of Medical Ozone Societies

www.ozone-association.com
An umbrella organization made up of the Austrian Mutual Interest Association of Ozone/Oxygen Therapists (Interessengemeinschaft der Ozon-Sauerstofftherapeuten), the Swiss Medical Society for Ozone and Oxygen Therapy Methods (Schweizerische Ärztegesellschaft für Ozon- und Sauerstofftherapien), the German Medical Society for Ozone Application in Prevention and Therapy (Ärztliche Gesellschaft für Ozonanwendung in Prävention und Therapie), and the new International Federation of Oxygen-Ozone Therapy, which includes Italy, Turkey, China, and India. Its goal is to develop and adopt universally accepted protocols for treatment as well as a European standard qualification for practitioners. Member organizations sponsor practitioner training, congresses, and seminars.

American Holistic Veterinary Medical Association

PO Box 630
Abingdon, MD 21009
USA
(410) 569-0795
www.ahvma.org
A professional organization devoted to promoting integrative veterinary medicine, including oxidative therapies. Publishes a peer-reviewed online journal.

Keep Hope Alive

PO Box 270041
West Allis, WI 53227
USA
www.keephopealive.org
An organization offering strategies related to diet, ozone, and other natural

therapies for those dealing with HIV and other immune disorders. The organization publishes occasional newsletters and the *Immune Restoration Handbook*. It has also assembled a collection of articles about medical ozone taken from medical journals, which is available for purchase.

Physicians Committee for Responsible Medicine
5100 Wisconsin Ave. NW, Ste. 400
Washington, DC 20016
USA
www.pcrm.org
While not involved with oxidative therapies, this group promotes preventive health strategies, higher standards for ethics and effectiveness in research, and alternatives to animal research. Publishes *Good Medicine*.

The Ann Wigmore Foundation
PO Box 399
San Fidel, NM 87049
USA
www.wigmore.org

Ann Wigmore Natural Health Institute
PO Box 429
Rincon, Puerto Rico 00677
www.annwigmore.org

Ann Wigmore was a major proponent of a natural lifestyle using raw foods and living foods (such as sprouts and wheatgrass) for maintaining and recovering good health. She worked with many patients with cancer, heart disease, and AIDS, often with impressive results. A number of oxidative practitioners have recommended her program for people undergoing therapy with ozone and hydrogen peroxide. Both the foundation and the institute teach people how to use living foods.

MANUFACTURERS AND DISTRIBUTORS OF OZONE GENERATORS AND SUPPLIES

There are dozens of companies that manufacture and distribute ozone generators and related equipment. Most can be found on the Internet. Some of these companies are listed in this section.

North America
Ozone Services
390 Silver Queen Road
Burton, BC V0G 1E0
Canada

(250) 265-4461

www.ozoneservices.com • www.ozonelab.com

Manufactures and distributes ozone generators, steam cabinets, shower equipment, ozonated oil, and supplies for water purification and medical use. Provides high-level training for ozone practitioners through the Ozone Therapy Training Program; website contains articles about ozone and other information.

Ven-Mar Scientific, Inc.

PO Box 974

Hempstead, TX 77445

USA

(979) 826-3863

Ven-Mar manufactures and distributes ozone generators and related equipment; sponsors educational seminars.

Longevity Resources

(877) 543-3398 • (250) 654-0092

www.ozonegenerator.com • info@ozonegenerator.com

Manufacturer and distributor of ozone generators, steam cabinets, pool ozonation systems, and air and water purifiers.

BiOzone Corporation

11026 East Crestline Circle

Englewood, CO 80111

USA

(303) 770-2095

www.biozone.com

Specializes in industrial and agricultural ozone generators.

Plasmafire

(604) 532-9596

www.plasmafire.com

Manufactures and distributes ozone generators, steam cabinets, and ozone supplies for water purification and medical use.

Ozone Safe Food Technologies, Inc.

951-228-2151

www.ozonesafefood.com

Manufacturer of the patented Ozone Safe Food MAC system for food process-ing and equipment sanitation.

Other Countries

Dr. J. Hänsler GmbH

Nordring 8
D-76473 Iffezheim
Germany
(49) 0-7229 3046-0
www.ozonosan.de
Founded by ozone pioneer Dr. Joaquim Hänsler, this is the world's oldest maker of medical ozone generators. Manufactures and distributes Ozonosan-brand generators for medical applications and water purification. Considered the "gold standard" in Europe, Ozonosan is used extensively in scientific research.

Kastner Praxisbedarf GmbH

Berliner Ring 40
D-76437 Rastatt
Germany
(49) 0-7222-53005
www.kastner-gmbh.de
Manufactures and distributes Ozomed ozone generators for medical applica-tions and water purification.

Sedecal

Medical Ozone Division
www.sedecal.com
Sedecal is a major designer and manufacturer of high-frequency X-ray genera-tors, X-ray systems, industrial power control and renewable energies, printed circuit boards, electronic systems, and electromechanical systems as well as high-quality medical ozone generators. The company is based in Spain and has sales offices in a number of countries, including the United States.

Medozons

Ul. B. Panina, 9
603089 Nizhni Novgorod
Russia
(7) 8312-167067, 383003

www.medozons.com

Russia's premier manufacturer of ozone generators and equipment. Sponsors educational programs; website includes scientific papers and instructional material.

Multiossigen Srl
Via Roma 26
24020 Gorle (Bg)
Italy
(39) 35 299573
www.multiossigen.com

Manufacturer and distributor of ozone generators and supplies; offers training programs for practitioners.

Wilhelm Schmidding & Co. GmbH
Emdener Strasse 10
50735 Cologne
Germany
(49) 0-221 717401

Manufactures industrial ozone equipment.

Ozonia International
North American Office
600 Willow Tree Road
Leonia, NJ 07605
USA
(201) 676-2525
www.ozonia.com

International Offices
Based in France, this manufacturer and distributor of industrial ozone equipment and UV technology has offices in Great Britain, Russia, Switzerland, North America, China, Japan, and South Korea. From the website, click on "Contacts" for international addresses.

PUBLICATIONS

Madrid Declaration on Ozone Therapy
International Scientific Committee of Ozone Therapy
www.isco3.org

Revised and updated periodically, this landmark publication contains the latest and most authoritative information about the scientific basis and therapeutic applications of ozone. It also includes detailed protocols for administering ozone therapy for practitioners. Available in many languages, the *Madrid Declaration on Ozone Therapy* can be purchased in either digital or hard copy form from the ISCO3 website.

Family Health News
9845 N.E. 2nd Ave.
Miami Shores, FL 33138
USA
(800) 284-6263 ● (305) 759-9500
www.familyhealthnews.com
Founded in 1989 by John Taggart, *Family Health News* is a tabloid newspaper/mail-order catalog devoted to oxidative therapies and related products. Articles on oxygen therapies, health, and nutrition can be found on the website.

VIDEOS

Ozone and the Politics of Medicine
Ozone: A Medical Breakthrough?
Geoffrey Rogers/Threshold Films
Professionally done, provocative documentaries on how government health agencies and traditional medicine view ozone in the treatment of AIDS and other diseases. Available from *Family Health News*.

BOOKS

On Oxygen Therapies
Bocci, Velio. *Oxygen-Ozone Therapy: A Critical Evaluation.* New York: Kluwer Academic Publishers, 2002.
> An exhaustive (and breakthrough) treatise on all aspects of ozone therapy written primarily for clinical researchers, physicians, and ozone therapists by the world's leading authority on oxidative medicine. Includes protocols and clinical guidance.

Bocci, Velio. *Ozone: A New Medical Drug.* New York: Springer, 2005.
> A somewhat simplified version of his previous book, better understood by lay readers with a solid scientific background. Includes protocols and clinical guidance.

Douglass, William Campbell. *Hydrogen Peroxide: Medical Miracle.* Atlanta, Ga.: Second Opinion Publishing, 1994.

A small book describing the original work with hydrogen peroxide by Drs. Farr, Douglas, and others. Many patient testimonials and case histories.

Menéndez, Silvia, and Mark T. Weiser. *Advances of Ozone Therapy in Medicine and Dentistry.* Havana: Editorial CENIC, 2016.

An updated and expanded English language edition of Dr. Menéndez's acclaimed book *Ozono: Aspectos básicos y aplicaciones clínicas.* Written primarily for physicians.

Neubauer, Richard A., and Morton Walker. *Hyperbaric Oxygen Therapy.* New York: Avery Publishing Group, 1998.

A comprehensive and definitive book about HBO and how it can be used to treat a wide variety of health conditions.

Reillo, Michelle. *AIDS under Pressure.* Cambridge, Mass.: Hogrefe & Huber Publishers, 1998.

A well-researched book documenting the success of HBO therapy in the clinical management of many HIV-related health problems.

Shallenberger, Frank. *The Principles and Applications of Ozone Therapy: A Practical Guideline for Physicians.* CreateSpace Independent Publishing Platform, 2011.

A small book exploring the theory and practical applications of ozone therapy written by America's most prominent ozone practitioner. Written primarily for health care providers.

Viebahn-Haensler, Renate. *The Use of Ozone in Medicine.* 4th English edition. Iffezheim, Germany: ODREI-Publishers, 2002.

A classic text by one of the world's most respected practitioners. Includes protocols and clinical guidance. New editions are published every few years.

On Holistic Health and Complementary Therapies (Including Diet)

Angelo, Jack. *Self-Healing with Breathing.* Rochester, Vt.: Healing Arts Press, 2012.

How the power of breathing can increase energy and help us achieve optimal wellness. Includes conscious breathing and visualization exercises.

Ballentine, Rudolph. *Radical Healing: Integrating the World's Great Therapeutic Traditions to Create a New Transformative Medicine.* New York: Three Rivers Press, 2000.

A well-researched book introducing the principles of holistic healing. The author presents an integrated system combining the awareness, tools, and practices taught by a variety of healing disciplines, including ayurveda, homeopathy, and herbal medicine. Written by the director of the Center for Holistic Medicine in New York City and the author of the classic book Diet and Nutrition.

Bohan, Suzanne, and Glenn Thompson. *50 Simple Ways to Live a Longer Life: Everyday Techniques from the Forefront of Science.* Naperville, Ill.: Sourcebooks, 2005.

An easy-to-read guide to a healthier life, covering both common illnesses and lifestyle issues. Well researched.

Dethlefsen, Thorwald, and Rüdiger Dahlke. *The Healing Power of Illness: Understanding What Your Symptoms Are Telling You.* London: Vega Books, 2002.

A provocative book on the inner meaning of disease symptoms and their psychological interpretations.

Epstein, Donald M. *Healing Myths, Healing Magic.* San Rafael, Calif.: Amber-Allen Publishing, 2000.

A revolutionary book. The author divides healing myths into four categories: social, biomedical, religious/spiritual, and new age. He discusses each myth individually—from "healing is expensive" to "every condition can be traced to a demonstrable physical cause." He then offers "healing magic" that the reader can meditate upon and declare out loud in order to open the door to healing.

Epstein, Donald M., with Nathaniel Altman. *The Twelve Stages of Healing.* San Rafael, Calif.: Amber-Allen Publishing, 1994.

A powerful self-help guide for achieving healing and personal transformation by traveling along the Twelve Stages of the healing process.

Gray, Robert. *The Colon Health Handbook.* Oakland, Calif.: Rockridge Publishing, 1982.

A booklet about colon cleansing and intestinal health.

Gregory, Scott J. *A Holistic Protocol for the Immune System*. Joshua Tree, Calif.: Tree of Life Publications, 1995.

A comprehensive manual for patients with HIV, AIDS-related complex, or AIDS, including advice on how to deal with opportunistic infections through natural means.

Harrison, John. *Love Your Disease*. Carlsbad, Calif.: Hay House, 1989.

A powerful book by a medical doctor that discusses the psychological basis for disease, including information on why people decide to become ill, what we do to prevent recovery, and how self-healing can take place.

Hay, Louise. *The AIDS Book*. Carlsbad, Calif.: Hay House, 1988.

A self-help manual to assist people facing AIDS and other life-threatening illnesses using Louise Hay's practical approaches for self-love and personal transformation. Her popular book You Can Heal Your Life is also a valuable resource.

Konlee, Mark, and Conrad LeBeau. *Immune Restoration Handbook*. 2nd edition. West Allis, Wis.: Keep Hope Alive, 2004.

An excellent resource about nutrition and alternative/complementary therapies for people infected with HIV. Available from Keep Hope Alive.

Kordich, Jay. *The Juiceman's Power of Juicing: Delicious Juice Recipes for Energy, Health, Weight Loss, and Relief from Scores of Common Ailments*. New York: Morrow Cookbooks, 2007.

A new edition of the popular book about fruit and vegetable juices.

Kunz, Dora (compiler). *Spiritual Aspects of the Healing Arts*. Wheaton, Ill.: Quest Books, 1985.

An excellent anthology from a variety of noted healers exploring many of the deeper aspects of healing.

Kurzweil, Ray, and Terry Grossman. *Fantastic Voyage: Live Long Enough to Live Forever*. New York: Plume, 2005.

Though the focus is on anti-aging, this comprehensive book presents cutting-edge scientific knowledge on diet, supplements, detoxification, lifestyle modification, and more.

Myss, Caroline. *Why People Don't Heal and How They Can.* New York: Three Rivers Press, 1998.

A practical and transformative book that helps us understand not only the mind–body connection in health and disease, but also how cultural and individual factors help determine our level of health.

Ornstein, Robert, and David Sobel. *The Healing Brain.* Cambridge, Mass.: Malor Books, 1999.

How the brain can keep us healthy.

Pamplona-Roger, George. *Healthy Foods.* Madrid: Editorial Safeliz, 2007.

A comprehensive and well-written illustrated guide about how food could be our best medicine, written by a board-certified general and digestive surgeon.

Pert, Candace. *Molecules of Emotion: The Science behind Mind–Body Medicine.* New York: Scribner, 1999.

A fascinating—and very personal—book by a neuroscientist who explores the mind–body connection in health and well-being.

Robbins, John. *Diet for a New America.* Tiburon, Calif.: H. J. Kramer, 1998.

A well-researched guide to eating low on the food chain.

Siegel, Bernie S. *Peace, Love and Healing.* New York: Harper, 1990.

An inspiring book about the body–mind connection and the path to self-healing.

Vogel, Alfred. *The Nature Doctor.* New Canaan, Conn.: Keats Publishing, 1992.

A comprehensive manual on traditional and complementary medicine by the ninety-year-old naturopath.

Walker, N. W. *Raw Vegetable Juices: What's Missing in Your Body.* Pomeroy, Wash.: Health Research, 2003.

This is a reprint of Walker's classic, first published in 1936. It is considered the bible of vegetable juicing.

Wigmore, Ann. *Overcoming AIDS.* San Fidel, N.Mex.: Ann Wigmore Foundation, 1987.

A holistic protocol for AIDS focusing on body cleansing, living food nutrition, and natural rejuvenation. Wigmore has also written dozens of other books on the living foods lifestyle, sprouting, wheatgrass, and related subjects. Available at natural food stores or from the Ann Wigmore Foundation. Other information about Ann Wigmore's approach to healing can be found in Be Your Own Doctor (Avery Books, 1990).

Wolfe, David. *Superfoods: The Food and Medicine of the Future*. Berkeley, Calif.: North Atlantic Books, 2009.

A comprehensive guide focusing on the role of superfoods in promoting nutritional excellence, health and well-being, beauty enhancement, and sustainable agriculture.

Notes

CHAPTER 1. FOUNDATIONS OF OXIDATIVE THERAPIES

1. R. Radel and M. H. Navidi, *Chemistry* (St. Paul, Minn.: West Publishing, 1990), 441, 445.
2. S. S. Hendler, *The Oxygen Breakthrough* (New York: Pocket Books, 1989), 79.
3. M. Barry and M. Cullen, "The Air You Breathe Up There," *Conde Nast Traveler* (December 1993): 110–12.
4. Otto Warburg, *The Prime Cause and Prevention of Cancer* (Wurzburg, Germany: K. Triltsch, 1966).
5. D. M. Considine, ed., *Van Nostrand's Scientific Encyclopedia,* 7th ed., vol. 2 (New York: Van Nostrand Reinhold, 1989), 2112.
6. Natalie Angier, "The Price We Pay for Breathing," *New York Times Magazine* (April 25, 1993): 64.
7. David Lin, *Free Radicals and Disease Prevention* (New Canaan, Conn.: Keats Publishing, 1993), 19–21.
8. Sara Shannon, *Good Health in a Toxic World: The Complete Guide to Fighting Free Radicals* (New York: Warner Books, 1994).
9. Stephen A. Levine and Parris Kidd, *Antioxidant Adaptation* (San Leandro, Calif.: Allergy Research Group, 1986), 63.
10. Natalie Angier, "The Price We Pay for Breathing," *New York Times Magazine* (April 25, 1993): 100.

CHAPTER 2. WHAT ARE OXIDATIVE THERAPIES?

1. Velio Bocci, *Ozone: A New Medical Drug* (Dordrecht, Netherlands: Springer, 2005), 28.
2. Ibid., 22–24, 27.

3. Marie Theres Jacobs, "Adverse Effects and Typical Complications in Ozone-Oxygen Therapy," *Ozonachrichten* 1982, no. 1: 193–201.

4. I. N. Love, "Peroxide of Hydrogen as a Remedial Agent," *Journal of the American Medical Association* (March 3, 1888): 262–65.

5. *Oxidative Therapy* (Oklahoma City, Okla.: IBOM, n.d.), 2–3.

6. International Scientific Committee of Ozone Therapy, *Madrid Declaration on Ozone Therapy*, 2nd ed. (Madrid: International Scientific Committee of Ozone Therapy, 2015): 29–31.

7. Frank Shallenberger, "Intravenous Ozone Therapy in HIV Related Disease," in *Proceedings of the 4th International Bio-Oxidative Medicine Conference* (Oklahoma City, Okla.: IBOM, 1993).

8. Robert Atkins, interview in *Ozone and the Politics of Medicine* (Vancouver: Threshold Film, 1993).

9. Michael T. F. Carpendale, interview in *Ozone and the Politics of Medicine* (Vancouver: Threshold Film, 1993).

10. Horst Kief, interview in *Ozone and the Politics of Medicine* (Vancouver: Threshold Film, 1993).

11. "Drug's Lucrative Sales, Some Danger Signals and Role of the F.D.A.," *New York Times* (June 10, 2005): A1, C6.

12. *The Value Line Investment Survey* (October 9, 2015), 1605–34.

13. Visit www.opensecrets.org (accessed November 2, 2015). Search for the term "pharmaceuticals/health products" for more articles on this topic.

14. See *Journal of the American Medical Association* 314, no. 15 (October 20, 2015).

15. See *Family Circle,* November 2015.

16. B. R. Cassileth, "Oxygen Therapies," *Oncology* 23, no. 13 (November 30, 2009): 1132, www.cancernetwork.com/oncology-journal/oxygen-therapies #sthash.KhyPOCEa.dpuf (accessed December 20, 2015).

17. National Institute on Drug Abuse,"Drug Facts: Heroin," revised October 2014, www.drugabuse.gov/publications/drugfacts/heroin (accessed December 20, 2015).

18. Center for Disease Control and Prevention, "Injury Prevention & Control: Prescription Drug Overdoses," November 4, 2015, www.cdc.gov/drugoverdose /data/overdose.html (accessed December 5, 2015).

19. National Institute on Drug Abuse, "America's Addiction to Opioids: Heroin and Prescription Drug Abuse," presented by Nora D. Volkow, M.D., Senate Caucus on International Narcotics Control, May 14, 2014, www.drugabuse .gov/about-nida/legislative-activities/testimony-to-congress/2015/americas -addiction-to-opioids-heroin-prescription-drug-abuse#_ftn2 (accessed December 20, 2015).

20. Agency for Healthcare Research and Quality (Rockville, Maryland), "Ending Health Care-Associated Infections," October 2014, www.ahrq.gov /research/findings/factsheets/errors-safety/haicusp/index.html (accessed December 20, 2015).

21. Agency for Healthcare Research and Quality (Rockville, Maryland), "Saving Lives and Saving Money: Hospital-Acquired Conditions Update," December 2015, www.ahrq.gov/professionals/quality-patient-safety/pfp /interimhacrate2014.html (accessed December 20, 2015), and "Appendix: Incidence of Hospital-Acquired Conditions in the Partnership for Patients: Estimates and Projected and Measured Impact," November 2015, www .ahrq.gov/professionals/quality-patient-safety/pfp/interimhac2014-ap1 .html (accessed December 20, 2015).

CHAPTER 3. OZONE:
PROPERTIES AND USES

1. *Chemical Technology: An Encyclopedic Treatment,* vol. 1 (New York: Barnes & Noble, 1968), 79.

2. Bernard M. Babior et al., "Investigating Antibody-Catalyzed Ozone Generation by Human Neutrophils," *Proceedings of the National Academy of Sciences USA* 100, no. 6 (March 18, 2003): 3031–34.

3. Renate Viebahn-Haensler, *The Use of Ozone in Medicine,* 4th English ed. (Iffezheim, Germany: ODREI-Publishers, 2002), 19.

4. *Chemical Technology: An Encyclopedic Treatment,* vol. 1 (New York: Barnes & Noble, 1968), 82–83.

5. *McGraw-Hill Encyclopedia of Science & Technology,* vol. 12, 6th ed. (New York: McGraw-Hill, 1987), 610.

6. Kirk Othmer, *The Encyclopedia of Chemical Technology,* vol. 16, 3rd ed. (New York: John Wiley & Sons, 1981), 705.

7. Ibid., 704.

8. Renate Viebahn-Haensler, *The Use of Ozone in Medicine,* 4th English ed. (Iffezheim, Germany: ODREI-Publishers, 2002), 18.

9. Ibid., 19–20.

10. James Dulley, "The Sensible Home: Ozone Is a Solid Pool, Spa Purifier," *Los Angeles Times* (May 12, 1996): 5.

11. *Chemical Technology: An Encyclopedic Treatment,* vol. 1 (New York: Barnes & Noble, 1968), 82.

12. Kirk Othmer, *The Encyclopedia of Chemical Technology,* vol. 16, 3rd ed. (New York: John Wiley & Sons, 1981), 710.

13. Ibid.; *Chemical Technology: An Encyclopedic Treatment,* vol. 1 (New York: Barnes & Noble, 1968), 82.

14. L. R. Beuchat, "Surface Disinfection of Raw Produce," *Dairy, Food and Environmental Sanitation* 12, no. 1 (1992): 6–9.
15. Liangji Xu, "Use of Ozone to Improve the Safety of Fresh Fruits and Vegetables," *Food Technology* (October 1999): 58–62.
16. M. M. Barth et al., "Ozone Storage Effects on Anthocyanin Content and Fungal Growth in Blackberries," *Journal of Food Science* 60, no. 6 (November 1995): 1286–88.
17. M. A. Khadre et al., "Microbiological Aspects of Ozone Applications in Food: A Review," *Journal of Food Science* 66, no. 9 (November 2001): 1242–52.
18. A. D. Prudente Jr. and J. M. King, "Efficacy and Safety Evaluation of Ozonation to Degrade Aflatoxin in Corn," *Journal of Food Science* 67, no. 8 (October 2002): 2866–72.
19. M. Balawejder et al., "Potential of Ozone Utilization for Reduction of Pesticide Residue in Food of Plant Origin: A Review," *Roczniki Państwowego Zakładu Higieny* 64, no. 1 (2013): 13–18.
20. Paul Eng, "Potato Technology May Protect Mail From Anthrax, ABC News, http://abcnews.go.com/Technology/CuttingEdge/story?id=98108&page=1 (accessed March 22, 2017).
21. Will Knight, "Ozone Tested as Anti-Anthrax Weapon," *New Scientist* (January 28, 2002): 44.
22. "Ozone Sterilization," *Self Study Series Lesson No. 83* (July 2005). Continuing Education Division, Purdue University.

CHAPTER 4. OZONE IN MEDICINE

1. S. R. Beckwith, *A New Therapeutics for the Cure of Disease by Sending Ozone, Oxygen and Medicine into Diseased Tissues* (New York: Thermo-Ozone Company, 1899).
2. Renate Viebahn-Haensler, *The Use of Ozone in Medicine,* 4th English ed. (Iffezheim, Germany: ODREI-Publishers, 2002), 24–25.
3. Paul Wentworth et al., "Evidence for Antibody-Catalyzed Ozone Formation in Bacterial Killing and Inflammation," *Science* (December 13, 2002): 2195–99.
4. Jean Marx, "Antibodies Kill by Producing Ozone," *Science* (November 15, 2002): 1319.
5. A. C. Baggs, "Are Worry-Free Transfusions Just a Whiff of Ozone Away?" *Canadian Medical Association Journal* (April 1, 1993): 1159.
6. Margaret Gilpin, "Update-Cuba: On the Road to a Family Medicine Nation," *Journal of Public Health Policy* 12, no. 1 (Spring 1991): 90–91.
7. Andres Oppenheimer, *Castro's Final Hour* (New York: Touchstone Books, 1993), 82–83.

8. V. Bocci and L. Paulesu, "Studies on the Biological Effects of Ozone 1: Induction of Interferon Gamma on Human Leucocytes," *Haematologica* 75 (1990): 510–15.

9. Renate Viebahn-Haensler, *The Use of Ozone in Medicine*, 4th English ed. (Iffezheim, Germany: ODREI-Publishers, 2002), 27.

10. Ibid., 42–47.

11. Ibid.; *Proceedings of the First Iberolatinamerican Congress on Ozone Application* (Havana, Cuba: National Center for Scientific Research, 1990); *Revista CENIC Ciencias Biologicas* 20, no. 1-2-3 (1989); Silvia Menendez, *Ozomed/Ozone Therapy* (Havana, Cuba: National Center for Scientific Research, 1993).

CHAPTER 5. HOW IS OZONE THERAPY APPLIED?

1. Renate Viebahn-Haensler, *The Use of Ozone in Medicine*, 4th English ed. (Iffezheim, Germany: ODREI-Publishers, 2002), 44–47.

2. Gerard Sunnen, "Ozone in Medicine: Overview and Future Direction," *Journal of Advancement in Medicine* 1, no. 3 (Fall 1988).

3. Velio Bocci, *Oxygen-Ozone Therapy: A Critical Evaluation* (Dordrecht, Netherlands: Kluwer Academic Publishers, 2002), 213–14.

4. Renate Viebahn-Haensler, *The Use of Ozone in Medicine*, 4th English ed. (Iffezheim, Germany: ODREI-Publishers, 2002), 45.

5. Horst Kief, *Therapeutic Significance of Intestinal Insufflation of Medical Ozone* (Ludwigshafen, Germany: Kief Clinic, n.d.).

6. Silvia Menéndez et al., *Ozono: Aspectos básicos y aplicaciones clínicas* (Havana: Centro de Investigaciones del Ozono, 2008), 129.

7. Ibid.

8. Renate Viebahn-Haensler, *The Use of Ozone in Medicine*, 4th English ed. (Iffezheim, Germany: ODREI-Publishers, 2002), 44.

9. Ibid.

10. Gerard Sunnen, "Ozone in Medicine: Overview and Future Direction," *Journal of Advancement in Medicine* 1, no. 3 (Fall 1988).

11. Velio Bocci, *Oxygen-Ozone Therapy: A Critical Evaluation* (Dordrecht, Netherlands: Kluwer Academic Publishers, 2002), 211–12.

12. Ed McCabe, *Flood Your Body with Oxygen* (Miami Shores, Fla.: Energy Publications, 2003), 297.

13. Frank Shallenberger, *The Principles and Applications of Ozone/UVB Therapy* (Carson City, Nev.: Frank Shallenberger, 1999), 13–14.

14. Velio Bocci, "Ozonetherapy Today," in *Ozone in Medicine*, vol. 3 of *Proceedings of the 12th World Congress of the International Ozone Association* (Zurich: International Ozone Association, 1995), 14.

15. Letter from Velio Bocci, August 31, 2005.

16. Letter from Velio Bocci, December 7, 2005.

17. International Scientific Committee of Ozone Therapy, *Madrid Declaration on Ozone Therapy,* 2nd ed. (Madrid: International Scientific Committee of Ozone Therapy, 2015), 27–28.

18. G. A. Boyarinov et al., "Dissolution of Ozone in Physiological Saline," in *Proceedings of the 3rd All-Russian Scientific-Practical Conference: Ozone & Methods of Efferent Therapy in Medicine* (Nizhny Novgorod, 1998), 6–9.

19. Ibid., 9–11.

20. Letter from Natalia Berdnikova, January 10, 2006.

21. Letters from Velio Bocci, December 7, 2005, and January 10, 2006.

22. Letter from Renate Viebahn-Haensler, February 8, 2006.

23. Letter from Velio Bocci, January 10, 2006.

24. Velio Bocci, *Oxygen-Ozone Therapy: A Critical Evaluation* (Dordrecht, Netherlands: Kluwer Academic Publishers, 2002), 189–97.

25. N. Di Paolo et al., "Extracorporeal Blood Oxygenation and Ozonation: Clinical and Biological Implications of Ozone Therapy," *Redox Report: Communications in Free Radical Research* 10, no. 3 (2005): 121–30.

26. International Scientific Committee of Ozone Therapy, *Madrid Declaration on Ozone Therapy,* 2nd ed. (Madrid: International Scientific Committee of Ozone Therapy, 2015), 26–27.

27. Velio Bocci, *Oxygen-Ozone Therapy: A Critical Evaluation* (Dordrecht, Netherlands: Kluwer Academic Publishers, 2002), 176–77.

28. Denise Grady, "Gain Reported in Combating Ovary Cancer," *New York Times* (January 5, 2006): A1.

29. Silvia Menéndez et al., *Ozono: Aspectos básicos y aplicaciones clínicas* (Havana: Centro de Investigaciones del Ozono, 2008), 116.

30. S. Schulz et al., "Ozone Therapy in a Cancer Model (VX2 Carcinoma: Head And Abdomen) in Rabbits: A Pilot Study," presented at the 4th International Symposia on Ozone Applications, Havana, Cuba, 2004; M. Bette et al., "Efficiency of Tazobactem/Piperacillan in Lethal Peritonitis Is Enhanced after Preconditioning of Rats with O_3/O_2-Pneumoperitoneum," *Shock* 25, no. 1 (January 2006): 23–29.

31. Silvia Menéndez et al., *Ozono: Aspectos básicos y aplicaciones clínicas* (Havana: Centro de Investigaciones del Ozono, 2008), 122.

32. S. N. Gorbunov et al., "The Use of Ozone in the Treatment of Children Suffered Due to Different Catastrophies," in *Ozone in Medicine,* vol. 3 of *Proceedings of the 11th Ozone World Congress* (Stamford, Conn.: International Ozone Association, Pan American Committee, 1993), M-3-31-33.

33. Horst Kief, *The Autohomologous Immune Therapy* (Ludwigshafen, Germany: Kief Clinic, 1992).

34. Velio Bocci, *Oxygen-Ozone Therapy: A Critical Evaluation* (Dordrecht, Netherlands: Kluwer Academic Publishers, 2002), 306.

35. Ibid., 139.

CHAPTER 6. HYDROGEN PEROXIDE

1. Ed McCabe, *Flood Your Body with Oxygen* (Miami Shores, Fla.: Energy Publications, 2003), 34.

2. Anthony di Fabio, *Supplement to the Art of Getting Well,* chap. 3 (Franklin, Tenn.: Rheumatoid Disease Foundation, 1989), 17.

3. C. H. Farr, *Protocol for the Intravenous Administration of Hydrogen Peroxide* (Oklahoma City, Okla.: International Bio-Oxidative Medicine Foundation, 1993), 29–31.

4. *McGraw-Hill Encyclopedia of Science and Technology,* vol. 12, 6th ed. (New York: McGraw-Hill, 1987), 596.

5. "Hydrogen Peroxide and Peroxyacetic Acid," *Pesticides: Topical & Chemical Fact Sheets* (Washington, D.C.: U.S. Environmental Protection Agency, 2005).

6. *Hydrogen Peroxide Power Sources* (China Lake, Calif.: Naval Air Warfare Center Weapons Division, 2005).

7. Letter from Randall Prue to Oxytherapy.com, March 15, 1996.

8. *Hydrogen Peroxide Uses in Agriculture* (Glencoe, Minn.: Farmgard Products, n.d.).

9. "Sterilization Methods and Impact on Electronics in Medical Devices," *EE Times* (July 8, 2011), www.eetimes.com/document.asp?doc_id=1278906 (accessed October 22, 2016).

10. David Godkin, "Tso3's Sterizone Seen as Revolutionary Weapon in the Treatment of Superbugs, Other Bacteria," Medical Device Daily, July 26, 2016, https://medicaldevicedaily.com/servlet/com.accumedia.web .Dispatcher?next=bioWorldHeadlines_article&forceid=93272 (accessed October 22, 2016); "STERIZONE VP4 Sterilizer," www.tso3.com/products /sterizone-vp4 (accessed October 22, 2016).

CHAPTER 7. HYDROGEN PEROXIDE IN MEDICINE

1. I. N. Love, "Peroxide of Hydrogen as a Remedial Agent," *The Journal of the American Medical Association* (March 3, 1888): 262–65.

2. P. R. Cortelyou, "80 Years Ago: Using Peroxide of Hydrogen in Diseases of the Throat and Nose," *Journal of the Medical Association of Georgia* (September 1968): 449–50. [Original article appeared in 1888.]

3. T. H. Oliver and D. V. Murphy, "Influenzal Pneumonia: The Intravenous Use of Hydrogen Peroxide," *Lancet* (February 21, 1920): 432–33.

4. Ed McCabe, *Flood Your Body with Oxygen* (Miami Shores, Fla.: Energy Publications, 2003), 132.

5. J. W. Finney et al., "Protection of the Ischemic Heart with DMSO Alone or DMSO with Hydrogen Peroxide," *Annals of the New York Academy of Sciences* 151 (1967): 231–41.

6. H. C. Urschel Jr., *Circulation* 31, supp. 2 (1965): 203–10.

7. H. C. Urschel Jr., "Cardiovascular Effects of Hydrogen Peroxide," *Diseases of the Chest* 51 (February 1967): 187–88.

8. Nathaniel Altman, *Oxygen Healing Therapies* (Rochester, Vt.: Healing Arts Press, 1998), x.

9. C. H. Farr, *Protocol for the Intravenous Administration of Hydrogen Peroxide* (Oklahoma City, Okla.: International Bio-Oxidative Medicine Foundation, 1993), 32.

10. Nathaniel Altman, *Oxygen Healing Therapies* (Rochester, Vt.: Healing Arts Press, 1998), x–xi.

11. C. H. Farr, *Protocol for the Intravenous Administration of Hydrogen Peroxide* (Oklahoma City, Okla.: International Bio-Oxidative Medicine Foundation, 1993), 32, 38–39.

12. S. P. Chaki and M. M. Misro, "Assessment of Human Sperm Function after Hydrogen Peroxide Exposure: Development of a Vaginal Contraceptive," *Contraception* (September 2002): 187–92.

13. K. Brudzynski, "Effect of Hydrogen Peroxide on Antibacterial Activities of Canadian Honeys," *Canadian Journal of Microbiology* 52 (2006): 1228.

14. Patricia E. Lusby et al., "Activity of Honeys against Medically Significant Bacteria," *Archives of Medical Research* 36, no. 5 (September–November 2005): 464.

15. K. L. Allen, P. C. Molan, and G. M. Reid, "A Survey of the Antibacterial Activity of Some New Zealand Honeys," *Journal of Pharmacy and Pharmacology* 43 (1991): 817–822.

CHAPTER 8. HOW IS HYDROGEN PEROXIDE ADMINISTERED?

1. Quoted in Anthony di Fabio, *Supplement to the Art of Getting Well,* chap. 3 (Franklin, Tenn.: Rheumatoid Disease Foundation, 1989), 15.

2. *Oxidative Therapy* (Oklahoma City, Okla.: International Bio-Oxidative Medicine Foundation, n.d.), 3.

3. Velio Bocci, *Oxygen-Ozone Therapy: A Critical Evaluation* (Dordrecht, Netherlands: Kluwer Academic Publishers, 2002), 355.

4. Betsy Russell-Manning, ed., *Self-Treatment for AIDS, Oxygen Therapies, Etc.* (San Francisco: Greensward Press, 1988), 19.

5. Kurt Donsbach, *Oxygen–Peroxides–Ozone* (Tulsa, Okla.: Rockland Corp., 1993), 44–45.

6. Conrad LeBeau, *Hydrogen Peroxide Therapy,* 9th ed. (Monterey, Calif.: Conrad LeBeau, 1993), 8–9.

7. Kurt Donsbach, *Oxygen–Peroxides–Ozone* (Tulsa, Okla.: Rockland Corp., 1993), 45.

8. Letter from Charles H. Farr, February 4, 1994.

9. Y. Oya et al., "The Biological Activity of Hydrogen Peroxide," *Mutation Research* 172 (1986): 245–53.

10. Letter from Velio Bocci, December 12, 2005.

11. Bill Thomson, "Do Oxygen Therapies Work?" *EastWest* (September 1989): 110.

12. C. H. Farr, *The Use of Hydrogen Peroxide to Inject Trigger Points, Soft Tissue Injuries and Inflamed Joints* (Oklahoma City, Okla.: C. H. Farr, 1993).

13. C. H. Farr, *Protocol for the Intravenous Administration of Hydrogen Peroxide* (Oklahoma City, Okla.: International Bio-Oxidative Medicine Foundation, 1993), 9.

CHAPTER 9. HYPERBARIC OXYGEN THERAPY AND OXYGEN MULTISTEP THERAPY

1. Felicity Barringer, "Under Strain, Towns Prepare for 12 Funerals," *New York Times* (January 8, 2006): 17; Paul H. B. Shin and Corky Siemaszko, "Using Meds & Music to Help Miner," *New York Daily News* (January 7, 2006): 2.

2. Richard A. Neubauer and Morton Walker, *Hyperbaric Oxygen Therapy* (Garden City Park, N.Y.: Avery Publishing Group, 1998).

3. Michelle Reillo, *AIDS under Pressure* (Seattle, Wash.: Hogrefe & Huber Publishers, 1998).

4. Pamela S. Grim et al., "Hyperbaric Oxygen Therapy," *Journal of the American Medical Association* (April 25, 1990): 216.

5. Velio Bocci, *Oxygen-Ozone Therapy: A Critical Evaluation* (Dordrecht, Netherlands: Kluwer Academic Publishers, 2002), 361.

6. Von Ardenne Institut für Angewandte Medizinische Forschung GmbH, "Oxygen Multistep Therapy," http://med.ardenne.de/?therapien=oxygen-multistep-therapy&lang=en (accessed February 15, 2016).

7. Exercise with Oxygen Training, www.ewot.com (accessed February 15, 2016).

PART 2. OXIDATIVE THERAPIES IN MEDICINE

1. Velio Bocci, *Oxygen-Ozone Therapy: A Critical Evaluation* (Dordrecht, Netherlands: Kluwer Academic Publishers, 2002), 371.
2. J. Varro, "Ozone Applications in Cancer Cases," in *Medical Applications of Ozone,* ed. Julius LaRaus (Stamford, Conn.: International Ozone Association, Pan American Committee, 1983), 98.
3. Paul A. Sergios, *One Boy at War: My Life in the AIDS Underground* (New York: Alfred A. Knopf, 1993), 84.
4. Ibid.
5. Sheryl Gay Stolberg, "U.S. AIDS Research Abroad Sets Off Outcry over Ethics," *New York Times* (September 18, 1997): A1.

CHAPTER 10. CARDIOVASCULAR DISEASES

1. E. Riva Sanseverino, E. Castellacci, and P. Castellacci, "Oxygen-Ozone Therapy and Physical Activity in Humans," in *Ozone in Medicine,* vol. 3 of *Proceedings of the 12th World Congress of the International Ozone Association* (Zurich: International Ozone Association, 1995), 65–72.
2. F. Hernández et al., "Decrease of Blood Cholesterol and Stimulation of Antioxidative Response in Cardiopathy Patients Treated with Endovenous Ozone Therapy," *Free Radical Biology & Medicine* 19 (July 1995): 115–19.
3. E. I. Sycheva et al., "[The influence of ozone therapy on oxygen metabolism kinetics and the microcirculation system during spa and resort treatment of the post-infarction patients]," *Voprosy kurortologii, fizioterapii, i lechebnoĭ fizicheskoĭ kultury* 58, no. 6 (November–December 2013): 9–13.
4. Davor Huic, "Nicaragua's Ortega in Cuba for Medical Check," Reuters News Service (February 1, 1996).
5. Velio Bocci, *Oxygen-Ozone Therapy: A Critical Evaluation* (Dordrecht, Netherlands: Kluwer Academic Publishers, 2002), 122.
6. R. T. Canoso et al., "Hydrogen Peroxide and Platelet Function" *Blood* 43, no. 5 (May 1974).
7. B. N. Setty et al., "Effects of Hydrogen Peroxide on Vascular Arachidonic Acid Metabolism," *Prostaglandins, Leukotrienes, and Medicine* 14 (1984): 205–13; P. H. Levine et al., "Leukocyte-Platelet Interaction," *Journal of Clinical Investigation* 57 (April 1976): 955–63.
8. C. H. Farr, "The Therapeutic Use of Hydrogen Peroxide," *Townsend Letter for Doctors* (July 1987): 185.
9. Renate Viebahn-Haensler, "The Biochemical Processes Underlying Ozone Therapy," *Ozonachrichten* (January 4, 1985): heft 1/2.
10. N. I. Zhulina et al., "Ozonotherapy Efficiency in the Treatment of Patients with Atherosclerosis of Coronary and Cerebral Vessels," in *Ozone in*

Medicine, vol. 3 of *Proceedings of the 11th Ozone World Congress* (Stamford, Conn.: International Ozone Association, Pan American Committee, 1993), M-2-9-11.

11. G. Martínez-Sánchez et al., "Effects of Ozone Therapy on Haemostatic and Oxidative Stress Index in Coronary Artery Disease," *European Journal of Pharmacology* 69 (September 15, 2012): 156–62.

12. Frank Hernández et al., "Decrease of Blood Cholesterol and Stimulation of Antioxidative Response in Cardiopathy Patients Treated with Endovenous Ozone Therapy," *Free Radical Biology and Medicine* (July 1995): 115–19.

13. G. Verrazzo et al., "Hyperbaric Oxygen, Oxygen-Ozone Therapy, and Rheologic Parameters of Blood in Patients with Peripheral Occlusive Arterial Disease," *Undersea & Hyberbaric Medicine* (March 1995): 17–22.

14. O. Rokitansky, "The Clinical Effects and Biochemistry of Ozone Therapy in Peripheral Arterial Circulatory Disorders," in *Medical Applications of Ozone,* ed. Julius LaRaus (Stamford, Conn.: International Ozone Association, Pan American Committee, 1983), 33–54.

15. A. Romero et al., "La Ozonoterapia en la Atersclerosis Obliterante," *Revista CENIC Ciencias Biologicas* 20, no. 1-2-3 (1989): 70–76.

16. J. Sroczynski et al., "[Various Parameters of Lipid Metabolism after Intra-arterial Injections of Ozone in Patients with Ischemia of the Lower Extremities and Diabetes Mellitus]," *Polski Tygodnik Lekarski* (November 19–26, 1990): 953–55. [In Polish.]

17. B. Turczynski et al., "[Ozone Therapy and Viscosity of Blood and Plasma, Distance of Intermittent Claudication and Certain Biochemical Plasma Components in Patients with Occlusive Arteriosclerosis of the Lower Limbs]," *Polski Tygodnik Lekarski* (September 9–30, 1991): 700–703. [In Polish.]

18. J. Sroczynski et al., "[Clinical Assessment of Treatment Results for Atherosclerotic Ischemia of the Lower Extremities with Intraarterial Ozone Injections]," *Polski Tygodnik Lekarski* (October 19, 1992): 964–66. [In Polish.]

19. S. N. Gorbunov et al., "Medical Ozone in the Treatment of Lower Extremities Peripheral Circulation Disorders," in *Ozone in Medicine,* vol. 3 of *Proceedings of the 12th World Congress of the International Ozone Association* (Zurich: International Ozone Association, 1995), 109–10.

20. O. V. Maslennikov et al., "[Effect of Ozone Therapy on Hemostatic Changes in Patients with Vascular Atherosclerosis]," *Klinicheskaia Meditsina* 75, no. 10 (1997): 35–37. [In Russian.]

21. Oleg V. Maslennikov et al., *Ozone Therapy in Practice: Health Manual*

(Nizhny Novgorod: Ministry of Health Service of the Russian Federation, 2008), 21–22.

22. A. Romero et al., "Arteriosclerosis Obliterans and Ozone Therapy: Its Administration by Different Routes," *Angiologia* (September–October 1993): 177–79.

23. R. Giunta et al., "Ozonized Autohemotransfusion Improves Hemorheological Parameters and Oxygen Delivery to Tissues in Patients with Peripheral Occlusive Arterial Disease," *Annals of Hematology* 80 (December 2001): 745–48.

24. B. Clavo et al., "Effect of Ozone Therapy on Muscle Oxygenation," *Journal of Alternative and Complementary Medicine* (April 2003): 251–56.

25. B. A. Korolyov et al., "Ozone Application by Cardiosurgical Patients in Correction of Heart Defects, Complicated by Infectious Endocarditis," *Ozone in Biology and Medicine* (Nizhny Novgorod: Ministry of Public Health of Russian Federation, 1992), 88.

26. J. W. Finney et al., "Removal of Cholesterol and Other Lipids from Experimental Animal and Human Atheromatous Arteries by Dilute Hydrogen Peroxide," *Angiology* 17 (April 1966): 223–28.

27. F. Hernandez et al., "Decrease of Blood Cholesterol and Stimulation of Antioxidative Response in Cardiopathy Patients with Endovenous Ozone Therapy," *Free Radical Biology & Medicine* (July 1995): 115–19.

28. H. C. Urschel Jr., "Cardiovascular Effects of Hydrogen Peroxide: Current Status," *Diseases of the Chest* 51 (February 1967): 187–88.

29. J. W. Finney et al., "Protection of the Ischemic Myocardium with DMSO Alone or in Combination with Hydrogen Peroxide," *Annals of the New York Academy of Sciences* (1967).

30. S. P. Peretyagin, "Mechanisms of Ozone Medicinal Effect in Case of Hypoxy," in *Ozone in Biology and Medicine* (Nizhny Novgorod: Ministry of Public Health of Russian Federation, 1992), 76.

31. F. Devesa et al., "Ozone Therapy in Ischemic Cerebro-Vascular Disease," in *Ozone in Medicine,* vol. 3 of *Proceedings of the 11th Ozone World Congress* (Stamford, Conn.: International Ozone Association, Pan American Committee, 1993), M-4-10-18.

32. Bernardino Clavo et al., "Ozone Therapy on Cerebral Blood Flow: A Preliminary Report," *Evidence-Based Complementary and Alternative Medicine* 1, no. 3 (2004): 315.

33. Bernardino Clavo et al., "Brain Ischemia and Hypometabolism Treated by Ozone Therapy," *Forsch Komplementmedizine* 18 (2011): 283–287.

34. Oleg V. Maslennikov et al., *Ozone Therapy in Practice: Health Manual*

(Nizhny Novgorod: Ministry of Health Service of the Russian Federation, 2008), 22–23.

35. Gerd Wasser, "Additional Therapy of Cerebro-Vascular Disorder (Here: Acute Brain Stroke) by Ozone Therapy," in *Ozone in Medicine,* vol. 3 of *Proceedings of the 12th World Congress of the International Ozone Association* (Zurich: International Ozone Association, 1995), 91–95.

CHAPTER 11. CANCER

1. S. Thomas, et al., "CD24 Is an Effector of HIF-1–Driven Primary Tumor Growth and Metastasis," *Cancer Research* 72, no. 21 (November 1, 2012): 5600–12.

2. J. Cui et al., "Hypoxia and Miscoupling between Reduced Energy Efficiency and Signaling to Cell Proliferation Drive Cancer to Grow Increasingly Faster," *Journal of Molecular Cell Biology* 4 (2012): 174–76.

3. Renate Viebahn-Haensler, *The Use of Ozone in Medicine,* 4th English ed. (Iffezheim, Germany: ODREI-Publishers, 2002), 89.

4. Otto Warburg, *The Prime Cause and Prevention of Cancer* (Wurzburg, Germany: K. Tritsch, 1966).

5. James D. Watson, *Molecular Biology of the Gene* (New York: W. A. Benjamin, 1965), 469.

6. J. Varro, "Die Krebsbehandlung mit Ozon," *Erfahrungsheilkunde* 23 (1974): 178–81.

7. F. Sweet et al., "Ozone Selectively Inhibits Growth of Cancer Cells," *Science* 209 (August 22, 1980): 931–32.

8. Betsy Russell-Manning, ed., *Self-Treatment for AIDS, Oxygen Therapies, Etc.* (San Francisco: Greensward Press, 1988), 23.

9. J. T. Mallams et al., "The Use of Hydrogen Peroxide as a Source of Oxygen in a Regional Intra-Arterial Infusion System," *Southern Medical Journal* (March 1962).

10. B. L. Aronoff et al., "Regional Oxygenation in Neoplasms," *Cancer* 18 (October 1965): 1250.

11. H. Sasaki et al., "Application of Hydrogen Peroxide to Maxillary Cancer," *Yonago Acta Medica* 11, no. 3 (1967): 149.

12. C. F. Nathan et al., "Extracellular Cytolysis by Activated Macrophages and Granulocytes," *Journal of Experimental Medicine* 149 (January 1979): 109.

13. C. F. Nathan and Z. A. Cohn, "Antitumor Effects of Hydrogen Peroxide in Vivo," *Journal of Experimental Medicine* 154 (November 1981): 1551.

14. M. K. Samoszuk et al., "In Vitro Sensitivity of Hodgkins Disease to Hydrogen Peroxide Toxicity," *Cancer* 63 (1989): 2114.

15. N. C. Nicholson et al., "Hydrogen Peroxide Inhibits Giant Cell Tumor and Osteoblast Metabolism In Vitro," *Clinical Orthopedics and Related Research* 347 (February 1998): 250–60.

16. M. C. Symonds et al., "Hydrogen Peroxide: A Potent Cytotoxic Agent Effective in Causing Cellular Damage and Used in the Possible Treatment for Certain Tumors," *Medical Hypotheses* 57 (July 2001): 56–58.

17. I. O. Farah and R. A. Begum, "Effect of Nigella sativa (N. sativa L.) and Oxidative Stress on the Survival Pattern of MCF-7 Breast Cancer Cells," *Biomedical Sciences Instrumentation* 39 (2003): 359–64.

18. M. Arnan and L. E. DeVries, "Effect of Ozone/Oxygen Gas Mixture Directly Injected into the Mammary Carcinoma of the Female C3H/HEJ Mice," in *Medical Applications of Ozone,* ed. Julius LaRaus (Norwalk, Conn.: International Ozone Association, Pan American Committee, 1983), 101–7.

19. F. Sweet et al., "Ozone Selectively Inhibits Growth of Cancer Cells," *Science* 209 (August 22, 1980).

20. J. Varro, "Die Krebsbehandlung mit Ozon," *Erfahrungsheilkunde* 23 (1974): 94–95.

21. Ibid., 97–98.

22. Kurt W. Donsbach and H. R. Alsleben, *Wholistic Cancer Therapy* (Tulsa, Okla.: Rockland Corporation, 1992), 49.

23. Kurt W. Donsbach, *Oxygen–Peroxides–Ozone* (Tulsa, Okla.: Rockland Corporation, 1993), 66.

24. Letter from Kurt W. Donsbach, December 30, 1993.

25. Interview with Jon Greenberg, December 21, 1993.

26. Interview with Horst Kief, December 15, 1993.

27. Ibid.

28. Horst Kief, *Treatment of Malignant Diseases with AHIT-aM* (Ludwigshafen, Germany: FBM-PHARMA GmbH, 2003), 9.

29. Luis Borrego et al., "Ozono Mas Cobaltoterapia en Pacientes con Adrenocarcinoma Prostatico," *Revista CENIC Ciencias Biologicas* 29, no. 3 (1998): 137–40.

30. Guennadi O. Gretchkanev et al., "Medical Ozone for Prophylaxis and Treatment of Complications Associated [with] Chemotherapy [for] Ovarian Cancer," in *Ozone in Medicine,* vol. 3 of *Proceedings of the 15th Ozone World Congress,* London (London: International Ozone Association, 2001).

31. N. A. Terekhina et al., "[The Activity of Adenosinetriphosphatase of Erythrocites in Peripheral Blood of Patients with Colorectal Cancer]," *Klinicheskaia Laboratornaia Diagnostika* 5 (May 2005): 20–22. [In Russian.]

32. B. Clavo et al., "Intravesical Ozone Therapy for Progressive Radiation-Induced Hematuria," *Journal of Alternative and Complementary Medicine* 11 (June 2005): 539–41.

33. B. Clavo et al., "Ozone Therapy in the Management of Persistent Radiation-Induced Rectal Bleeding in Prostate Cancer Patients," *Evidence-Based Complementary and Alternative Medicine* (2015): 1–7.

34. Lionel Resnick et al., "Topical Sulindac Combined with Hydrogen Peroxide in the Treatment of Actinic Keratoses," *Journal of Drugs in Dermatology* 8, no. 1 (2009): 29–32.

35. V. Bocci et al., "Restoration of Normoxia by Ozone Therapy May Control Neoplastic Growth: A Review and a Working Hypothesis," *Journal of Alternative and Complementary Medicine* 11 (April 2005): 257–65.

36. Letter from Velio Bocci, December 28, 2005.

37. International Scientific Committee of Ozone Therapy, *Madrid Declaration on Ozone Therapy,* 2nd ed. (Madrid: International Scientific Committee of Ozone Therapy, 2015): 30.

38. Carl Franklin, "Oxygen Is Key to Tumor Treatment," *New Scientist* (May 7, 1994): 17.

39. S. Schulz et al., "Ozone Therapy in a Cancer Model (VX2 Carcinoma: Head and Abdomen) in Rabbits: A Pilot Study," presented at the 4th International Symposia on Ozone Applications, Havana, Cuba, 2004.

CHAPTER 12. HIV/AIDS

1. *Resource Needs for an Expanded Response to AIDS in Low- and Middle-Income Countries* (New York: Joint United Nations Programme on HIV/AIDS, 2005), 3.

2. Velio Bocci, *Oxygen-Ozone Therapy: A Critical Evaluation* (Dordrecht, Netherlands: Kluwer Academic Publishers, 2002), 253.

3. Siegfried Rilling and Renate Viebahn, *The Use of Ozone in Medicine* (Heidelberg, Germany: Haug Publishers, 1987), 41–44.

4. "HIV Clue Announced," *American Medical News* (March 1, 1993): 25.

5. *Health Facts* (July 1992): 4.

6. Interview with Juliane Sacher, January 26, 1994.

7. Letter from Velio Bocci, January 6, 2006.

8. Letter from Frank Shallenberger, December 9, 1993.

9. M. T. Carpendale and J. K. Freeberg, "Ozone Inactivates HIV at Non-Cytotoxic Concentrations," *Antiviral Research* 16 (1991): 281–92.

10. K. H. Wells et al., "Inactivation of Human Immunodeficiency Virus Type I by Ozone In Vitro," *Blood* 78, no. 7 (October 1, 1991): 1882.

11. G. V. Kornilaeva et al., "Ozone Influence on HIV Infection In Vitro," in

Ozone in Biology and Medicine (Nizhny Novgorod, Russia: Ministry of Public Health of Russia Federation, 1992), 86.

12. A. C. Baggs, "Are Worry-Free Transfusions Just a Whiff of Ozone Away?" *Canadian Medical Association Journal* (April 1, 1993): 1159.

13. M. E. Shannon, interview in *Ozone and the Politics of Medicine* (Vancouver: Threshold Film, 1993).

14. Horst Kief, "Die Biologischen Grundlagen der Autohomologen Immunotherapie," *Erfahrungsheilkunde* 37, no. 7 (July 1988): 175–80.

15. Horst Kief, interview in *Ozone and the Politics of Medicine* (Vancouver: Threshold Film, 1993).

16. Alexander Pruess, "Positive Treatment Results in AIDS Therapy," *Ozonachrichten* 5 (1986): 1, 2, 3–5.

17. Horst Kief, *Ozone and the Auto-homologous Immune Therapy in AIDS Patients* (Ludwigshafen, Germany: Kief Clinic, 1993).

18. M. T. Carpendale and J. Griffiss, "Is There a Role for Medical Ozone in the Treatment of HIV and Associated Infections?" in *Ozone in Medicine*, vol. 3 of *Proceedings of the 11th Ozone World Congress* (Stamford, Conn.: International Ozone Association, Pan American Committee, 1993), M-1-38-43.

19. M. T. Carpendale et al., "Does Ozone Alleviate AIDS Diarrhea?" *Journal of Clinical Gastroenterology* 17 (1993): 142–45.

20. Frank Shallenberger, "Intravenous Ozone Therapy in HIV-related Disease," in *Proceedings of the 4th International Bio-Oxidative Medicine Conference* (Oklahoma City, Okla.: IBOM, 1993).

21. *Case Studies* (Salisbury, N.C.: Cure AIDS Now, 1993).

22. John C. Pittman, *Introduction* (Salisbury, N.C.: Cure AIDS Now, 1993), 2.

23. Michelle Reillo, *AIDS under Pressure* (Seattle, Wash.: Hogreve & Huber Publishers, 1997), 24.

24. Ibid., 6.

25. Ibid., 94–96.

26. Ibid., 98.

27. G. E. Garber et al., "The Use of Ozone Treated Blood in the Therapy of HIV Infection and Immune Disease," *AIDS* 5 (1991): 981–84.

28. Letter from Michael E. Shannon, January 21, 1994.

29. Letter from M. E. Shannon to Ed McCabe, January 13, 1995.

30. Interview with Silvia Menendez, January 6, 1994.

31. G. P. Miley et al., "Ultraviolet Blood Irradiation Therapy of Apparently Intractable Bronchial Asthma," *Archives of Physical Medicine* 27 (1946): 24–29; G. P. Miley and J. A. Christensen, "Ultraviolet Blood Irradiation Therapy in Acute Virus and Virus-Like Infections," *Review of*

Gastroenterology 15, no. 4 (1948): 271–77; V. P. Wasson et al., "Ultraviolet Blood Irradiation Therapy (Knott Technic) in Rheumatic Fever in Children," *Experimental Medicine and Surgery* 8 (1950): 15–33; and R. C. Olney et al., "Treatment of Viral Hepatitis with the Knott Technic of Blood Irradiation," *American Journal of Surgery* 90, no. 3 (1955): 402–9.

32. P. Morel et al., "Photochemical Inactivation of Viruses and Bacteriophage in Plasma and Plasma Fractions," *Blood Cells* 18 (1992): 27–41; F. Knutson et al., "Photochemical Inactivation of Bacteria and HIV in Buffy-Coat-Derived Platelet Concentrates under Conditions That Preserve In Vitro Platelet Function," *Vox Sanguinis* 78, no. 4 (2004): 209–16; C. T. Jordan et al., "Photochemical Treatment of Platelet Concentrates with Amotosalen Hydrochloride and Ultraviolet A Light Inactivates Free and Latent Cytomegaovirus in a Murine Transfusion Model," *Transfusion* 44, no. 8 (August 2004): 1159–65; and L. Lin et al., "Inactivation of Viruses in Platelet Concentrates by Photochemical Treatment with Amotosalen and Long-Wavelength Ultraviolet Light," *Transfusion* 45, no. 4 (April 2005): 580–90.

33. Robert Jay Rowan, "Ultraviolet Blood Irradiation Therapy (Photo-Oxidation): The Cure That Time Forgot," *International Journal of Biosocial Medical Research* 14, no. 2 (1996): 128.

34. *A Special Report from Keep Hope Alive* no. 4 (December 13, 1993), 2.

35. M. T. Carpendale and J. Griffiss, "Is There a Role for Medical Ozone in the Treatment of HIV and Associated Infections?" in *Ozone in Medicine,* vol. 3 of *Proceedings of the 11th Ozone World Congress* (Stamford, Conn.: International Ozone Association, Pan American Committee, 1993), M-1-38.

36. Mark Konlee and Conrad LeBeau, *Immune Restoration Handbook,* 2nd ed. (West Allis, Wis.: Keep Hope Alive, 2004), 206.

37. Velio Bocci, "A Reasonable Approach for the Treatment of HIV Infection in the Early Phase with Ozonetherapy (Autohaemotherapy): How 'Inflammatory' Cytokines May Have a Therapeutic Role," *Mediators of Inflammation* 3 (1994): 315–21.

38. Velio Bocci, Iacopo Zanardi, and Valter Travagli, "Ozonation of Human HIV-infected Plasmas for Producing a Global Vaccine: How HIV-patients May Help Fight the HIV Pandemia," *Virulence* 1, no. 3 (2010): 215–17.

39. Statement by Randolph F. Wykoff before the Committee on the Judiciary, Subcommittee on Crime and Criminal Justice, U.S. House of Representatives, May 23, 1993.

40. Testimony by Richard Schrader on AIDS fraud before the Committee on the Judiciary, Subcommittee on Crime and Criminal Justice, U.S. House of Representatives, May 23, 1993.

CHAPTER 13. INFECTIOUS DISEASES

1. P. Madej et al., "Ozonotherapy," *Materia Medica Polona* 27 (April–June 1995): 53–56.
2. Kenneth Bock, "Oxidative Therapies in Lyme Disease," presentation at the 8th International Bio-Oxidative Medicine Conference, Anchorage, Alaska (May 18, 1997).
3. I. T. Vasilyev, "Perspectives of Ozone Application in the Treatment of Diffused Peritonitis," in *Ozone in Biology and Medicine* (Nizhny Novgorod, Russia: Ministry of Public Health of Russia Federation, 1992), 89.
4. V. I. Bulynin and A. A. Glukhov, "[Treatment of Peritonitis Using Ozone and Hydropressive Technology]," *Khirirgiia* 7 (1999): 9–11. [In Russian.]
5. H. Konrad, "Ozone vs. Hepatitis and Herpes," in *Medical Applications of Ozone,* ed. Julius LaRaus (Norwalk, Conn.: International Ozone Association, Pan American Committee, 1983), 140–41.
6. Y. Betancourt et al., "Ozone Therapy: A Useful Alternative on Virulent Hepatitis Treatment," in *Abstracts: 2nd International Symposium on Ozone Applications* (Havana, Cuba: Ozone Research Center/National Center for Scientific Research, 1997), 61–62.
7. Ronald M. Davis, untitled monograph, 5002 Todville, Seabrook, TX 77586.
8. Velio Bocci, *Ozone: A New Medical Drug* (Dordrecht, Netherlands: Springer, 2005), 112–13.
9. M. Nabil Mawsouf et al., *Ozone Therapy in Patients with Hepatitis "C": A Clinical Study* (Cairo: First International Congress of Ozone and Medicine, 2006).
10. Oleg V. Maslennikov et al., *Ozone Therapy in Practice: Health Manual* (Nizhny Novgorod: Ministry of Health Service of the Russian Federation, 2008), 29.
11. S. Zaky et al., "Preliminary Results of Ozone Therapy as a Possible Treatment for Patients with Chronic Hepatitis C," *Journal of Alternative and Complementary Medicine* 17, no. 3 (March 2011): 259–63.
12. X. B. Gu et al., "Effect of Medical Ozone Therapy on Renal Blood Flow and Renal Function of Patients with Chronic Severe Hepatitis," *Chinese Medical Journal* 123, no. 18 (September 2010): 2510–13.
13. C. H. Farr, *Rapid Recovery from Type A/Shanghai Influenza Treated with Intravenous Hydrogen Peroxide* (Oklahoma City, Okla.: C. H. Farr, 1993).
14. Joseph Mercola, website citation, Optimal Wellness Center, www.mercola.com (accessed January 2006).

15. C. H. Farr, *The Therapeutic Use of Intravenous Hydrogen Peroxide* (Oklahoma City, Okla.: Genesis Medical Center, 1987), 18–19.

16. D. A. Blaine and M. A. Frable, "Mucormycosis: Adjunctive Therapy with Hydrogen Peroxide," *Virginia Medical Quarterly: VMQ* 123, no. 1 (Winter 1996): 30–32.

17. Silvia Menendez et al., "Onicomycosis Treated with Ozonized Oil," in *Ozone in Medicine,* vol. 3 of *Proceedings of the 12th World Congress of the International Ozone Association* (Zurich: International Ozone Association, 1995), 279–82.

18. Silvia Menéndez et al., "Therapeutic Efficacy of Topical OLEOZON® in Patients Suffering from Onychomycosis," *Mycoses* 54, no. 5 (September 2011): 272–77.

19. J. O. Sardina et al., "Tratamiento de la Giardiasis Recidivante con Ozono," *Revista CENIC Ciencias Biologicas* 20, no. 1-2-3 (1989): 61–64.

20. Silvia Menendez et al., "Application of Ozonized Oil in the Treatment of Infantile Giardiasis," in *Ozone in Medicine,* vol. 3 of *Proceedings of the 12th World Congress of the International Ozone Association* (Zurich: International Ozone Association, 1995), 297–300.

21. H. M. Dockrell and H. L. Playfair, "Killing of Blood-Stage Murine Malaria Parasites by Hydrogen Peroxide," *Infection and Immunity* (January 1983): 456–59.

22. Bertram Lell et al., "The Activity of Ozone against *Plasmodium falciparum,*" *Ozone Science & Engineering* 23 (2001): 89.

23. Adriana Schwartz, "A Possible Solution to Ebola: Ozone Therapy" (Madrid: International Medical Ozone Association, October 7, 2014).

24. Silvia Menéndez Cepero, letter to the author, January 31, 2016.

CHAPTER 14. MUSCULOSKELETAL PROBLEMS

1. R. I. Gracer and V. Bocci, "Can the Combination of Localized 'Proliferative Therapy' with 'Minor Ozonated Autohemotherapy' Restore the Natural Healing Process?" *Medical Hypotheses* 65, no. 4 (2005): 752–59.

2. C. H. Siemsen, "The Use of Ozone in Orthopedics," in *Ozone in Medicine,* vol. 3 of *Proceedings of the 12th World Congress of the International Ozone Association* (Zurich: International Ozone Association, 1995), 125–30.

3. Lamberto Re et al., "Clinical Evidence of Ozone Interaction with Pain Mediators," *Saudi Medical Journal* 32, no. 12 (2011): 1363–67.

4. *Proceedings of the 10th Ozone World Congress* (Monaco, 1991), 87–93.

5. R. Wong et al., "Ozonoterapia Analgesica," *Revista CENIC Ciencias Biologicas* 20, no. 1-2-3 (1989): 143.

6. C. F. Andreula et al., "Minimally Invasive Oxygen-Ozone Therapy for Lumbar Disc Herniation," *ANJR American Journal of Neuroradiology* 24, no. 5 (May 2003): 996–1000.

7. M. Gallucci et al., "Sciatica: Treatment with Intradiscal and Intraforaminal Injections of Steroid and Oxygen-Ozone versus Steroid Only," *Radiology* 242, no. 3 (March 2007): 907–13.

8. Wei Lu et al., "Treatment of Large Lumbar Disc Herniation with Percutaneous Ozone Injection via the Posterior-lateral Route and Inner Margin of the Facet Joint," *World Journal of Radiology* 2 (March 28, 2010): 109–12.

9. L. Xu et al., "Evaluation of the Clinical Curative Effect of an O_2-O_3 mixture to Treat Lumbar Disc Herniation with Different Treatment Sessions," *Journal of Interventional Neurology* 15 (2009): 159–63.

10. Z. Yu et al., "[Targeted Injection of Ozone through the Posterior Approach via the Spinal Canal and Dural Sac for Treating Lumbar Disc Herniation]," [*Journal of Southern Medical University*] 32, no. 2 (February 2012): 243–46. [In Chinese.]

11. M. Perri et al., "MRI DWI/ADC Signal Predicts Shrinkage of Lumbar Disc Herniation after O_2–O_3 Discolysis," *Neuroradiology Journal* 2 (April 28, 2015): 198–204.

12. M. Paolini et al., "Intramuscular Oxygen-Ozone Therapy in the Treatment of Acute Back Pain with Lumbar Disc Herniation," *Spine* 34, no. 13 (2009): 1337–44.

13. M. Dall'Olio et al., "Oxygen-Ozone Therapy for Herniated Lumbar Disc in Patients with Subacute Partial Motor Weakness Due to Nerve Root Compression," *Interventional Neuroradiology* 20 (2014): 547–54.

14. V. Eslami and V. Rahimi-Movaghar, "The Major Efficient Mechanisms of Ozone Therapy Are Obtained in Intradiscal Procedures," *Pain Physician* 15 (November/December 2012): 1007.

15. M. D'Erme et al., "[Ozone Therapy in Lumbar Sciatic Pain]," *La Radiologia Medica* 95, no. 1–2 (January–February 1998): 21–24. [In Italian.]

16. M. Muto et al., "Treatment of Herniated Lumbar Disc by Intradiscal and Intraforaminal Oxygen-Ozone (O_2-O_3) Injection," *Journal de Neuroradiologie* 31, no. 3 (June 2004): 183–89.

17. M. Bonetti et al., "Intraforaminal O_2-O_3 versus Periradicular Steroidal Infiltrations in Lower Back Pain: Randomized Controlled Study," *ANJR American Journal of Neuroradiology* 26, no. 5 (May 2005): 996–1000.

18. M. Bonetti et al., "CT-Guided Oxygen-Ozone Treatment for First Degree Spondylolisthesis and Spondylolysis," *Acta Neurochirurgica* 92 (2005): 87–92.

19. K. Gu et al., "Safety and Efficacy Study of an Ozone Laser Combined Therapy Using Puncture Needle in the Treatment of Patients with Cervical Spondylosis," *Journal of Spinal Disorders & Techniques* (August 20, 2014).

20. Frank Shallenberger, *The Principles and Applications of Ozone/UVB Therapy* (Carson City, Nev.: Frank Shallenberger, 1999).

21. Frank Shallenberger, *Prolozone Therapy* (Carson City, Nev.: Frank Shallenberger, 2003).

22. V. S. Agapov et al., "[Ozone Therapy of Chronic Mandibular Osteomyelitis]," *Stomatologiia* 80, no. 5 (2001): 14–17. [In Russian.]

23. A. Ceballos, "Tratamiento de la Osteoartritis con Ozono," *Revista CENIC Ciencias Biologicas* 20, no. 1-2-3 (1989): 152.

24. J. H. Li, "[Treatment of Middle-Aged and Aged Patients with Knee Osteoarthritis of Yang-Deficiency Induced Cold-Damp Syndrome by Ozone Combined Chinese Materia Medica: A Clinical Research]," [*Chinese Journal of Integrated Traditional and Western Medicine*] 33, no. 4 (April 2013): 471–75.

25. American College of Rheumatology (ACR), "Ozone Gas Injections May Do the Trick for Knee Osteoarthritis Sufferers," *ScienceDaily* (November 8, 2015), www.sciencedaily.com/releases/2015/11/151108084632.htm (accessed September 15, 2016).

26. Interview with Horst Kief, December 15, 1993.

27. S. Menendez et al., "Ozonoterapia en la Artritis Reumatoidea," *Revista CENIC Ciencias Biologicas* 20, no. 1-2-3 (1989): 144–51.

28. Jon Greenberg, "An Auto-Vaccine for Human Use Produced with the Aid of Ozone Gas," in *Ozone in Medicine,* vol. 3 of *Proceedings of the 11th Ozone World Congress* (Stamford, Conn.: International Ozone Association, Pan American Committee, 1993), M-3-21.

29. Mansur Doğan et al., "Effects of High-Frequency Bio-Oxidative Ozone Therapy in Temporomandubular Disorder-related Pain," *Medical Principles and Practice* 23 (2014): 507–10.

30. F. Nêuton de Oliveira Magalhães et al. "Effects of Ozone Applied by Spinal Endoscopy in Patients with Chronic Pain Related to Failed Back Surgery Syndrome: A Pilot Study," *Neuropsychiatric Disease and Treatment* 9 (2013): 1759–66.

31. Javier Hidalgo-Tallón et al., "Ozone Therapy as Add-on Treatment in Fibromyalgia Management by Rectal Insufflation: An Open-Label Pilot Study," *Journal of Alternative and Complementary Medicine* 18 (2012): 1–5.

CHAPTER 15. NEURODEGENERATIVE DISORDERS

1. M. Rodriguez et al., "Ozone Therapy in the Treatment of Elderly Patients Suffering from Parkinson's Syndromes," in *Abstracts: 2nd International Symposium on Ozone Applications* (Havana, Cuba: Ozone Research Center/National Center for Scientific Research, 1997), 43–44.

2. M. Rodriguez et al., "Ozone Therapy for Senile Dementia," in *Ozone in Medicine,* vol. 3 of *Proceedings of the 11th Ozone World Congress* (Stamford, Conn.: International Ozone Association, Pan American Committee, 1993), M-4-19-25.

3. M. Casas et al., "Ozone Therapy in Demential Syndrome in the Elderly," in *Abstracts: 2nd International Symposium on Ozone Applications* (Havana, Cuba: Ozone Research Center/National Center for Scientific Research, 1997), 42–43.

4. Interview with Josué García, January 6, 1994.

5. F. Molinari et al., "Ozone Autohemotherapy Induces Long-Term Cerebral Metabolic Changes in Multiple Sclerosis Patients" *International Journal of Immunopathology and Pharmacology* 27, no. 3 (July–September 2014): 379–89.

CHAPTER 16. DIABETES

1. N. Velasco, "Valor de la Ozonoterapia en el Tratamiento del Pie Diabetico Neuroinfeccioso," *Revista CENIC Ciencias Biologicas* 20, no. 1-2-3 (1989): 64–70.

2. E. Pavlovskaya et al., "Effectiveness of Ozone Therapy in the Process of Diabetes Treatment," in *Abstracts: 2nd International Symposium on Ozone Applications* (Havana, Cuba: Ozone Research Center/National Center for Scientific Research, 1997), 50.

3. A. G. Kulikov et al., "[Efficacy of Different Methods of Ozone Therapy in Vascular Complications of Diabetes Mellitus]," *Voprosy Kururtologii Fizioterapii* 5 (September–October 2002): 17–20. [In Russian.]

4. Oleg V. Maslennikov et al., *Ozone Therapy in Practice: Health Manual* (Nizhny Novgorod: Ministry of Health Service of the Russian Federation, 2008), 23–24.

5. Ibid.

6. Ibid.

7. Gregorio Martinez-Sanchez et al., "Therapeutic Efficacy of Ozone in Patients with Diabetic Foot," *European Journal of Pharmacology* (October 31, 2005): 151.

8. Ibid., 156.

9. M. R. Hayden et al., "Type 2 Diabetes Mellitus as a Conformational Disease," *JOP: Journal of the Pancreas* (Online) 6, no. 4 (2004): 28.

10. Velio Bocci et. al., "It Is Time to Integrate Conventional Therapy by Ozone Therapy in Type-2 Diabetes Patients," *Annals of Translational Medicine* 2 no. 12 (December 2014): 117.

CHAPTER 17. GYNECOLOGY AND OBSTETRICS

1. T. de la Cagigas et al., "Use of Ozonized Oil on Patients with Vulvovaginitis," in *First Iberolatinamerican Congress on Ozone Applications* (Havana, Cuba: National Center on Scientific Research, 1990), 66.

2. T. S. Kachalina et al., "Some Aspects of Ozone Therapy Application in Gynecological Practice," in *Ozone in Biology and Medicine* (Nizhny Novgorod: Ministry of Public Health of Russia Federation, 1992), 90.

3. N. M. Pobedinsky et al., "Effectiveness of Ozone Therapy in the Treatment of Condilomatosis in Women," in *Ozone in Biology and Medicine* (Nizhny Novgorod: Ministry of Public Health of Russia Federation, 1992), 90.

4. S. J. Winceslaus and G. Calver, "Recurrent Bacterial Vaginosis: An Old Approach to a New Problem," *International Journal of STD & AIDS* 7, no. 4 (July 1996): 284–87.

5. G. O. Grechkanyov and T. S. Kachalaina, "Ozone Therapy in a Complex Treatment of Threatened Abortion," in *Ozone in Medicine,* vol. 3 of *Proceedings of the 12th World Congress of the International Ozone Association* (Zurich: International Ozone Association, 1995), 291–94.

6. V. M. Andikyan et al., "Morphological Changes in the Placenta after Ozone Therapy," *Bulletin of Experimental Biology and Medicine* 130, no. 7 (July 2000): 715–18.

7. Guennadi O. Gretchkanev, "Ozonetherapy as the Main Component of the Complex Treatment of Threatened Abortion," in *Proceedings of the 15th World Ozone Congress* (London: International Ozone Association, 2001), 229–36.

8. C. He and X. Ma, "Distal Fallopian Tube Recanalization Using Ozone Treatment: A Clinical Study in Two Hundred Tubal Obstruction Chinese Patients," *International Journal of Clinical and Experimental Medicine* 9, no. 2 (2015): 2958–61.

CHAPTER 18. LUNG AND BRONCHIAL DISEASES

1. Velio Bocci, *Ozone: A New Medical Drug* (Dordrecht, Netherlands: Springer, 2005), 193–95.

2. Gilbert Glady, "Diverse Pathology Treated in Medical Ozone Clinic," in

Ozone in Medicine, vol. 3 of *Proceedings of the 11th Ozone World Congress* (Stamford, Conn.: International Ozone Association, Pan American Committee, 1993), M-3-3.

3. Horst Kief, "Die Behandlung des Asthma Bronchiale mit der Autohomologen Immuntherapie (AHIT)," *Erfahrungsheilkunde* 9 (1990): 534.

4. Frank A. Hernandez Rosales et al., "Ozone Therapy Effects on Blood Biomarkers and Lung Function in Asthma," *Archives of Medical Research* 36, no. 5 (September–October 2005): 549–54.

5. Silvia Menéndez et al., *Ozono: Aspectos básicos y aplicaciones clínicas* (Havana: Centro de Investigaciones del Ozono, 2008), 188.

6. A. A. Priimak, "[The Effect of an Ozone-Oxygen Mixture on Mycobacterium Tuberculosis and Conditionally Pathogenic Microorganisms]," *Problemy Tuberkuleza* 4 (1991): 7–10. [In Russian.]

7. V. G. Dobkin et al., "[Local Ozone Therapy in the Complex Surgical Treatment of Pulmonary and Pleural Tuberculosis Patients]," *Problemy Tuberkuleza* 7 (2001): 18–20. [In Russian.]

8. Z. Antoszewski et al., "[Ozone Therapy in the Management of Respiratory Failure after Long-Term Mechanical Respiration]," *Polski Merkuriusz Lekarski* 11, no. 62 (August 2001): 180–81. [In Polish.]

9. J. Calunga et al., "Rectal Ozone Therapy for Patients with Pulmonary Emphysema," *La Revista Médica de Chile* 139 (2011): 439–47.

CHAPTER 19. DISEASES OF THE SKIN

1. Velio Bocci, *Ozone: A New Medical Drug* (Dordrecht, Netherlands: Springer, 2005), 192–93.

2. S. L. Krivatkin, "The Experience of Ozone Therapy in Dermatovenereological Dispensary," in *Ozone in Medicine,* vol. 3 of *Proceedings of the 11th Ozone World Congress* (Stamford, Conn.: International Ozone Association, Pan American Committee, 1993), M-3-5-11.

3. S. L. Krivatkin et al., "Ozonetherapy in Out-Patient Dermatological Practice," in *Ozone in Medicine,* vol. 3 of *Proceedings of the 12th World Congress of the International Ozone Association* (Zurich: International Ozone Association, 1995), 157–63.

4. M. Miulani et al., "Efficacy and Safety of Stabilized Hydrogen Peroxide Cream (Crystacide) in Mild-to-Moderate Acne Vulgaris: A Randomised, Controlled Trial versus Benzoyl Peroxide Gel," *Current Medical Research and Opinion* 19, no. 2 (2003): 135–38.

5. R. Capizzi et al., "Skin Tolerability and Efficacy of Combination Therapy with Hydrogen Peroxide Stabilized Cream and Adapalene Gel

in Comparison with Benzoyl Peroxide Cream and Adapalene Gel in Common Acne: A Randomised, Investigator-Masked, Controlled Trial," *British Journal of Dermatology* 151, no. 2 (2004): 481–84.

6. E. Riva Sanseverino et al., "Effects of Ozonized Autohemotherapy on Human Hair Cycle," *Panminerva Medica* 37 (September 1995): 129–32.

7. Letter from Velio Bocci, January 17, 2006.

8. T. de las Cagigas et al., "Ozonized Oil and Its Efficacy in Epidermophitosis," in *First Iberolatinamerican Congress on Ozone Applications* (Havana, Cuba: National Center on Scientific Research, 1990), 63.

9. Heinz Konrad, "Ozone vs. Hepatitis and Herpes," in *Medical Applications of Ozone,* ed. Julius LaRaus (Norwalk, Conn.: International Ozone Association, Pan American Committee, 1983), 144.

10. R. Mattassi et al., "Ozone as Therapy in Herpes Simplex and Herpes Zoster Diseases," in *Medical Applications of Ozone,* ed. Julius LaRaus (Norwalk, Conn.: International Ozone Association, Pan American Committee, 1983), 136.

11. Ibid., 134.

12. J. Delgado, "Tratamiento con Ozono del Herpes Zoster," *Revista CENIC Ciencias Biológicas* 20, no. 1-2-3 (1989): 160–62.

13. Heinz Konrad, "Ozone vs. Hepatitis and Herpes," in *Medical Applications of Ozone,* ed. Julius LaRaus (Norwalk, Conn.: International Ozone Association, Pan American Committee, 1983), 147.

14. Ibid., 189.

15. M. Franzini et al., "Subcutaneous Oxygen-Ozone Therapy in Indurative Hypodermatitis and in Localized Lipodystrophies: A Clinical Study of Efficiency and Tolerability," in *Ozone in Medicine,* vol. 3 of *Proceedings of the 12th World Congress of the International Ozone Association* (Zurich: International Ozone Association, 1995), 131–43.

16. Horst Kief, "Die Behandlung der Neurodermatitis mit Autohomologer Immuntherapie (AHIT)," *Erfahrungsheilkunde* 1 (1989).

17. Horst Kief, "Die Behandlung der Neurodermatitis mit AHIT," *Erfahrungsheilkunde* 3a (March 1993): 166–89.

18. O. B. Christiansen and S. Anehus, "Hydrogen Peroxide Cream: An Alternative to Topical Antibiotics in the Treatment of Impetigo Contagiosa," *Acta Dermato-venereologica* 74 (November 1994): 460–62.

19. S. I. Ahmad, "Control of Skin Infections by a Combined Action of Ultraviolet A (from Sun or UV Lamp) and Hydrogen Peroxide (HUVA Therapy) with Special Emphasis on Leprosy," *Medical Hypotheses* 57 (October 2001): 484–86.

20. Felipe J. J. Reis et al., "The Use of Ozone in High Frequency Device to

Treat Hand Ulcers in Leprosy: A Case Study," *Tropical Medicine and Health* 43, no. 3 (2015): 195–99.

21. M. Manok, "[On a Simple and Painless Treatment of Warts]," *Hautarzt* 12 (September 1961): 425. [In German.]

22. T. de la Cagigas et al., "Therapy with Ozonized Oil in Ulcers in Lower Limbs," in *First Iberolatinamerican Congress on Ozone Applications* (Havana, Cuba: National Center on Scientific Research, 1990), 64.

23. Lamberto Re et al., "Stevens-Johnson Syndrome Treated with Ozone Hemo Therapy: A Case Report," *International Journal of Medical and Pharmaceutical Case Reports* 4, no. 4 (2015): 92–96.

24. R. Zanardi et al., "What Is the Best Strategy for Enhancing the Effects of Topically Applied Ozonated Oils in Cutaneous Infections?" *BioMed Research International,* article ID 702949 (2013): 6 pages.

CHAPTER 20. EYE DISEASES

1. A. Gierek-Lapinska et al., "[Preliminary Report on Using General Ozone Therapy in Diseases of the Posterior Segment of the Eye]," *Klinika Oczna* (May–June 1992): 139–40. [In Polish.]

2. Silvia Menendez et al., "Ozone Therapy and Magneto Therapy: New Methods for the Rehabilitation of Patients with Simple Chronic Glaucoma," in *Ozone in Medicine,* vol. 3 of *Proceedings of the 12th World Congress of the International Ozone Association* (Zurich: International Ozone Association, 1995), 99–106.

3. Rosaralis Santiesteban et al., "Ozone Therapy in Optic Nerve Dysfunction," in *Ozone in Medicine,* vol. 3 of *Proceedings of the 11th Ozone World Congress* (Stamford, Conn.: International Ozone Association, Pan American Committee, 1993), M-4-1-9.

4. Rosaralis Santiesteban et al., "Ozone Therapy in Patients Suffering from Optic Nerve Dysfunction," in *Abstracts: 2nd International Symposium on Ozone Applications* (Havana, Cuba: Ozone Research Center/National Center for Scientific Research, 1997), 40.

5. E. Riva Sanseverino et al., "Effects of Oxygen-Ozone Therapy on Age-Related Degenerative Retinal Maculopathy," *Panminerva Medica* (April–June 1990): 77–84.

6. Silvia Menendez et al., "Aplicacion de la Ozonoterapia en la Retinosis Pigmentaria," *Revista CENIC Ciencias Biologicas* 20, no. 1-2-3 (1989): 84–90.

7. E. C. Diaz et al., "Ozone Therapy in Different Ophthalmologic Diseases," in *Abstracts: 2nd International Symposium on Ozone Applications* (Havana, Cuba: Ozone Research Center/National Center for Scientific Research, 1997): 38–39.

8. M. Copello et al., "Ten Year Study in Patients Suffering from Retinitis Pigmentosa and Treated with Repeated Cycles of Ozone Therapy," in *Abstracts: 2nd International Symposium on Ozone Applications* (Havana, Cuba: Ozone Research Center/National Center for Scientific Research, 1997), 36.

9. Interview with Rosaralis Santiesteban, January 5, 1994.

10. V. V. Neroev et al., "[Effects of Ozone Therapy on the Functional Activity of the Retina in Patients with Involutional Central Chorioretinal Dystrophy]," *Vesnik Oftalmologii* 119, no. 6 (November–December 2003): 18–21. [In Russian.]

11. Letter from Velio Bocci, January 19, 2006.

12. Velio Bocci, *Oxygen-Ozone Therapy: A Critical Evaluation* (Dordrecht, Netherlands: Kluwer Academic Publishers, 2002), 287.

13. E. Borrelli and V. Bocci, "Visual Improvement Following Ozonetherapy in Dry Age Related Macular Degeneration; a Review," *Medical Hypotheses, Discovery & Innovation: Opthamology* 2 (2013): 47–51.

CHAPTER 21. DISEASES OF THE EAR

1. Ernesto Basabe et al., "Ozone Therapy Like a Favoring Element in the Rehabilitation of Children with Hearing Loss," in *Ozone in Medicine*, vol. 3 of *Proceedings of the 12th World Congress of the International Ozone Association* (Zurich: International Ozone Association, 1995), 275–78.

2. P. D. Spraggs et al., "A Prospective Randomized Trial of the Use of Sodium Bicarbonate and Hydrogen Peroxide Ear Drops to Clear a Blocked Tympanostomy Tube," *International Journal of Pediatric Otorhinolaryngology* 31 (March 1995): 207–14.

3. I. Ovchinnikov and E. V. Sinkov, "[Use of Gaseous Ozone and Ozonized Solutions in the Treatment of Chronic Suppurative Otitis Media]," *Vestnik Otorinolaringologii* 6 (1998): 11–12. [In Russian.]

4. K. Pawlak-Osinska et al., "Ozone Therapy and Pressure-Pulse Therapy in Ménière's Disease," *International Tinnitus Journal* 10, no. 1 (2004): 54–57.

5. R. Persaud, "A Novel Approach to the Removal of Superglue from the Ear," *Journal of Laryngology and Otology* 115, no. 11 (November 2001): 901–2.

CHAPTER 22. OTHER HEALTH PROBLEMS

1. Velio Bocci, "Ozone as a Bioregulator: Pharmacology and Toxicology of Ozonetherapy Today," *Journal of Biological Regulators and Homeostatic Agents* 10 (April–September 1996): 31–53.

2. R. Behar et al., "Tratamiento de la Ulcera Gastrodoudenal con Ozono," *Revista CENIC Ciencias Biologicas* 20, no. 1-2-3 (1989): 60–61.

3. S. Schulz, "The Role of Ozone/Oxygen in Clindamycin-Associated Enterocolitis in the Djungarian Hamster (*Phodopus sungorus sungorus*)," *Laboratory Animals* 20 (1986): 41–48.

4. Letter from Siegfried Schulz, January 9, 2006.

5. Y. Geng et al., "[Ozonetherapy Combined with Sulfasalazine Delivered via a Colon Therapy System for Treatment of Ulcerative Colitis]." [*Journal of Southern Medical University*], 30, no. 12 (December 2010): 2683–85. [In Chinese.]

6. R. A. Mayer, "Experiences of a Pediatrician Using Ozone as a Chemotherapeutic Agent for the Treatment of Diseases of Children," in *Medical Applications of Ozone,* ed. Julius LaRaus (Norwalk, Conn.: International Ozone Association, Pan American Committee, 1983), 210.

7. Silvia Menendez et al., "Application of Ozone Therapy in Children with Humoral Immunity Deficiency," in *Ozone in Medicine,* vol. 3 of *Proceedings of the 12th World Congress of the International Ozone Association* (Zurich: International Ozone Association, 1995), 271–74.

8. I. Parkhisenko and S. V. Bil'chenko, "[The Ozone Therapy in Patients with Mechanical Jaundice of Tumorous Genesis]," *Vestnik Khirurgii Imeni I. I. Grekova* 162, no. 5 (2003): 85–87. [In Russian.]

9. S. A. Kotov, "[Ozone Therapy of Migraine]," *Zhurnal Nevrologii I Psikhiatrii Imeni S.S. Korsakova* 110, no. 11 (2000): 35–37. [In Russian.]

10. B. Clavo et al., "Long-Term Improvement in Refractory Headache Following Ozone Therapy," *Journal of Alternative and Complementary Medicine* 19, no. 5 (2013): 453–58.

11. M. E. Shannon, interview in *Ozone and the Politics of Medicine* (Vancouver: Threshold Film, 1993).

12. Silvia Menendez et al., "Application of Medical Ozone Therapy in Patients with Sickle Cell Anemia: Preliminary Report," in *Ozone in Medicine,* vol. 3 of *Proceedings of the 11th Ozone World Congress* (Stamford, Conn.: International Ozone Association, Pan American Committee, 1993), M-3-12-17.

13. Velio Bocci and Carlo Aldinucci, *Rational Bases for Using Oxygen-Ozone Therapy in Sickle-Cell Anemia and ß-Thalassaemia: A Therapeutic Perspective* (Siena, Italy: Department of Physiology, Ozonetherapy Centre, University of Siena, 2001), 10.

14. A. I. Muminov and N. Zh. Khushvakova, "[Ozone Therapy in Patients with Chronic Purulent Rhinosinusitis]," *Vestnik Otorinolaringologii* 6 (2001): 48–49. [In Russian.]

15. G. Bonforte et al., "Ozone Therapy: A Potential Adjunct Approach to Lower Urinary Tract Infection? A Case Series Report," *Giornale Italiano de Nefrologia* 30, no. 4 (2013): 1–6.

CHAPTER 23. ACCIDENTS, INJURIES, AND WOUND HEALING

1. J. Ramos et al., "Estudio Imunologico de 25 Pacientes Grandes Quemados Tratados con Ozono," *Revista CENIC Ciencias Biologicas* 20, no. 1-2-3 (1989): 116–20.

2. W. Xie et al., "[The Role of Ozone Solution on Debridement and Sterilization of Burn Wound]," *Zhonghua Shao Shang Za Zhi* 16, no. 3 (June 2000): 163–65. [In Chinese.]

3. S. I. Ahmad and O. G. Iranzo, "Treatment of Post-Burns Bacterial Infections by Fenton Reagent, Particularly the Ubiquitous Multiple Drug Resistant Pseudomonas Spp.," *Medical Hypotheses* 61, no. 4 (October 2003): 431–34.

4. A. Campanati et al., "Topical Ozonated Oil versus Hyaluronic Gel for the Treatment of Partial- to Full-Thickness Second-Degree Burns: A Prospective, Comparative, Single-Blind, Non-randomised, Controlled Clinical Trial," *Burns* 39, no. 6 (September 2013): 1178–83.

5. H. Kawalsky et al., "The Use of Ozonotherapy in Nose Correction Operations," *Acta Chirirgiae Plasticae* 34, no. 3 (1992): 182–84.

6. E. P. Kudriavtsev et al., "[Ozone Therapy of Diffuse Peritonitis in the Early Postoperative Period]," *Khirurgiia* no. 3 (1997): 36–41. [In Russian.]

7. H. Al-Saadi et al., "Ozonated Saline Shows Activity against Planktonic and Biofilm Growing *Staphylococcus aureus* In vitro: A Potential Irrigant for Infected Wounds," *International Wound Journal* 13, no. 5 (January 14, 2015): 936–42.

8. H. Calvo et al., "Experiencias Preliminares en la Utilizacion del Ozono en Pacientes de Terapia Intensiva del Hospital 'Carlos J. Finlay,'" *Revista CENIC Ciencias Biologicas* 20, no. 1-2-3 (1989): 128–35.

9. M. Bette et al., "Efficiency of Tazobactam/Piperacillan in Lethal Peritonitis Is Enhanced after Preconditioning of Rats with O_3/O_2-Pneumoperitoneum," *Shock* 25, no. 1 (January 2006): 23–29.

10. R. A. Mayer, "Experiences of a Pediatrician Using Ozone as a Chemotherapeutic Agent for the Treatment of Diseases of Children," in *Medical Applications of Ozone*, ed. Julius LaRaus (Norwalk, Conn.: International Ozone Association, Pan American Committee, 1983), 205.

11. S. N. Gorbunov et al., "The Use of Ozone in the Treatment of Children Suffered Due to Different Catastrophies," in *Ozone in Medicine*, vol. 3 of *Proceedings of the 11th Ozone World Congress* (Stamford, Conn.:

International Ozone Association, Pan American Committee, 1993), M-3-31-33.

12. G. A. Balla et al., "Use of Intra-arterial Hydrogen Peroxide to Promote Wound Healing," *American Journal of Surgery* 108 (November 1964).

13. A. A. Daulbaeva and G. T. Baizakova, "[Effect of Ozone on Antibiotic Sensitivity of Microorganisms]," *Stomatologiia* 82, no. 2 (2003): 36–38. [In Russian.]

14. J. Wainstein et al.,"Efficacy of Ozone-Oxygen Therapy for the Treatment of Diabetic Foot Ulcers," *Diabetes Technology & Therapeutics* 13, no. 12 (December 2011): 1255–60.

15. World Health Organization, "Buruli Ulcer Fact Sheet," updated February 2016, www.who.int/mediacentre/factsheets/fs199/en (accessed September 15, 2016).

16. A. Bertolotti et al., "The Use of Ozone Therapy in Buruli Ulcer Had an Excellent Outcome," *BMJ Case Reports* (2013), doi:10.1136/bcr-2012 -008249 (accessed September 15, 2016).

17. A. Thabusum et al., "Ozone: The New Nemesis of Canker Sore," *Journal of Clinical and Diagnostic Research* 9, no. 3 (March 2015): ZC01–4.

CHAPTER 24. ATHLETIC PERFORMANCE, PREVENTIVE HEALTH, AND HEALTHY AGING

1. Velio Bocci, *Oxygen-Ozone Therapy: A Critical Evaluation* (Dordrecht, Netherlands: Kluwer Academic Publishers, 2002), 341.

2. M. Nabil Mawsouf, *Ozone in Athletes,* presentation at the First International Congress of Ozone in Medicine, Cairo, 2006.

3. Terry O'Hanlon, "Queen Mum Is Staying Young with Ozone Jabs," *Sunday Mirror* (May 13, 2001).

4. Shadia Barakat, *Role of Medical Ozone in Angiogenesis: To Promote Healthy Aging,* presentation at the First International Congress of Ozone in Medicine, Cairo, 2006.

CHAPTER 25. DENTISTRY

1. Renate Viebahn-Haensler, *Ozone in Medicine* (Iffezheim, Germany: ODREI-Publishers, 2002), 24.

2. M. V. Marshall et al., "Hydrogen Peroxide: A Review of Its Use in Dentistry," *Journal of Periodontology* 66, no. 9 (September 1995): 786–96.

3. Fritz Kramer, "Ozone in Dental Practice," in *Medical Applications of Ozone,* ed. Julius LaRaus (Norwalk, Conn.: International Ozone Association, Pan American Committee, 1983), 258–65.

4. C. G. Nogales et al., "Comparison of the Antimicrobial Activity of Three

Different Concentrations of Aqueous Ozone on *Pseudomonas aeruginosa, Staphylococcus aureus,* and *Enterococcus faecalis*—In Vitro Study," *Revista Española de Ozonoterapia* 4, no. 1 (2014): 9–15.

5. G. Gupta and M. Bansal, "Ozone Therapy in Periodontics," *Journal of Medicine and Life* 5, no. 1 (January–March 2012): 59–67.

6. J. Wennstrom and J. Lindhe, "Effect of Hydrogen Peroxide on Developing Plaque and Gingivitis in Man," *Journal of Clinical Periodontology* 6 (1979): 115–30.

7. M. V. Marshall et al., "Hydrogen Peroxide: A Review of Its Use in Dentistry," *Journal of Periodontology* 66, no. 9 (September 1995).

8. G. Klinger et al., "Bacteriological Studies during Conservative Treatment of Periapical Inflammations," *Stomatol-DDR* (December 25, 1975): 801–8.

9. S. J. Meraw and C. M. Reeve, "A Case Report: Treating Localized Refractory Idiopathic Gingivitis with Superoxol," *Journal of the American Dental Association* 129, no. 4 (April 1998): 470–72.

10. V. S. Agapov et al., "[Ozone Therapy in Treatment of Local Sluggish Suppurative Inflammation of Maxillofacial Soft Tissues]," *Stomatologiia* 80, no. 3 (2001): 23–27. [In Russian.]

11. H. Hasturk et al., "Efficacy of a Fluoridated Hydrogen Peroxide–Based Mouthrinse for the Treatment of Gingivitis: A Randomized Clinical Trial," *Journal of Periodontology* 75, no. 1 (January 2004): 57–65.

12. I. Khatriet al., "Evaluation of Effect of Topical Ozone Therapy on Salivary Candidal Carriage in Oral Candidiasis," *Indian Journal of Dental Research* 26, no. 2 (March–April 2015): 158–62.

13. Julian Holmes, "New Technologies for Dental Care," *Dentistry* (May 16, 2002): 14.

14. Aylin Baysan and Edward Lynch, "Effect of Ozone on the Oral Microbiota and Clinical Severity of Primary Root Caries," *American Journal of Dentistry* 17 (February 2004): 56.

15. Aylin Baysan and Edward Lynch, "The Use of Ozone in Dentistry and Medicine," *Primary Dental Care* 12 (April 2005): 51.

16. Julian Holmes, "Clinical Reversal of Root Caries Using Ozone, Double-Blind, Randomised, Controlled 18-Month Trial," *Gerodontology* 20 (December 2003): 106–14.

17. Russell Beggs, "Reliable Caries Reversal: Another Paradigm Shift?" *Dentistry Today* 23 (February 2004): 16.

18. R. Noites et al., "Synergistic Antimicrobial Action of Chlorhexidine and Ozone in Endodontic Treatment," *BioMed Research International,* article ID 592423 (2014): 6 pages, doi:10.1155/2014/592423 (accessed September 15, 2016).

19. F. Kaptan et al., "*In vitro* Assessment of the Recurrent Doses of Topical Gaseous Ozone in the Removal of *Enterococcus faecalis* Biofilms in Root Canals," *Nigerian Journal of Clinical Practice* 17, no. 5 (September–October 2014): 573–78.

20. Philip Mollica and Robert E. Harris Jr., "Integrating Oxygen/Ozone Therapy into Your Practice, www.ozonefordentistry.com/Doc.html (accessed August 10, 2015).

21. H. O. Kazancioglu et al., "Effects of Ozone Therapy on Pain, Swelling, and Trismus Following Third Molar Surgery," *International Journal of Oral and Maxillofacial Surgery* 43, no. 5 (May 2014): 644–48.

22. D. F. McKenna, "The Effect of Subgingival Ozone and/or Hydrogen Peroxide on the Development of Peri-implant Mucositis: A Double-Blind Randomized Controlled Trial," *International Journal of Oral & Maxillofacial Implants* 28, no. 6 (November–December 2013): 1483–89.

23. Rajiv Saini, "Ozone Therapy in Dentistry: A Strategic Review," *Journal of Natural Science, Biology and Medicine* 2, no. 2 (July–December 2011): 151–53.

24. William C. Domb, "Ozone Therapy in Dentistry," *Interventional Neuroradiology* 20 (2014): 634.

CHAPTER 26. VETERINARY MEDICINE

1. Margo Roman, "Ozone Therapy in the Veterinary Practice," *IVC Journal,* Fall 2013, http://ivcjournal.com/ozone-therapy-in-the-veterinary-practice (accessed September 15, 2016).

2. Kathy Backus and Jonathan Lowe, "Ozone & Biophotonic Therapy," *IVC Journal,* Summer 2014, http://ivcjournal.com/ozone-biophotonic-therapy (accessed September 15, 2016).

3. Gerald M. Buchoff, "Alternative Veterinary Pain Control for Surgeries and Injuries," *IVC Journal,* Summer 2015, http://ivcjournal.com/alternative-veterinary-pain-control-for-surgeries-and-injuries (accessed September 15, 2016).

4. Robert Smatt, *The Use of Ozone and Oxygen Therapies in Veterinary Medicine* (San Diego, Calif.: Genesee Bird and Pet Clinic, n.d.).

5. Ibid.

6. Ibid.

7. Interview with Robert Smatt, December 12, 2005.

8. Martin Goldstein, *The Nature of Animal Healing* (New York: Random House, 1999), 158–59.

9. Ibid., 198.

10. Ibid., 202.

11. Ibid., 230–31.

12. Ibid., 247.

13. Ibid., 274–75.

14. C. T. Liou et al., "Effect of Ozone Treatment in *Eimeria colchici* Oocysts," *Journal of Parasitology* 88 (February 2002): 159–62.

15. N. Terasaki et al., "Changes of Immunological Response after Experimentally Ozonated Autohemnoadministration in Calves," *Journal of Veterinary Medical Sciences* 63, no. 12 (2001): 1327–30.

16. K. S. McKenzie et al., "Aflatoxicosis in Turkey Poults Is Prevented by Treatment of Naturally Contaminated Corn with Ozone Generated by Electrolysis," *Poultry Science* 77, no. 8 (August 1998): 1094–102.

17. A. Otaga and H. Nagahata, "Intramammary Application of Ozone Therapy to Acute Clinical Mastitis in Dairy Cows," *Journal of Veterinary Medical Sciences* 62, no. 7 (2000): 681–86.

18. Velio Bocci, *Oxygen-Ozone Therapy: A Critical Evaluation* (Dordrecht, Netherlands: Kluwer Academic Publishers, 2002), 338–39.

19. Y. Shinozuka et al., "Comparison of the Amounts of Endotoxin Released from Escherichia coli after Exposure to Antibiotics and Ozone: An In Vitro Evaluation," *Journal of Veterinary Medical Science* 70, no. 4 (April 2008): 419–22.

PART 3. A HOLISTIC PROTOCOL

1. Janet F. Quinn, "The Healing Arts in Modern Health Care," in *Spiritual Aspects of the Healing Arts,* ed. Dora Kunz (Wheaton, Ill.: Quest Books, 1985), 121.

2. John C. Pittman, *Comprehensive HIV/AIDS Protocol* (Salisbury, N.C.: Cure AIDS Now, 1993).

CHAPTER 27. BODY CLEANSING

1. Robert Gray, *The Colon Health Handbook* (Oakland, Calif.: Rockridge Publishing, 1982), 29.

2. Horst Kief, *Therapeutic Significance of Intestinal Insufflation of Medical Ozone* (Ludwigshafen, Germany: The Kief Clinic, n.d.).

3. Robert Gray, *The Colon Health Handbook* (Oakland, Calif.: Rockridge Publishing, 1982), 37, 44.

4. Max Gerson, *A Cancer Therapy* (Bonita, Calif.: Gerson Institute/Pulse, 1990), 216–17.

5. *Keep Hope Alive Newsletter* (September 27, 1993).

6. Alfred Vogel, *The Nature Doctor* (New Canaan, Conn.: Keats Publishing, 1991), 482–83.

7. Interview with Juliane Sacher, January 26, 1994.

8. Velio Bocci, *Ozone: A New Medical Drug* (Dordrecht, Netherlands: Springer, 2005), 58.

CHAPTER 28. AN OXYGENATION DIET

1. David Pimental, *Handbook of Pest Management in Agriculture*, 2nd ed. (Boca Raton, Fla.: CRC Press, 1990).

2. Nathaniel Altman, *Nathaniel Altman's Total Vegetarian Cooking* (New Canaan, Conn.: Keats Publishing, 1980).

3. Sara Shannon, *Good Health in a Toxic World: The Complete Guide to Fighting Free Radicals* (New York: Warner Books, 1994).

4. Monica H. Carlsen et al., "The Total Antioxidant Content of More Than 3100 Foods, Beverages, Spices, Herbs and Supplements Used Worldwide," *Nutrition Journal* 9, no. 3 (2010), doi:10.1186/1475-2891-9-3.

5. *The New Four Food Groups* (Washington, D.C.: Physicians Committee for Responsible Medicine, 1991).

6. *Dietary Guidelines for Americans 2005* (Washington, D.C.: Department of Health and Human Services and the United States Department of Agriculture, 2005), chapter 5.

7. U.S. Department of Health and Human Services and U.S. Department of Agriculture. *2015–2020 Dietary Guidelines for Americans,* 8th ed., December 2015, http://health.gov/dietaryguidelines/2015/guidelines (accessed September 15, 2016).

8. C. H. Farr, *Workbook on Free Radical Chemistry and Hydrogen Peroxide Metabolism* (Oklahoma City, Okla.: International Bio-Oxidative Medicine Foundation, 1993), 46.

9. S. S. Hendler, *The Oxygen Breakthrough* (New York: Pocket Books, 1989), 150.

10. Letter from Kurt Donsbach, December 30, 1993.

11. S. Pulugurtha, "Foods to Increase Oxygen in the Blood," www.livestrong .com/article/344130-foods-to-increase-the-oxygen-in-the-blood (accessed November 6, 2015).

12. P. Sexton et al., "Influence of Mediterranean Diet on Asthma Symptoms, Lung Function, and Systemic Inflammation: A Randomized Controlled Trial," *Journal of Asthma* 50, no. 1 (2013): 75–81.

13. Mark Konlee and Conrad LeBeau, *Immune Restoration Handbook,* 6th ed. (West Allis, Wis.: Keep Hope Alive, 2004), 230–31.

14. Ann Wigmore, *Overcoming AIDS* (Boston: Ann Wigmore Foundation, 1987), 96.

CHAPTER 29. NUTRITIONAL SUPPLEMENTS
AND HEALING HERBS

1. John C. Pittman, *Comprehensive HIV/AIDS Protocol* (Salisbury, N.C.: Cure AIDS Now, 1993).

2. Letter from Velio Bocci, February 1, 2006.

3. M. J. Stampfer et al., "Vitamin E Consumption and the Risk of Coronary Disease in Women," *New England Journal of Medicine* 328 (1993): 1444–49.

4. E. J. Jacobs et al., "Vitamin C and Vitamin E Supplement Use and Bladder Cancer Mortality in a Large Cohort of U.S. Men and Women," *American Journal of Epidemiology* 156 (2002): 1002–10.

5. T. Tankova et al., "Treatment for Diabetic Mononeuropathy with alpha-Lipoic Acid," *International Journal of Clinical Practice* 59, no. 6 (June 2005): 645.

6. G. Zimmer et al., "Dose/Response Curves of Lipoic Acid R- and S-Forms in the Working Rat Heart during Reoxygenation: Superiority of the R-Entantiomer in the Enhancement of Aortic Flow," *Journal of Molecular and Cellular Cardiology* 27 (1995): 1895–903.

7. S. Sola et al., "Irbesartan and Lipoic Acid Improve Endothelial Function and Reduce Markers of Inflammation in the Metabolic Syndrome: Results of the Irbesartan and Lipoic Acid in Endothelial Dysfunction (ISLAND) Study," *Circulation* 111 (January 25, 2005): 343–48.

8. Parris M. Kidd, "Glutathione: Systemic Protection against Oxidative and Free Radical Damage," *Alternative Medicine Review* 2 (1997): 153–76.

9. International Scientific Committee of Ozone Therapy, *Madrid Declaration on Ozone Therapy*, 2nd ed. (Madrid: International Scientific Committee of Ozone Therapy, 2015): 15.

10. Z. L. Zhou et al., "[Study on Effect of Astragalus Injection in Treating Congestive Heart Failure]," *Zhongguo Zhing Xi Yi Jie He Za Zhi* 21 (October 2001): 747–49. [In Chinese.]

11. J. Dong et al., "[Effects of Large Dose of Astragalus membranaceus on the Dendritic Cell Induction of Peripheral Mononuclear Cell and Antigen Presenting Ability of Dendritic Cells in Children with Acute Leukemia]," *Zhongguo Zhing Xi Yi Jie He Za Zhi* 25 (October 2005): 872–75. [In Chinese.]

12. L. L. Agnew et al., "Echinacea Intake Induces an Immune Response through Altered Expression of Leucocyte hsp70, Increased White Cell Counts and Improved Erythrocyte Antioxidant Defences," *Journal of Clinical Pharmacy & Therapeutics* 30 (August 2005): 363.

13. T. Heinenn-Kammerer et al., "[Effectiveness of Echinacea in Therapy

of Chronic Recurrent Respiratory Disease]," *Gesundheitswesen* 67 (April 2005): 296–301. [In German.]

14. V. Goel et al., "Efficacy of a Standardized Echinacea Preparation (Echinilin™) for the Treatment of the Common Cold: A Randomized, Double-Blind, Placebo-Controlled Trial," *Journal of Clinical Pharmacy & Therapeutics* 29 (February 2004): 75.

15. Ellen Tattleman, "Health Effects of Garlic," *American Family Physician* 72 (July 2005): 103–6.

16. H. S. Chung et al., "Ginkgo biloba Extract Increases Ocular Blood Flow Velocity," *Journal of Ocular Pharmacology and Therapeutics* 15 (June 1999): 233–40.

17. M. R. Lyon et al., "Effect of the Herbal Extract Combination Panax quinquefolium and Ginkgo biloba on Attention-Deficit Hyperactivity Disorder: A Pilot Study," *Journal of Psychiatry & Neuroscience* 26 (May 2001): 221–28.

18. P. L. LeBars et al., "Influence of the Severity of Cognitive Impairment on the Effect of the Ginkgo biloba Extract EGb 761 in Alzheimer's Disease," *Neuropsychobiology* 45 (2002): 19–26.

19. D. L. McKay and Jeffrey B. Blumberg, "The Role of Tea in Human Health: An Update," *Journal of the American College of Nutrition* 21, no. 1 (2002): 1–12.

20. T. Nagao et al., "Ingestion of a Tea Rich in Catechins Leads to a Reduction in Body Fat and Malondialdehyde-Modified LDL in Men," *American Journal of Clinical Nutrition* 81, no. 1 (January 2005): 122–29.

21. H. J. Woo and Y. H. Choi, "Growth Inhibition of A549 Human Lung Carcinoma Cells by Beta-Lapachone through Induction of Apoptosis and Inhibition of Telomerase Activity," *International Journal of Oncology* 26 (April 2005): 1017–23.

22. J. H. Lee et al., "Down-Regulation of Cyclooxygenase-2 and Telomerase Activity by Beta-Lapachone in Human Prostate Carcinoma Cells," *Pharmacological Research* 51 (June 2005): 553–60.

CHAPTER 30. EXERCISE AND BREATHING: OXYGENATION AND OXIDATION

1. *Physical Activity and Health: A Report of the Surgeon General* (Atlanta, Ga.: Centers for Disease Control and Prevention, National Center for Chronic Disease Prevention and Health Promotion, 1999).

2. G. W. Davison et al., "Manipulation of Systemic Oxygen Flux by Acute Exercise and Normobaric Hypoxia: Implications for Reactive Oxygen Species Generation," *Clinical Science* (London) 111, no. 1 (January 2006): 133–41.

3. P. G. Peters et al., "Short-Term Isometric Exercise Reduces Systolic Blood Pressure in Hypertensive Adults: Possible Role of Reactive Oxygen Species (R1)," *International Journal of Cardiology* (October 17, 2005).

4. N. B. Vollaard et al., "Exercise-Induced Oxidative Stress: Myths, Realities and Physiological Relevance," *Sports Medicine* 35, no. 12 (2005): 1045–62.

5. *Physical Activity and Health: A Report of the Surgeon General* (Atlanta, Ga.: Centers for Disease Control and Prevention, National Center for Chronic Disease Prevention and Health Promotion, 1999).

6. U. Wisløff et al., "Superior Cardiovascular Effect of Aerobic Interval Training versus Moderate Continuous Training in Heart Failure Patients," *Circulation* 115 (2007): 3086–94.

7. Conor McLean et al., "Effects of Exercise Intensity on Postexercise Endothelial Function and Oxidative Stress," *Oxidative Medicine and Cellular Longevity*, article ID 723679 (2015): 8 pages, doi:10.1155/2015/723679.

8. S. S. Hendler, *The Oxygen Breakthrough* (New York: Pocket Books, 1989), 220.

9. Yogi Ramacharaka, *The Science of Breath* (Chicago: Yogi Publication Society, 1905), 40–41.

10. Majid Ali, "Your Health: One Way to Breathe," *Easy English News* 21 (February 2016): 5.

CHAPTER 31. EMOTIONS, MIND, AND SPIRIT

1. Donald M. Epstein, "There Is No Cure for Healing," *Association for Network Chiropractic Newsletter* (Summer 1993): 1.

2. Larry Dossey, *Space, Time & Medicine* (Boulder, Colo.: Shambhala Publications, 1982), 183.

3. Sara Shannon, *Good Health in a Toxic World: The Complete Guide to Fighting Free Radicals* (New York: Warner Books, 1994).

4. T. Dethlefsen and R. Dahlke, *The Healing Power of Illness* (Rockport, Mass.: Element Books, 1990), 7.

5. O. Carl Simonton, Stephanie Matthews-Simonton, and James L. Creighton, *Getting Well Again* (New York: Bantam Books, 1980), 61–62.

6. Jason Serenus, ed., *Psychoimmunity and the Healing Process* (Berkeley, Calif.: Celestial Arts, 1986), 72.

7. C. Mikluscak-Cooper and E. E. Miller, *Living in Hope* (Berkeley, Calif.: Celestial Arts, 1990), 250.

8. Scott J. Gregory, *A Holistic Protocol for the Immune System* (Joshua Tree, Calif.: Tree of Life Publications, 1989), 83–84.

9. Candace B. Pert, *Molecules of Emotion* (New York: Scribner, 1997), 192–93.
10. Norman Cousins, *Anatomy of an Illness* (New York: W. W. Norton, 1979).
11. Karen Shultz, "Laughter and Smiling: Good Medicine," in *The Essence of Healing* (Tucson, Ariz.: Theosophical Order of Service, 1984), 62.
12. Diane Chun, "Experts Dismiss Scare over Bird Flu," *Gainesville* [Fla.] *Sun* (November 3, 2005).
13. Donald M. Epstein, *Healing Myths, Healing Magic* (San Rafael, Calif.: Amber-Allen Publishing, 2000), 12–13.
14. Louise L. Hay, *The AIDS Book* (Santa Monica, Calif.: Hay House, 1988), 132.
15. Swami Sivananda Radha, *The Divine Light Invocation* (Portholl, Idaho: Timeless Books, 1966).

CONCLUSION. THE FUTURE OF OXYGEN THERAPIES

1. "Pharmaceuticals/Health Products, Industry Profile: Summary 2015," www.opensecrets.org/lobby/indusclient.php?id=h04 (accessed February 24, 2016).
2. Zdenek Rasplicka, website citation, OzoneLab Instruments, www .ozone services.com (accessed January 2006).
3. Ibid.

APPENDIX 1. OXYGEN PRODUCTS, SERVICES, AND APPLICATIONS

1. "The AAO Position on DIV (Direct I.V. Injection of Ozone/Oxygen)," http://aaot.us/?page=PostitionPapers (accessed December 24, 2015); American Academy of Ozonotherapy, *AAO Guidelines for Medical, Dental, "UltraPure" Laboratory Research Ozone Generators,* 3rd ed. (n.p.: American Academy of Ozonotherapy, 2013), 1–7.
2. Letters from Zdenek Rasplicka of Ozone Services, September 1997.
3. U.S. Environmental Protection Agency, *2015 National Ambient Air Quality Standards (NAAQS) for Ozone,* www.epa.gov/ozone-pollution/2015 -national-ambient-air-quality-standards-naaqs-ozone (accessed March 21, 2017).
4. U.S. Food and Drug Administration, *Code of Federal Regulations,* Title 21, Volume 8 (Medical Devices). April 1, 2016, www.accessdata.fda.gov /scripts/cdrh/cfdocs/cfcfr/CFRSearch.cfm?fr=801.415 (accessed March 21, 2017).

5. Bradford Cook, "Ozone Treatment Gains Popularity," *New Hampshire Business Review* 18 (May 24, 1996): 19.
6. Letters from Zdenek Rasplicka of Ozone Services, September 1997.
7. Anthony DePalma, "Just When You Thought Air Was Free," *New York Times* (June 12, 1997): 27, 30.
8. Press release for Oxygen Station, September 1997.

Index

486